The PREVENTION of SUDDEN CARDIAC DEATH

Editors

John B. Kostis, M.D.
John G. Detwiler Professor of Cardiology
Professor of Medicine and Pharmacology and
Chief, Division of Cardiovascular Diseases and Hypertension
UMDNJ-Robert Wood Johnson Medical School
New Brunswick, New Jersey

Michael Sanders, M.D.
Associate Professor of Clinical Medicine
Division of Cardiovascular Diseases and Hypertension
UMDNJ-Robert Wood Johnson Medical School
New Brunswick, New Jersey

WILEY-LISS

A JOHN WILEY & SONS, INC., PUBLICATION
New York • Chichester • Brisbane • Toronto • Singapore

Address all Inquiries to the Publisher
Wiley-Liss, Inc., 41 East 11th Street, New York, NY 10003

Printed in United States of America

Library of Congress Cataloging-in-Publication Data
The Prevention of sudden cardiac death / editors, John B. Kostis, Michael Sanders.
p. cm.
Includes bibliographical references.
ISBN 0-471-56679-9
1. Cardiac arrest—Prevention. I. Kostis, John B. II. Sanders, Michael, 1943–
[DNLM: 1. Death, Sudden. 2. Heart Arrest—prevention & control. WG 205 P944]
RC685.C173P74 1989
616.1′23—dc20
DNLM/DLC
for Library of Congress 89-13136
CIP

Contents

Contributors

Robert Allan, Ph.D., Assistant Professor of Psychology in Medicine, Division of Cardiology, The New York Hospital-Cornell Medical Center, New York, NY 10021 **[261]**

Keaven Anderson, Ph.D., Statistician, Framingham Heart Study, Framingham, MA 01701 **[1]**

Gail Aylmer, Cardiology Section, New England Deaconess Hospital, and Administrative Assistant, Cardiovascular Division, Brigham and Women's Hospital, Harvard Medical School, Boston, MA 02115 **[21]**

J. Thomas Bigger, Jr., M.D., Professor of Medicine and Pharmacology, and Arrhythmia Control Unit, Columbia-Presbyterian Medical Center, New York, NY 10032 **[155]**

Ross Brooks, M.D., M.Sc., Clinical and Research Fellow, Cardiac Unit, Massachusetts General Hospital, Harvard Medical School, Boston, MA 02104 **[221]**

William P. Castelli, M.D., Medical Director, Framingham Heart Study, Framingham, MA 01701 **[1]**

Nabil El-Sherif, M.D., Professor of Medicine and Physiology, Cardiology Division, State University of New York Health Science Center, and Chief, Cardiology Division, Veterans Administration Medical Center, Brooklyn, NY 11203 **[109]**

William H. Frishman, M.D., Professor of Medicine, Epidemiology, and Social Medicine, Albert Einstein College of Medicine, and Director of Medicine, Hospital of the Albert Einstein College of Medicine, Bronx, NY 10461 **[139]**

Hasan Garan, M.D., Co-Director, Cardiac Arrhythmia Services, Cardiac Unit, Massachusetts General Hospital, Harvard Medical School, Boston, MA 02104 **[221]**

George J. Klein, M.D., F.R.C.P.(C), F.A.C.C., Professor of Medicine and Director of Electrophysiology Laboratories, University of Western Ontario, London, Ontario N6A 5A5, Canada **[197]**

Paul Kligfield, M.D., Associate Professor of Medicine, Division of Cardiology, Department of Medicine, The New York Hospital–Cornell Medical Center, New York, NY 10021 **[43]**

The numbers in brackets are the opening page numbers of the contributors' articles.

John B. Kostis, M.D., John G. Detwiler Professor of Cardiology, Professor of Medicine and Cardiology, and Chief, Division of Cardiovascular Diseases and Hypertension, UMDNJ–Robert Wood Johnson Medical School, New Brunswick, NJ 08903-0019 **[ix, 83]**

Daniel Levy, M.D., Director of Cardiology, Framingham Heart Study, Framingham, MA 01701 **[1]**

James E. Muller, M.D., Chief of Cardiology, New England Deaconess Hospital, and Associate Professor of Medicine and Associate Physician in Medicine, Cardiovascular Division, Brigham and Women's Hospital, Harvard Medical School, Boston, MA 02115 **[21]**

William C. Roberts, M.D., Chief of Pathology Branch, National Heart, Lung, and Blood Institute, National Institutes of Health, Bethesda, MD 20285 **[13]**

Jeremy N. Ruskin, M.D., Director, Cardiac Arrhythmia Services, Cardiac Unit, Massachusetts General Hospital, Harvard Medical School, Boston, MA 02104 **[221]**

Michael Sanders, M.D., Associate Professor of Clinical Medicine, Division of Cardiovascular Diseases and Hypertension, UMDNJ–Robert Wood Johnson Medical School, New Brunswick, NJ 08903-0019 **[1, 83]**

Stephen Scheidt, M.D., Professor of Clinical Medicine and Assistant Dean for Continuing Medical Education, Division of Cardiology, The New York Hospital–Cornell Medical Center, New York, NY 10021 **[261]**

Arjun D. Sharma, M.D., Associate Professor of Medicine, University of Western Ontario, London, Ontario N6A 5A5, Canada **[197]**

Peter N. Smith, M.D., Clinical and Research Fellow, Cardiac Unit, Massachusetts General Hospital, Harvard Medical School, Boston, MA 02104 **[221]**

Peter H. Stone, M.D., Assistant Professor of Medicine, Cardiovascular Division, Brigham and Women's Hospital, Harvard Medical School, Boston, MA 02115 **[21]**

Geoffrey H. Toffler, M.B., Cardiology Section, New England Deaconess Hospital, and Instructor in Medicine, Cardiovascular Division, Brigham and Women's Hospital, Harvard Medical School, Boston, MA 02115 **[21]**

Gioia Turitto, M.D., Clinical Electrophysiology Fellow, Cardiology Division, Department of Medicine, State University of New York Health Science Center, and Veterans Administration Medical Center, Brooklyn, NY 11203 **[109]**

Carole A. Warnes, M.D., Pathology Branch, National Heart, Lung, and Blood Institute, National Institutes of Health, Bethesda, MD 20285; present affiliation: Consultant in Cardiovascular Diseases and Internal Medicine, Mayo Clinic, Rochester, MN 55905 **[13]**

Stefan N. Willich, M.D., Research Fellow in Medicine, Cardiovascular Division, Brigham and Women's Hospital, Harvard Medical School, Boston, MA 02115 **[21]**

Peter W.F. Wilson, M.D., Director of Laboratories, Framingham Heart Study, Framingham, MA 01701 **[1]**

Raymond Yee, M.D., F.R.C.P.(C), F.A.C.C., Assistant Professor of Medicine, University of Western Ontario, London, Ontario N6A 5A5, Canada **[197]**

Introduction

Despite vast leaps in knowledge and technology in the diagnosis and treatment of cardiovascular disease, sudden cardiac death (SCD) remains a vexing problem to today's cardiologist. The death rate from coronary heart disease has declined by more than 35% over the past 20 years; nevertheless, the incidence of SCD still remains appalling. However, recent research has begun to illuminate the problem in its unexpected complexity. Earlier simplistic assumptions have given way to a more thorough understanding of the epidemiology and pathophysiology of SCD, and new technologies have allowed a more scientifically based approach to risk stratification. New as well as established treatments, both pharmacologic and interventional, can now be applied in a more rational manner, with the hope of reducing the terrible toll of SCD on our patients, their families, and their communities.

In this book, we have gathered the latest thinking of experts in this multifaceted area to address these problems with an approach different from that of previously published collections in this field. Our focus is on the prevention of sudden cardiac death based on risk stratification techniques for the application of promising treatment modalities.

Dr. Castelli reviews the vast epidemiologic data from the Framingham Study as it pertains to SCD, with special emphasis on identifying clinical risk factors and the relationship of coronary heart disease to SCD. Dr. Roberts and Dr. Warnes present pathologic data to help explain this relationship in our present day population by providing convincing evidence of unexpectedly extensive coronary disease. Drs. Muller and Tofler give new insights into how coronary ischemia can lead to SCD by examining the tell-tale morning increase in its occurrence. Dr. Kligfield extensively reviews new information on SCD in noncoronary heart disease, including mitral valve prolapse. The chapters by Drs. Sanders and Kostis and Drs. El-Sherif and Turitto give us the background for risk stratification based on the well-established techniques of exercise testing and ambulatory electrocardiography as well as the newer methods of electrophysiologic testing and signal average electrocardiography. The different therapeutic modalities to prevent SCD are reviewed by Drs. Bigger, Frishman, Ruskin, Yee, and Klein; the importance of multicenter prospective drug trials are discussed as well as the early disappointments in this area. Nonpharmacologic interventions, both surgical and by implantable devices, are discussed in depth.

Finally, an original approach to this important clinical problem is given by Drs. Allan and Scheidt as they discuss the relationship of lifestyle to SCD and the possibility of lifestyle alteration for its prevention.

We hope that this collection will both stimulate and inform our readers on this important and timely problem of which we are just on the frontier.

John B. Kostis, M.D

Chapter 1

Sudden Death: The View From Framingham

William P. Castelli, M.D., Daniel Levy, M.D., Peter W.F. Wilson, M.D., Keaven Anderson, Ph.D., and Michael Sanders, M.D.

Framingham Heart Study, Framingham, Massachusetts 01701 (W.P.C., D.L., P.W.F.W., K.A.); Division of Cardiovascular Diseases and Hypertension, UMDNJ—Robert Wood Johnson Medical School, New Brunswick, New Jersey 08903-0019 (M.S.)

INTRODUCTION

Today the Framingham Study, initiated in 1948, stands as a major resource for epidemiologic information concerning death and disability from heart disease in the U.S. population. Our discussion on the prevention of sudden cardiac death begins with a compilation of the insights gained by the Framingham investigators from their large volume of epidemiologic data.

DEFINITION

Although many definitions of sudden death have been proposed to meet the needs of various studies, the following definition was chosen: For inclusion into our analysis subgroup of sudden death, a person who is observed to be alive experiences the onset of symptoms and is dead in less than 1 hour. Included in this definition is abrupt or near instantaneous death without other presenting symptoms. The initial presentation may be the sudden or rapidly progressive loss of consciousness, but cardiovascular death must ensue within 60 minutes of the onset. Usually, these are healthy, free-living people

The Prevention of Sudden Cardiac Death, pages 1–12

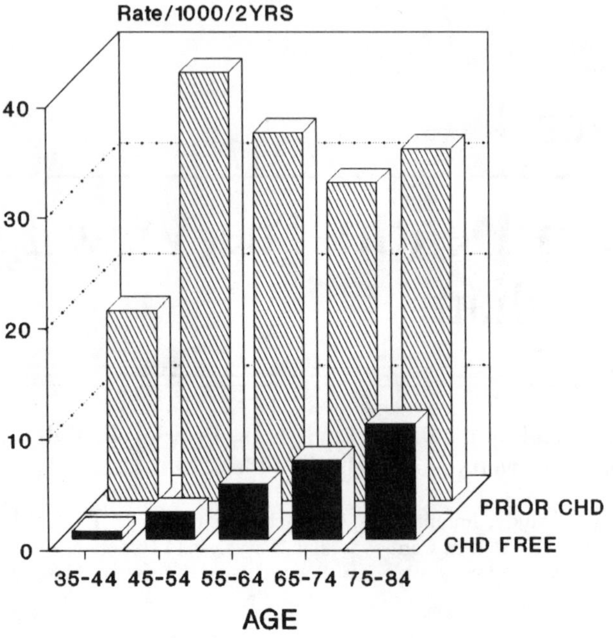

Fig. 1–1. Sudden CHD death data for men from the Framingham Heart Study.

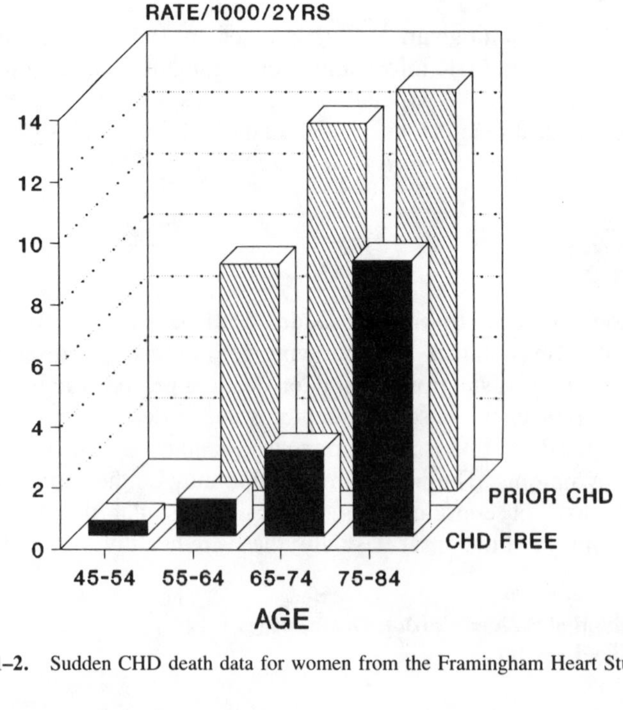

Fig. 1–2. Sudden CHD death data for women from the Framingham Heart Study.

who collapse at work or at home during the normal course of their activities. Many, if not most, have never been ill before. Seventy percent are dead within 15 minutes, and 92% were brought "dead on arrival" to the Framingham Union Hospital.

When sudden death is the first episode of illness, it is referred to as sudden "unexpected" death; it is more difficult to classify sudden death occurring in persons with the established diagnosis of coronary heart disease (CHD) who may be clinically stable. Patients with angina, for example, can qualify under the category of sudden death, although not "unexpected." Those who are admitted to the hospital for acute myocardial infarction can present even greater difficulties in classification.

1. Someone dying within several days following acute myocardial infarction is classified as CHD death, nonsudden.
2. For the purpose of this study, 1 month of uneventful survival following myocardial infarction is required for a person to again become eligible for inclusion under our sudden death definition.
3. Classification for the purpose of study may be impossible in patients with a stormy course following myocardial infarction in whom sudden cardiovascular collapse and death occur after months of continual crises, hypotension, or severe ventricular failure. It is possible that the exclusion of such patients has altered the conclusions of this study.

One reason for restricting our inclusion criteria to 1 hour as opposed to the 24 hour definition used by the World Health Organization [1] is to limit the possible mechanisms of death in our study cohort. The interpretation and usefulness of our epidemiologic data are facilitated by this etiologic limitation. Hinkle and Thaler [2] reported that in a series of patients in whom death occurred within 1 hour, 93% were due to arrhythmias, primarily ventricular fibrillation.

METHODS

The Framingham Study, begun in 1948, was initially a volunteer study; a major step was taken in 1951 when a two-thirds random sample of the entire town was drawn, from whom the majority of the subsequent 5,209 participants were derived. They were aged 30–62 years at entry and have been followed with examinations every 2 years. At these examinations, medical histories were taken and examinations designed to establish the health status of the participant were performed. Specific protocols were used to assess the cardiological endpoints; these have been described previously [3].

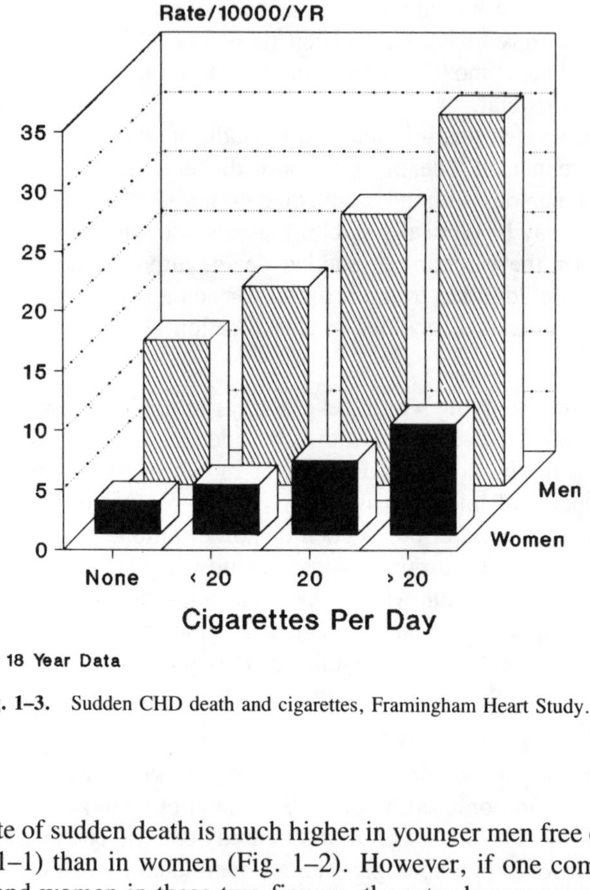

Fig. 1–3. Sudden CHD death and cigarettes, Framingham Heart Study.

RESULTS

The rate of sudden death is much higher in younger men free of clinical CHD (Fig. 1–1) than in women (Fig. 1–2). However, if one compares the oldest men and women in these two figures, the rates become very similar. The rates of sudden death are much higher in people who have had a prior episode of CHD; this appears to eradicate the age effect in men. The proportion of coronary deaths that are sudden decreases with age falling from greater than 50% in subjects under age 65 years to less than 50% in subjects over age 65 years [4]. Of first episodes of CHD, slightly over 10% are sudden death; another 10% are CHD death nonsudden; and the remainder are divided among angina, myocardial infarction, and coronary insufficiency.

THE RISK FACTORS FOR SUDDEN DEATH

Cigarette smoking is a powerful risk factor for sudden death. As Figure 1–3 shows, in men and women aged 45–74 years, cigarette smoking is statistically related to sudden death in men on multivariate analysis at $P < .005$ although not significantly in women; this may be related to the fact that so few women inhaled in the early days of the Framingham experience. Vital

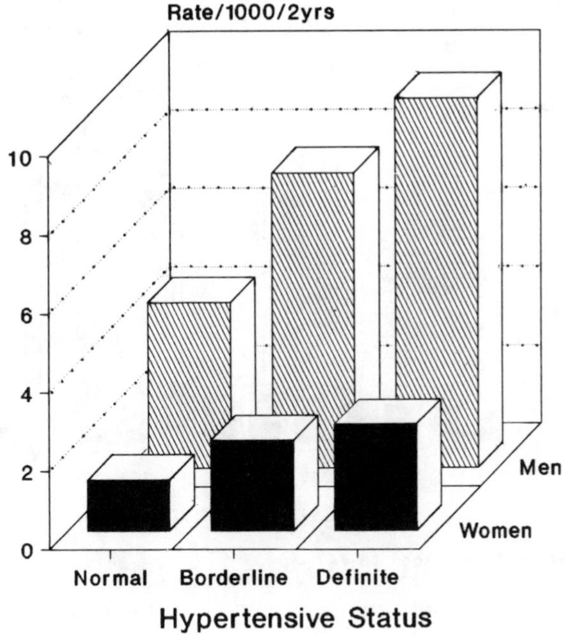

Fig. 1–4. Sudden CHD death and hypertension, Framingham Heart Study.

capacity is strongly related in women to sudden death in this age group, whereas it is not in men.

As systolic or diastolic blood pressure rise, there is a rise in sudden death; Figure 1–4 shows significant ($P < .001$) trends of sudden death related to hypertensive status in men and women.

The total serum cholesterol (Fig. 1–5) is related in a very smooth linear fashion to sudden death. This is significant on multivariate analysis in men and just misses the .05 level in women. It represents, with cigarettes and blood pressure, one of the three major risk factors for CHD. In subjects with prior CHD, it is a major force in sudden death, and one must be concerned with the indirect as well as the direct relationships seen here.

Figure 1–6 shows the significant relationship of glucosuria to the subsequent development of sudden death. Although these differences are significant in men and women in the univariate analysis, they remain significant on multivariate analysis in women only.

Measures of cardiac enlargement are highly significantly related to the development of sudden death. Whether by X-ray (Fig. 1–7) or electrocardiogram (ECG) (Fig. 1–8), significant trends are seen in men and women, but these may be more important in men, since only in men do these trends remain significant on multivariate analysis.

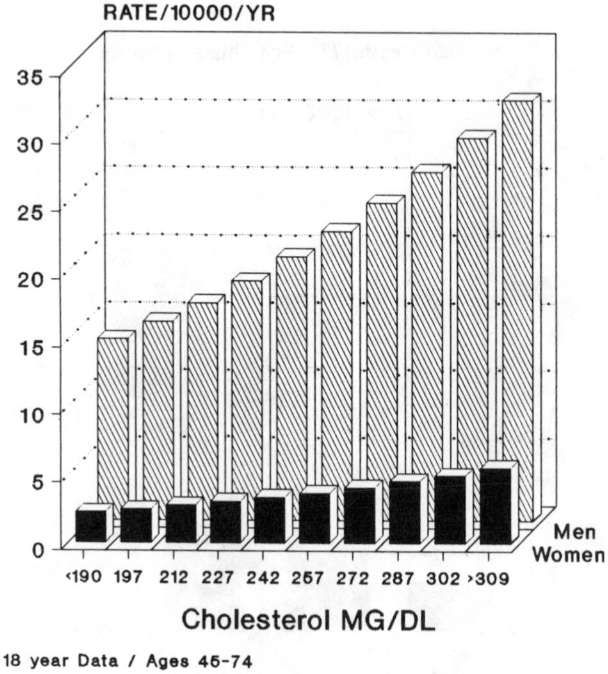

Fig. 1–5. Sudden CHD death and cholesterol level, Framingham Heart Study.

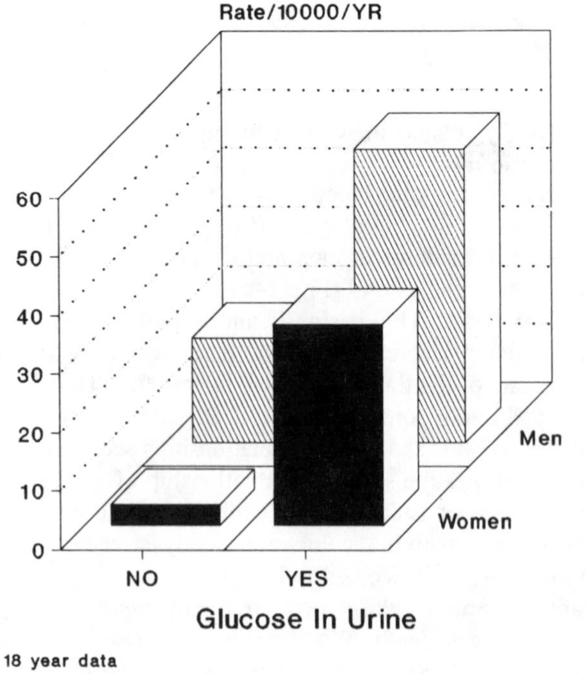

Fig. 1–6. Sudden CHD death and glucose in urine, Framingham Heart Study. Age-adjusted, ages 45–74 years.

ECG abnormalities such as intraventricular block (Fig. 1–9) show striking trends in men and women, which are significant by multivariate analysis in men. On the other hand, nonspecific T-wave or ST-segment abnormalities (Fig. 1–10) are related in men and women but reach statistical significance only in women on multivariate analysis.

Obesity, which shows a strong link in young men to sudden death risk, appears less striking in the older male cohort. Obesity, however, remains statistically significantly related to sudden death in all men, and, although the trends are seen in women, they do not reach statistical significance [5].

Pulse rate is significantly related to sudden death in men (Fig. 1–11) but not in women. A rapid heart rate can triple the risk of sudden death compared to a slower pulse.

Ventricular premature beats (VPBs) have always been considered as precursors for the kind of arrhythmias that lead to ventricular fibrillation. Only one case of sudden death occurred in the Framingham cohort while an individual was being monitored. This man had just completed a treadmill exercise test; he had finished 12.4 minutes of a Bruce protocol without any change in his ST segment or ectopy. About 1 hour later, he had his first VPB, which was late cycle. VPBs started to appear progressively earlier in the cardiac cycle and finally culminating in an R on T wave, which initiated a run of ventricular tachycardia, which in turn quickly degenerated to ventricular fibrillation and death within minutes [6]. VPBs in the Framingham study were significantly related to sudden death in men ($P = .001$) but, surprisingly, not in women (Fig. 1–12).

Combining coronary risk factors improves the predictability of sudden death. As Figure 1–13 shows, almost half of the sudden deaths in men and women occurred in those from the upper decile for multiple risk factors. Essentially, the message of our epidemiological data suggests that there is a soil of high CHD risk from which grows the susceptibility for sudden death.

DISCUSSION

If one holds to the 1 hour definition of sudden death as used in the Framingham study, the risk factors described in this discussion may allow the identification of people who are at high risk for death from ventricular fibrillation. Among these factors for sudden death are the familiar triad: cigarette smoking, high blood pressure, and elevated cholesterol. These not surprisingly are the same three major risk factors recognized for CHD in general. Add to this obesity and glycosuria and one may have reasons for postulating a continuing growth of atherosclerotic coronary lesions in subjects destined to experience sudden death. Among these risk factors, both obesity and uncontrolled hypertension are also powerful contributors to the two objective parameters related to sudden death, namely, ECG left ventricular hypertrophy (LVH) and X-ray evidence of cardiac enlargement.

Most cholesterol intervention studies have shown an effect on total CHD death as well as myocardial infarction rate. For example, the LRC study [7] demonstrated a close relationship between the decrease in coronary events and the fall in cholesterol. Will the current campaign to identify and control cholesterol levels significantly contribute to a decrease in sudden death? None of the intervention trials so far have been large enough to factor out sudden death specifically. However, it is reasonable to assume that the overall decrease in CHD death in these studies also reflects sudden death and that the general decrease seen in nonfatal CHD endpoints removes one of the most important risk factors for sudden death from our society, namely, prior CHD.

In addition to the traditional risk factors for atherosclerosis that appear related to sudden death, we have observed some other predictors. These are factors presumably related to end-organ damage: ECG LVH, X-ray cardiac enlargement, and nonspecific T-wave and ST-sgement abnormalities. Since these are powerful predictors for sudden death, these patients have already lost much of the potential benefit of our otherwise timely intervention. Prior CHD is the ultimate expression of the added risk from this end-organ damage

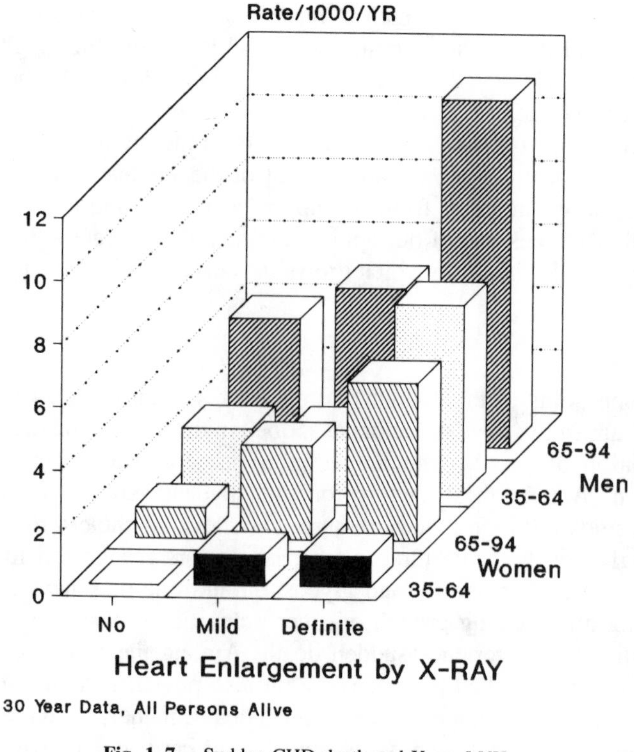

Fig. 1–7. Sudden CHD death and X-ray LVH.

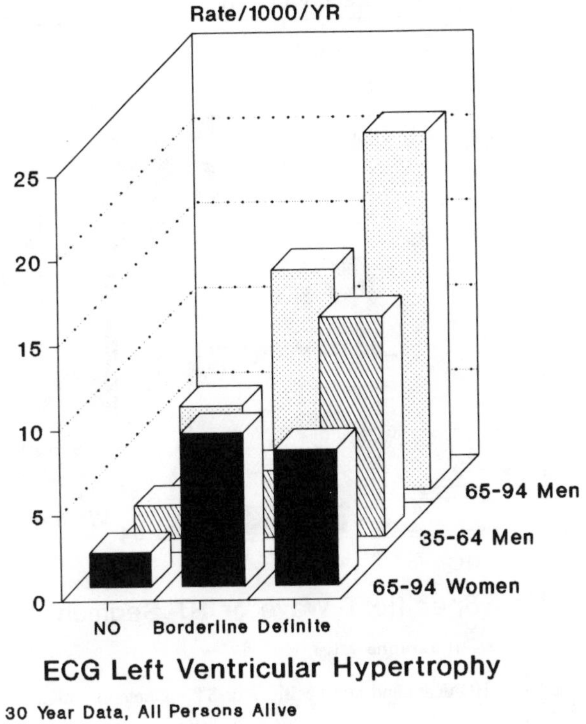

Fig. 1–8. Sudden CHD death and ECG LVH.

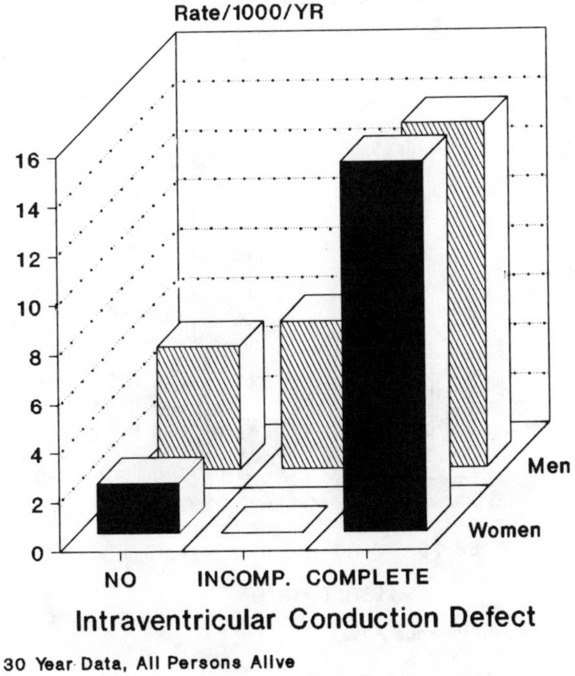

Fig. 1–9. Sudden CHD death and intraventricular conduction defect. Subjects aged 65–94 years.

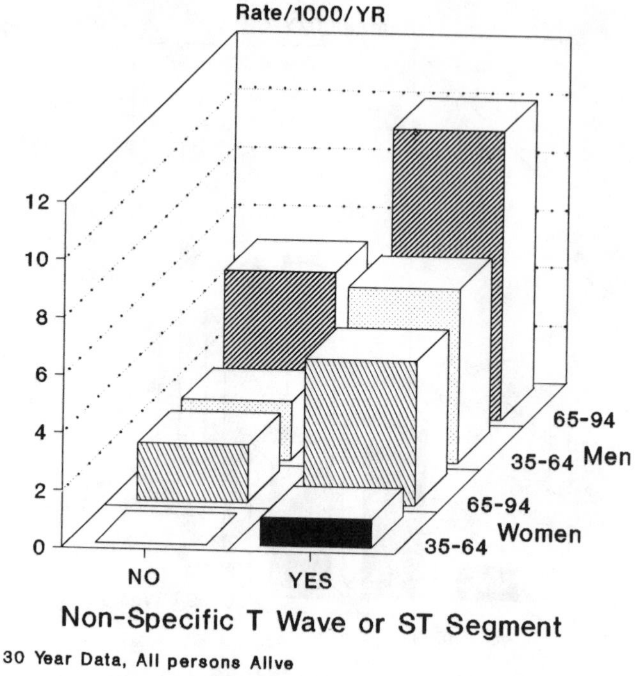

Fig. 1–10. Sudden CHD death and nonspecific T or ST segment elevation. Age-adjusted.

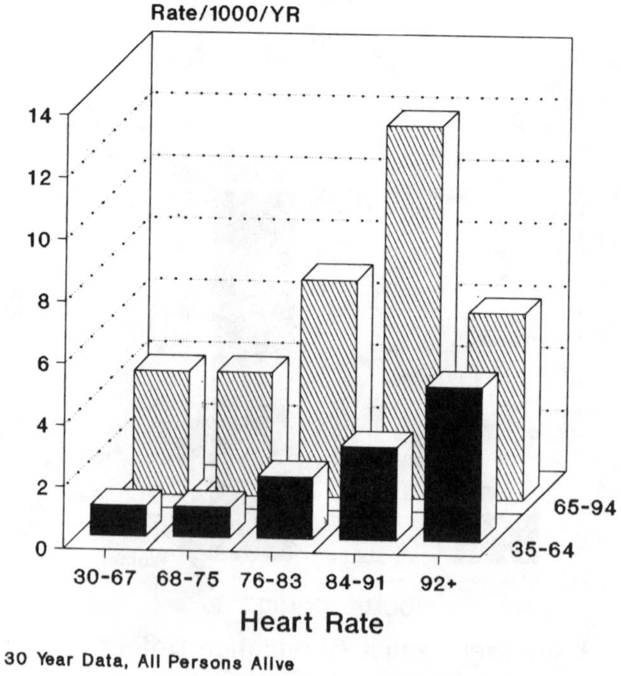

Fig. 1–11. Sudden CHD death and pulse rate (men).

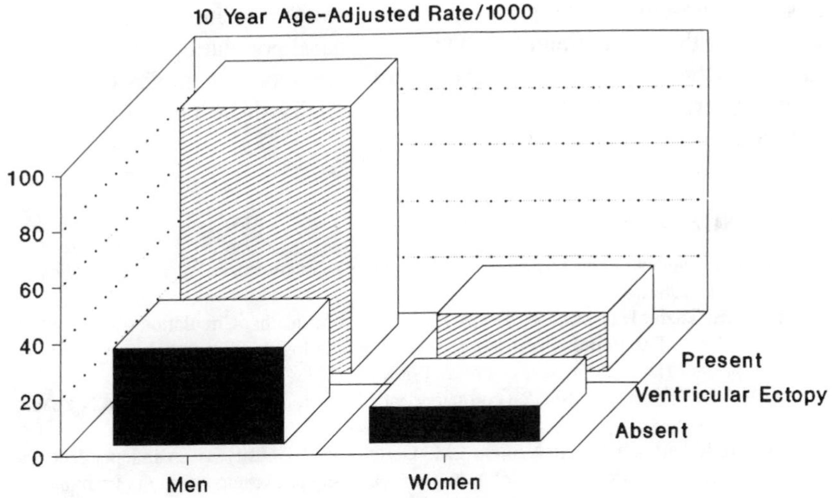

Fig. 1–12. Sudden CHD death and VPBs.

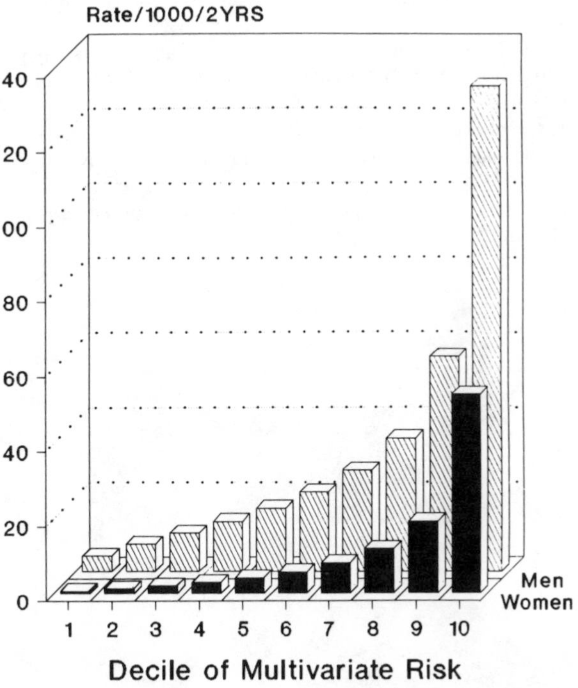

Fig. 1–13. Sudden CHD death and multiple risk factors.

and should present an even stronger incentive to physicians to institute early therapies for the prevention of CHD in the general population. With patients with established CHD, consideration must be given to therapies that could potentially prevent cardiac arrhythmias, especially those known to lead to ventricular fibrillation [8, 9,10].

REFERENCES

1. Kuller LH: Sudden death: Definitions and epidemiologic considerations. Prog Cardiovasc Dis 23:1, 1980.
2. Hinkle LE, Thaler HT: Clinical classification of cardiac deaths. Circulation 65:457, 1982.
3. Dawber TR: ''The Framingham Study. The Epidemiology of Atherosclrotic Disease.'' Cambridge: Harvard University Press. 1980.
4. Kannel WB, Thomas HE: Sudden coronary death: The Framingham Study. Ann N Y Acad Sci 382:3, 1982.
5. Hubert HB, Feinleib M, McNamara PM, Castelli WP: Obesity as an independent risk factor for cardiovascular disease: A 26-year follow-up of participants in the Framingham Heart Study. Circulation 67:968–977, 1983.
6. Savage DD, Castelli WP, Anderson SJ, Kannel WB: Sudden unexpected death during ambulatory electrocardiographic monitoring: The Framingham Study. Am J Med 74: 148–152, 1983.
7. Lipid Research Clinics Program: The Lipid Research Clinics Coronary Primary Prevention Trial results. I. Reduction in incidence of coronary heart disease. II. The relationship of reduction in incidence of coronary heart disease to cholesterol lowering. JAMA 251:351–374, 1984.
8. Kannel WB, McGee DL: Epidemiology of sudden death: Insights from the Framingham Study. In Josephson ME (ed): ''Sudden Cardiac Death.'' Philadelphia: F.A. Davis Co., 1985, pp 93–105.
9. Kannel WB, Cupples LA, D'Agostino RB, Stokes J III: Hypertension, antihypertensive treatment, and sudden coronary death. The Framingham Study. Hypertension 3[Suppl II]:1145–1150, 1988.
10. Kannel WB, Schatzkin A: Sudden death: Lessons froom subsets in population studies. J Am Coll Cardiol 5: 141B-149B,1985

Chapter 2

Relation of Amount and Distribution of Coronary Arterial Narrowing in Sudden Coronary Death to Previous Symptoms of Myocardial Ischemia

Carole A. Warnes, M.D., and William C. Roberts, M.D.

Pathology Branch, National Heart, Lung, and Blood Institute, National Institutes of Health, Bethesda, Maryland 20285

INTRODUCTION

We studied at necropsy 70 victims of sudden coronary death (SCD) to determine the amount and distribution of cross-sectional area (CSA) luminal narrowing in each 5-mm segment of the four major coronary arteries and compared the amount of narrowing both qualitatively and quantitatively in those with and without previous clinical evidence of myocardial ischemia.

PATIENTS, STUDIES, AND METHODS

All patients fulfilled the following criteria: 1) Death was known to occur within 6 hours of the previously witnessed usual state of health. 2) Although the patient may have died in a hospital, he or she was not a patient

The Prevention of Sudden Cardiac Death, pages 13–19

in a hospital at the onset of symptoms suggestive of myocardial ischemia. 3) At necropsy, at least one of the four major (left main [LM], left anterior descending [LAD], left circumflex [LC] and right) coronary arteries was narrowed 76–100% in CSA. 4) Ventricular myocardial coagulation necrosis was absent at necropsy. 5) A cause of death, cardiac or noncardiac, other than coronary artery disease was absent. 6) Chronic congestive heart failure had never been present. 7) A cardiovascular operation had never been performed. Review of clinical and necropsy records in the Pathology Branch, National Heart, Lung, and Blood Institute, yielded 63 men and seven women aged 22–81 years (mean 50 years) fulfilling these criteria. Of the 70 victims, 46 died outside the hospital. The other 24 had chest pain outside the hospital and had fatal cardiac arrest shortly after being brought to the hospital. The intact formalin-fixed heart in all 70 patients was submitted for detailed examination. The clinical information was obtained from the hospital where the patient had been hospitalized previously and/or from the patient's private physician, and often surviving family members were contacted for additional information.

The hearts were fixed for ≥24 hours in formalin. The four major coronary arteries were exicsed intact, X-rayed, and decalcified if necessary. Each artery was then cut transversely into 5 mm segments and labeled sequentially, either from the aortic ostium or from its origin from the LM coronary artery. The segments were then dehydrated with alcohol and xylene and embedded in paraffin, and at least two histologic sections were cut from the paraffin block. Each histologic section was stained by the Movat technique [1]. The amount of luminal narrowing by atherosclerotic plaque was determined by visual inspection of these histologic sections magnified 25–50 times. The percent of CSA narrowing of each 5-mm segment was categorized into five groups: 0–25, 26–50, 51–75, 76–95, and 96–100. All sections were examined, and the accuracy of the assessment of luminal narrowing was spot checked by videoplanimetry. The agreement between these two techniques is approximately 95% [2]. A total of 3,484 5 mm segments from the 70 victims were examined (mean number of segments per patient = 50). X^2 analysis was utilized for comparison of amounts of coronary narrowing by quantitative means.

RESULTS

Qualitative Studies

Of the 70 patients, one major coronary artery was narrowed 76–100% in CSA *at some point* in 11 patients (16%), two arteries in 19 (27%), three arteries in 33 (47%), and four arteries in seven (10%). Of the 280 major epicardial coronary arteries in the 70 patients (four per patient), 176 (63%) were narrowed at some point 76–100% in CSA, a mean of 2.5/4.0 major coronary arteries per patient. Excluding the LM coronary artery, 167 (80%)

of the other 210 major coronary arteries were narrowed 76–100% in CSA, an average of 2.4/3.0 coronary arteries per patient. Of the individual major coronary arteries, the LM was severely (76–100% in CSA) narrowed in 13% (9/70), the LAD in 86% (60/70), the LC in 74% (52/70), and the right in 79% (55/70).

Comparison of the number of coronary arteries narrowed 76–100% CSA in the 39 previously *asymptomatic* patients to the 31 with *previous acute myocardial infarction and/or angina pectoris* disclosed the following: one major artery so narrowed in eight (21%) vs. three (10%) (NS); two arteries in 11 (28%) vs. eight (26%) (NS); three arteries in 18 (46%) vs. 15 (48%) (NS); and four arteries in two (5%) vs. five (16%) (NS).

Comparison of the number of arteries narrowed 76–100% in CSA in the 39 patients without to the 31 with *healed* myocardial infarcts revealed the following: one major artery so narrowed in nine (23%) vs. 2 (7%) (NS); two arteries in 11 (28%) vs. eight (26%) (NS); three arteries in 13 (33%) vs. 20 (64%) ($P < .02$); and four arteries in six (15%) vs. (3%) (NS).

Quantitative Studies

Analysis of the 3,484 five-mm coronary segments showed that 950 (27%) were narrowed 76–100% in CSA; 1,127 (32%), 51–75%; 689 (20%), 26–50%, and 718 (21%), 0–25%. The percent of segments severely narrowed per patient, however, varied enormously; from 2% (1 of 50) to 88% (86 of 98). Sixteen patients had ≤10% of their 5 mm segments narrowed 76–100% in CSA; 15 patients had 11–20% of the segments so narrowed; 11 patients 21–30% of the segments; 16 patients 31–40% of the segments; seven patients 41–50% of the segments; two patients 51–60% of the segments; two patients 61–70% of the segments, and one patient 81–90% of the segments. Comparison of the mean percent of 5-mm segments narrowed 76–100% in CSA in the proximal and distal halves of the LAD, LC, and right coronary arteries disclosed a significantly higher percent of severely narrowed segments proximally in the LAD and LC arteries. A similar distribution of severe narrowing in the proximal and distal halves of these three arteries also was observed in the patients with and without previous symptoms of myocardial ischemia and in the patients with and without healed myocardial infarcts.

Of the 39 patients who had been asymptomatic, 502 (25%) of 1,991 five-mm segments were narrowed 76–100% in CSA compared to 448 (30%) of 1,493 five-mm segments in the 31 patients who had had either a clinical acute myocardial infarct and/or angina pectoris previously ($P < .005$). Comparison of the mean percent of segments in all five categories of CSA coronary narrowing between the previously *asymptomatic and symptomatic groups* disclosed significant differences in the category of minimal (0–25%) CSA narrowing (25% vs. 15%, $P < .001$). Comparison of the amounts of narrowing in each of the four major coronary arteries disclosed a higher mean percent of 5-mm segments narrowed 76–100% in CSA in the symptomatic versus the asymptomatic victims in the LM, LAD, and LC but not in the right coronary artery and a lower mean percent of segments narrowed 0–25% in CSA in all four coronary arteries in the symptomatic group.

Comparison of the mean percent of 5-mm segments in the five categories of narrowing between the 31 patients with and the 39 patients without *left ventricular scars* disclosed a higher mean percent of segments narrowed 76–100% in the healed myocardial infarct group (33% vs. 24%, $P < .001$) and a lower mean percent of segments narrowed 0–25% (13% vs. 26%, $P < .001$) compared to those without healed myocardial infarcts. A higher mean percent of 5-mm segments was minimally narrowed in those with no healed infarct, and a higher mean percent of segments were severely (76–100%) narrowed when a healed infarct was present. Severe narrowing of the LM coronary artery, however, occurred more frequently in those without healed infarct.

Of the 70 patients, 13 at necropsy had a thrombus in one coronary artery. In six patients, the thrombus consisted primarily of fibrin and erythrocytes and, in seven patients, nearly entirely of platelets. In all 13 patients, the thrombi were superimposed on atherosclerotic plaques, which had already narrowed the lumina 26–50% (one patient), 51–75% (four patients), or 76–100% (eight patients) in CSA.

DISCUSSION

A major findings in our study was that the sudden death victims had severe and extensive narrowing of their four major (LM, LAD, LC and right) extramural coronary arteries by atherosclerotic plaque. Of the 70 patients, 59 (84%) had two or more major arteries narrowed 76–100% in CSA, and 11 (16%) had only one artery so narrowed by atherosclerotic plaque. Of the 59 patients with multivessel coronary artery disease (CAD), two arteries were severely (76–100% in CSA) narrowed in 19 patients (27%), three arteries in 33 (47%), and four arteries in seven (10%). Of the four major coronary arteries per patient, 2.5/4.0 were severely narrowed. Of the 280 major coronary arteries in the 70 patients, 176 (63%) were narrowed severely, and, of them, the LAD was the most frequently (60/70, 86%) narrowed artery. The 11 patients with one-vessel CAD (one artery narrowed 76–100% in CSA) were significantly younger than the 59 patients with multivessel CAD (mean age 41 years vs. 51 years). The artery severely narrowed in these 11 patients was the LAD in five, right in four, LC in one, and LM in one.

Qualitative studies describing, from gross inspection, the number of four major coronary arteries severely narrowed in nontraumatic sudden death victims have been performed by others [3–7]. Of the 720 necropsy patients included in five studies, 499 (69%) patients had two or more major coronary arteries narrowed severely, and 132 (18%) had only one coronary artery so narrowed. One difficulty in comparing any of these five previous necropsy studies with the present study is the varying criteria for inclusion of cases. To be included in our study, a patient had to have at least one of the four major coronary arteries narrowed 76–100% in CSA by atherosclerotic plaque. In the five previously reported studies, however, 89 (12%) of the 720 patients had none of the four coronary arteries narrowed to this extent; all apparently had at least one artery narrowed 51–75% in CSA. Another major problem in comparing our findings with those in previously reported studies concerns different temporal definitions of the term ''sudden.'' We used a time period ≤6 hours from the time of previously witnessed usual health to death, whereas the studies both by Kuller and associates [3] and by Friedman and colleagues [4] used a time period of <24 hours. The time frame utilized in the other three studies was not defined [5–7]. Our study also included only patients without histologic evidence of left ventricular myocardial coagulation necrosis, whereas 126 (18%) of the 720 patients included in the five previous studies cited had acute myocardial infarcts at necropsy.

Although four of the five previously reported studies mentioned the number and percent of patients with previous clinical evidence of heart disease and with left ventricular scars at necropsy, none compared the amount of coronary narrowing in the group with to that in the group without clinical evidence of myocardial ischemia, or the group with to the group without left ventricular scars. We found the number of coronary arteries to be severely narrowed at some point (the qualitative approach) in the groups of patients with and without previous angina pectoris and/or myocardial infarcts and the groups with and without grossly visible left ventricular scars at necropsy to be roughly similar. Of our 70 patients, 31 (44%) had had previous clinical acute myocardial infarct (which healed) and/or angina, and 39 did not. Comparison of those with previous clinical evidence of myocardial ischemia to those without disclosed similar percentages of total coronary arteries (four per patient) severely narrowed (84/124 [68%] vs. 92/156 [59%] and roughly similar percents of two or more coronary arteries severely narrowed (28/31 [90%] vs. 31/39 [79%]). Comparison of the 31 patients with to the 39 without left ventricular scars disclosed similar percentages of total coronary arteries severely narrowed (82/124 [66%] vs. 94/156 [60%]) and similar percents of two or more coronary arteries severely narrowed (29/31 [94%] vs. 30/39 [77%]).

Cardiomegaly (heart weight >400 g) is frequently found at necropsy in individuals dying suddenly from coronary artery disease. Of the 64 patients studied by Kuller and associates [3], 37 (58%) had hearts weighing >450 g. Of the 208 victims studied by Baroldi and colleagues [7], 157 (75%) had hearts weighing >400 g. In the 220 patients studied by Liberthson and associates [5], the mean heart weight for 190 men was 460 g, and for the 30 women 374 g. Only one of these previous necropsy studies [7] correlated the number of coronary arteries severely narrowed to heart weight. Comparison of our 35 patients with the 35 patients without hearts weighing >450 g disclosed similar percentages of total coronary arteries severely narrowed (89/140 [64%] vs. 87/140 [62%]) and similar percents of two or more coronary arteries severely narrowed (30/35 [86%] vs. 29/35 [83%]).

None of the previously reported five necropsy studies [3–7] provided *quantitative* information on the amount and distribution of coronary narrowing in sudden death victims. In our study, a total of 3,484 five-mm segments were examined from the 70 patients: 27% of the segments were narrowed 76–100% in CSA, including 5% narrowed 96–100%. The 96–100% CSA narrowing group is probably equivalent to angiographic total occlusion. Not a single 5 mm segment was entirely free of atherosclerotic plaque. A higher mean percent of segments was severely narrowed in the proximal compared to the distal halves of the three (LAD, LC, and right) major coronary arteries. A previous report from this laboratory [8], which included 12 of the 70 patients included in the present study, also emphasized the diffuse extent of atherosclerosis in sudden death victims. Although a control group was not examined in the present study, the previous study [8] included 25 control subjects (mean age 49 years) and only 3% of the 5-mm segments of the four major coronary arteries were narrowed 76–100% in CSA by atherosclerotic plaque.

Of our 39 patients who had no clinical evidence of previous myocardial ischemia (asymptomatic group), 25% of 5-mm segments were narrowed 76–100% in CSA compared to 30% in those who had had symptoms of ischemia (acute infarcts that healed and/or angina pectoris) ($P < .05$). The asymptomatic group also had a higher mean percent of segments minimally narrowed (25% vs. 15%, $P < .001$).

Similar differences were apparent in the quantitative comparisons between those victims who had a healed myocardial infarcts at necropsy and those who did not. More 5-mm segments were narrowed 76–100% in those with than in those without a left ventricular scar (33% vs. 24%, $P < .001$); fewer 5-mm segments were minimally narrowed in those with compared to those without healed infarcts (13% vs. 26%, $P < .001$). Although a higher percentage of the 5-mm segments from the sum of all four major coronary arteries were severely narrowed in the patients with compared to those without healed infarcts, analysis of the individual arteries disclosed that the LM coronary artery was different from the other three. In the 31 patients with healed infarcts, only 4% of the 57 five-mm segments of LM were severely narrowed; in contrast, in the 39 patients without healed infarcts, 12% of the 78 five-mm segments were severely narrowed.

Although our study patients as a group had severe and extensive coronary narrowing by atherosclerotic plaque, considerable variation in the percent of 5 mm segments narrowed severely was observed. The range was from 2% to 86%: 16 patients (23%) had fewer than 10% of their coronary segments narrowed 76–100% in CSA, and 12 patients (17%) had >40% of their 5 mm segments severely narrowed. Thus, the extent of the severe narrowing is difficult to predict in the individual patient, but it is predictable in groups of patients dying suddenly from coronary artery disease. The previously symptomatic patients clearly had more severe narrowing and less minimal narrowing than the asymptomatic group, as did those patients with healed myocardial infarcts.

REFERENCES

1. Movat HZ: Demonstration of all connective tissue elements in a single section. Pentachrome stains. Arch Pathol 60:289–295, 1955.
2. Isner J, Wu M, Virmani R, Jones AA, Roberts WC: Comparison of degrees of coronary arterial luminal narrowing determined by visual inspection of histologic sections under magnification among three independent observers and comparison to that obtained by videoplanimetry. An analysis of 559 five-millimeter segments of 61 coronary arteries from eleven patients. Lab Invest 42:566–570, 1980.
3. Kuller L, Cooper M, Perper J: Epidemiology of sudden death. Arch Intern Med 129: 714–719, 1972.
4. Friedman M, Manwaring JH, Rosenman RH, Donlon G, Ortega P, Grube SM: Instantaneous and sudden deaths. Clinical and pathological differentiation in coronary artery disease. JAMA 225:1319–1328, 1973.
5. Liberthson RR, Nagel EL, Hirschman JC, Nussenfeld SR, Blackbourn BD, Davis JR: Pathophysiologic observations in prehospital ventricular fibrillation and sudden cardiac death. Circulation 49:790–798, 1974.
6. Perper JA, Kuller LH, Cooper M: Arteriosclerosis of coronary arteries in sudden, unexpected deaths. Circulation 51/52 [Suppl III]:III-27–III-33, 1975.
7. Baroldi G, Falzi G, Mariani F: Sudden coronary death. A postmortem study in 208 selected cases compared to 97 "control" subjects. Am Heart J 98:20–31, 1979.
8. Roberts WC, Jones AA: Quantitation of coronary arterial narrowing at necropsy in sudden coronary death. Analysis of 31 patients and comparison with 25 control subjects. Am J Cardiol 44:39–45, 1979.

Chapter 3

Triggers of Sudden Coronary Death: The Morning Increase

**James E. Muller, M.D., Geoffrey H. Tofler, M.B.,
Stefan N. Willich, M.D., Gail Aylmer, and Peter H. Stone, M.D.**

Cardiology Section, New England Deaconess Hospital (J.E.M., G.H.T., G.A.) and Cardiovascular Division, Brigham and Women's Hospital, Harvard Medical School (J.E.M., G.H.T., S.N.W., G.A., P.H.S.), Boston, Massachusetts 02115

INTRODUCTION

Although sudden cardiac death is the leading cause of death in industrialized countries [1–4], the mechanisms triggering this common catastrophic event remain obscure. Attempts to identify precipitating mechanisms have been hampered by the rarity of intensive medical observation in the critical moments prior to its onset. Although frequent in a population, sudden cardiac death is difficult to study because it is impossible to predict in which individual it will occur, and it often occurs without warning in an out-of-hospital setting. Retrieval of physiologic data from those who die is impossible; in those who are resuscitated, the period of arrest and the techniques of resuscitation obscure the events that preceded the arrest. Of necessity, therefore, our present, limited insight into the mechanism of sudden cardiac death is based primarily on knowledge of predisposing factors gained from extensive epidemiologic and pathologic studies.

A new approach to identification of the mechanisms precipitating sudden cardiac death is suggested by the recent demonstration that nonfatal myocardial infarction, a disease closely associated with sudden cardiac death and sharing its unexpected onset, is more likely to occur in the morning than at other times of day [5]. In addition, episodes of rest angina [6], silent

The Prevention of Sudden Cardiac Death, pages 21–41

myocardial ischemia [7], and the onset of stroke [8] have all been reported to show similar morning increases.

Because of the close relationship between myocardial infarction and sudden coronary death, the demonstration that myocardial infarction was three times more likely to occur at peak than at trough times led to efforts to determine if sudden cardiac death also had a similar pattern of occurrence.

The first step in such studies was to address several methodologic problems in determining the time of occurrence of sudden cardiac death. The apparently simple task of determining time of sudden cardiac death is complicated because 1) it is difficult, in certain cases, to determine if a sudden cardiac event is actually the cause of death; 2) unwitnessed deaths occur, for which determination of time of death, as well as cause of death, is uncertain; 3) there is an increased likelihood that such unwitnessed deaths will occur at night; and 4) a large number of cases is needed to detect a statistically significant morning increase. The assertion that sudden coronary death shows an increased incidence in the morning rests on the attempts to resolve these methodologic problems in studies of two large data bases—mortality records for Massachusetts for 1983 [9] and the Framingham Heart Study [10].

THE MASSACHUSETTS DEATH CERTIFICATE STUDY

Methods

Mortality records of the Massachusetts Department of Public Health were utilized to determine the time of occurrence of sudden coronary death in a large cohort of individuals. Massachusetts law requires that a death certificate be completed for each person dying in the state. Completed certificates are recorded locally and sent to the central office of the Department of Public Health, where internal consistency checks are performed. A portion of the data on the death certificates is entered into the central computer (Amdahl-5860) of the Department of Public Health.

For the study, the portions of the death certificates utilized were the sections describing the age, sex, location of death, date and time of death, interval from onset of symptoms to death, and cause of death as indicated by the physician signing the death certificate. Cause of death information is obtained from a three-line section of the death certificate asking for designation of the immediate cause of death and two underlying conditions leading to death. The time interval from onset of symptoms to death for each of the three conditions is also requested. The three conditions listed by the physician completing the form are manually assigned codes by the Department of Public Health using the Ninth Revision of the International Classification of Disease (ICD), adapted for use in the United States [11].

Identification of the primary analysis group. For the sudden cardiac death study, as a first step, it was necessary to identify a large number of individuals dying of sudden coronary death, defined as death from cardiac

TABLE 3–1. Deaths in Massachusetts in 1983

	No.	Percent of total deaths[a]
Total deaths in Massachusetts in 1983	54,742	100.0
Diseases of the circulatory system (ICD-390 to ICD-459)	26,798	49.0
Ischemic heart disease (ICD-410 to ICD-414)	16,861	30.8
Acute myocardial infarction (ICD-410)	8,620	15.7
Chronic ischemic heart disease (ICD-414)	8,172	14.9
Cardiac dysrhythmias (ICD-427)	1,235	2.3

[a]Percentages do not total 100% because only selected ICD codes are presented.

disease occurring ≤1 hour after onset of symptoms. It was decided to conduct the primary analysis on sudden coronary death occurring out of hospital (including death on hospital arrival) since out of hospital deaths occur in the presence of normal endogenous and exogenous circadian rhythms, which are altered in hospitalized patients. Furthermore, Hinkle and Thaler [12] have noted that "arrhythmic deaths," the focus of the present study, account for 88% of out-of-hospital cardiac deaths, but only 29% of in-hospital cardiac deaths, for which "circulatory failure" was found to be the most frequent cause.

Since previous epidemiologic studies indicated that sudden coronary death accounts for a substantial portion of total mortality, the overall mortality breakdown for Massachusetts was surveyed as a first step in selecting the primary analysis group (Table 3–1). There were 54,742 deaths in Massachusetts in 1983. Classification by cause of death indicated that "Diseases of the Circulatory System" (ICD-390 to ICD-459) were the leading cause of death, accounting for 49% of all deaths. "Ischemic heart disease" (ICD-410 to ICD-414) accounted for 30.8% of all deaths. The numbers of deaths assigned to the individual codes of interest are shown in Table 3–1.

The Department of Public Health generated a list of the names and death certificate numbers of the 18,027 individuals classified as ICD-410, ICD-414, or ICD 427 (32.9% of all deaths) including the variables age, sex, location of death, and date of death. Since the time of death and the interval from onset of symptoms to death were not routinely entered into the Department of Public Health computer, the death certificates of individuals in these three ICDs who were selected for study were manually reviewed, the times recorded, and entered into a new data file.

ICD-410, "acute myocardial infarction," contained most of the out-of-hospital cardiac deaths occurring ≤1 hour after onset of symptoms. Therefore, the *primary analysis group* for determination of the time of occurrence of sudden coronary death was defined as the group of 2,203 individuals within ICD-410 who died an out-of-hospital death from ischemic heart disease ≤1 hour after onset of symptoms.

Other analysis groups. To determine the time of occurrence of sudden coronary deaths classified under ICD codes other than ICD-410, we also studied patients listed under ICD-427, "cardiac dysrhythmias," and a random sample of ICD-414 "chronic ischemic heart disease." (All data presented for ICD-414 are multiplied by six to account for a one-sixth sampling fraction.) Only an estimated 685 out-of-hospital sudden coronary deaths were found in these two categories. Only 102 deaths were classified under ICD-798, "sudden death, cause unknown."

To permit a comparison of the incidence of sudden coronary death observed in the present study with that previously reported by others, we calculated age- and sex-specific incidence rates for the total sudden coronary death population identified (i.e., deaths occurring in or out of hospital classified under ICD codes 410, 414, or 427 and known to have occurred, or estimated to have occurred, ≤1 hour after onset of symptoms. To investigate the possibility that death certificate data underestimate the incidence of sudden coronary death during the night because deaths during sleep are reported to have occurred at the normal time of awakening, a literature search was conducted to determine the frequency of sudden coronary death during sleep in previously published detailed epidemiologic studies.

Statistical methods. To quantify the periodic structure of the frequency of occurrence of sudden coronary death, single-harmonic regression models were fitted to the data. Since the pattern of occurrence of sudden coronary death suggested bimodality, a double-harmonic regression model was also fitted to the data. The period of the oscillation was taken to be 24 hours. Model goodness of fit was evaluated by t tests (two-tailed) on the estimated coefficients, by F tests on the overall model, and by R^2 and adjusted R^2 statistics [13,14].

Results

Primary analysis group. The time of day of sudden coronary death of individuals in the primary analysis group is shown in Figure 3–1. A statistically significant ($P < 0.01$) morning increase is present, with a primary peak from 10 to 11 AM and a secondary peak from 5 to 6 PM. There is a strong similarity between this pattern of sudden coronary death and the previously reported morning increase of nonfatal myocardial infarction [5] (Fig. 3–2).

Characteristics of patients classified as dying of ICD-410, who were excluded from the primary analysis group because of missing data, were analyzed to assess the possibility that the primary analysis group was a biased subset of ICD-410 deaths. A total of 1,593 of the 8,620 ICD-410 individuals were excluded from the primary analysis group because the interval from onset of symptoms to death was not reported or was reported to be greater than 4 months, although time of death was reported. The time of day of

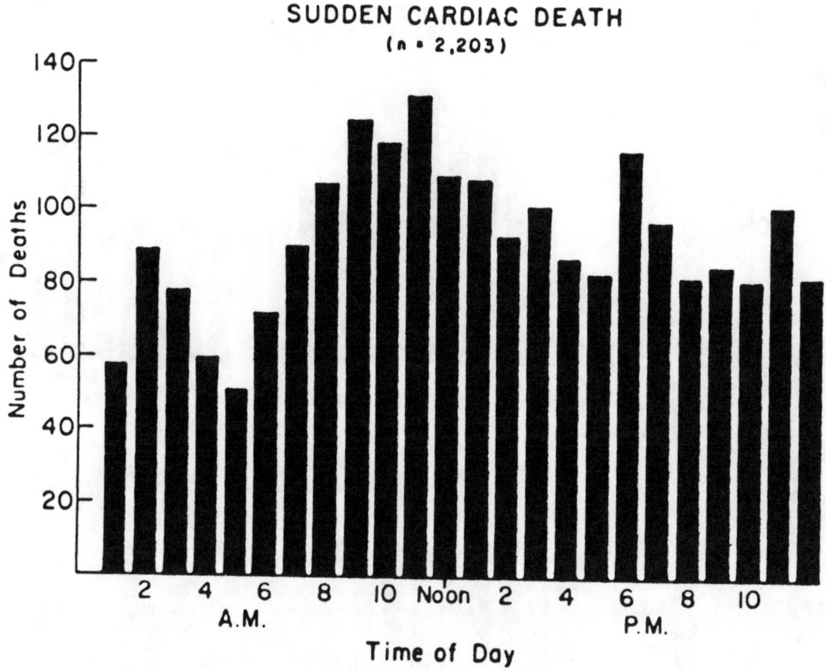

Fig. 3–1. Time of day of out-of-hospital sudden cardiac death (ICD-410; ≤1 hour from onset of symptoms to death) for 2,203 individuals dying in Massachusetts in 1983. A statistically significant ($P < 0.001$) morning increase is present, with a primary peak between 7 and 11 AM and a secondary peak between 5 and 6 PM.

cardiac death in this group demonstrated a pattern parallel to that of the primary analysis group.

Although 390 additional individuals were excluded from analysis because their time of death was not reported, in 283 of these cases the physician indicated on the death certificate that the interval from onset of symptoms to death was ≤1 hour. This level of information suggests that the omission of the time of death was more likely due to a clerical error than to selective lack of observation during the night. Finally, there were 75 individuals (0.9%) in the ICD-410 category for whom neither interval from onset of symptoms to death nor time of death was reported. Assumption that all of those deaths occurred from 11 PM to 6 AM did not abolish the low frequency of sudden coronary death during the night. A statistically significant variation similar to that observed for the group as a whole was also observed for males and females and for the older and younger halves of the population.

Other analysis groups. Review of the time of occurrence of the estimated 685 out-of-hospital sudden coronary deaths attributed to "chronic ischemic heart disease" (ICD-414) and to "cardiac dysrhythmias" (ICD-

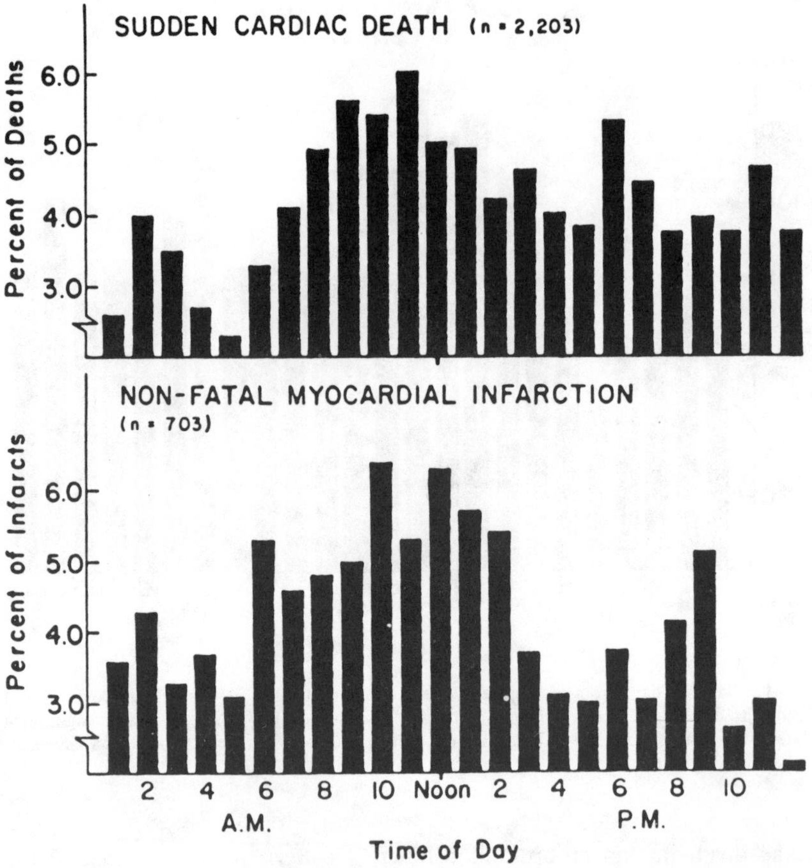

Fig. 3–2. Comparison between the morning increase of sudden cardiac death and the previously reported morning increase of nonfatal myocardial infarctions. The percent of total events for the 24 hour period occurring during each hour of the day is plotted. Both rhythms show a trough during the night (midnight to 4 AM), a primary peak between 6 AM and noon, and a secondary peak between 5 and 9 PM.

427) revealed that the sudden coronary deaths in these categories also demonstrated a pattern similar to that shown in Figure 3–1.

To eliminate a potential influence of errors in determination of the interval from onset of symptoms to death, and of errors in assignment to the three codes, an analysis of time of death was conducted regardless of the interval from onset of symptoms to death, for ICD codes 410, 414, and 427 combined. For out-of-hospital cardiac deaths, there was a prominent morning increase similar to that observed for the primary analysis group (Fig. 3–3). For the in-hospital deaths, the likelihood of occurrence of cardiac death was almost randomly distributed over the 24 hours of the day.

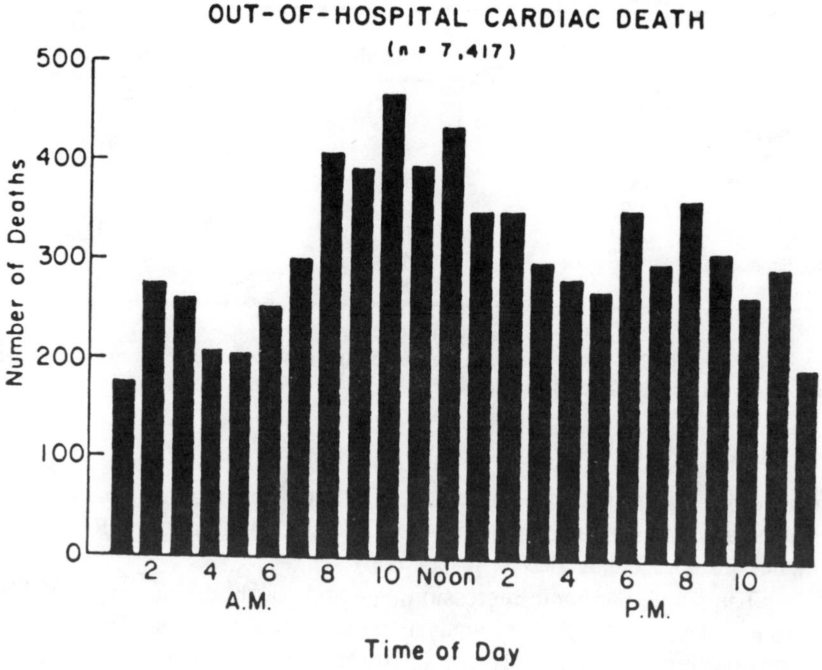

Fig. 3–3. Time of day of out-of-hospital cardiac death (ICD codes 410, 414, 427), regardless of the interval from onset of symptoms to death, for 7,417 individuals dying in Massachusetts in 1983. A statistically significant ($P < 0.001$) morning increase is present with a primary peak from 7 to 11 AM.

The sudden coronary deaths identified in the present study accounted for 10.1% of all deaths in Massachusetts in 1983. Age-specific and sex-specific incidence rates were similar to those obtained in previous population-based studies of sudden coronary death.

Results of the review of previous studies to determine the frequency of sudden coronary death during sleep are presented in Table 3–2 [12,15–20]. Only 85 of the 689 patients studied experienced sudden coronary death during sleep. This 12.3% incidence during sleep is significantly ($P < 0.001$) below the 29% that would be expected if the time of occurrence of sudden coronary death were randomly distributed throughout a 24 hour period with a 7 hour period of sleep.

Statistical assessment of the morning increase of sudden coronary death. All regression fits to the three sets of data were statistically significant as assessed by F tests, indicating the periodic nature of sudden and nonsudden coronary death. For the primary analysis group, the single-harmonic fit to the data was statistically significant (F test, $P < 0.01$). For this model, the estimated coefficient for the cosine term was significantly differ-

TABLE 3–2. Incidence of Sudden Cardiac Death During Sleep

Study	No. of deaths	No. of deaths during sleep (percent)
Hinkle and Thaler [12]	82	12 (15)
Bean [15]	88	16 (18)
French and Dock [16]	80	8 (10)
Moritz and Zamcheck [17]	115	15 (15)
Myers and Dewar [18]	100	9 (9)
Baroldi [19]	208	22 (11)
Roelandt et al. [20][a]	16	3 (19)
Total	689	85[b](12.3)

[a]Time of death determined by Holter monitoring.
[b]$P < 0.001$ vs. the 201 (29%) expected if sudden cardiac death were randomly distributed over a 24 hour period with 7 hours of sleep.

ent from zero (t test, $P < 0.01$), whereas the coefficient of the sine term was statistically indistinguishable from zero. The R^2 and adjusted R^2 for this model are 43.3% and 37.9%, respectively.

The single-harmonic regression equation for the frequency of sudden coronary death in the primary analysis group is as follows: sudden coronary deaths per hour $= 91.8 - 18 \cos (2\pi t/24) - 5.1 \sin (2\pi t/24)$, where t = time of day in hours. The double-harmonic regression equation for the frequency of sudden coronary death is: sudden coronary deaths per hour $= 91.8 - 18.0 \cos (2\pi t/24) - 5.1 \sin (2\pi t/24) + 7.7 \cos (4\pi t/24) - 11.7 \sin (4\pi t/24)$.

Although the coefficient of the second harmonic cosine term is not statistically significant (t test, $P > 0.5$), the coefficient of the second harmonic sine term is (t test, $P < 0.01$), indicating the value of the second harmonic. This double-harmonic equation demonstrated an improved fit to the data (F test, $P < 0.01$). There is a 24.3% improvement in the R^2 and a 22.8% improvement in the adjusted R^2 as compared with the single harmonic fit to the same data. The in-hospital and out-of-hospital cardiac death groups also showed significant improvements in the fit of the regression model when a second harmonic was added.

Discussion

These data from the Massachusetts Death Certificate Study demonstrate a prominent morning increase in the frequency of sudden coronary death, with a low frequency during the night and a peak frequency of occurrence from 7 to 11 AM. This rhythm is remarkably similar to that demonstrated for the frequency of onset of nonfatal myocardial infarction [5], the recognition of which provided the impetus for the study. A similar morning increase is present for the larger group of individuals dying out-of-hospital from cardiac disease (sudden and nonsudden) classified under any of the three ICD codes studied. For those who died in hospital, the hourly frequency of death from cardiac disease is almost equal, as might be expected in a setting in which daily variations in activity are markedly reduced.

Death certificates, which formed the base for the study, are known to have serious inadequacies, especially with regard to accuracy of cause of death determination [21,22]. Such inadequacies of death certificate diagnosis were not insurmountable obstacles to the study for several reasons. First, the study was not primarily an attempt to define the incidence of sudden coronary death in a community—our goal of studying the time of occurrence of sudden coronary death required only that a large number of cases of sudden coronary death with known onset time be identified. Second, although death certificate diagnoses of specific causes of death are unreliable, general categories such as death from "ischemic heart disease" are reliable [23,24]. The use of such larger categories (ICD-410, ICD-414, and ICD-427 combined), together with the requirement that deaths occurred 1 hour or less after onset of symptoms, permitted identification of a group of deaths occurring with approximately the same frequency, age distribution, and sex distribution as sudden coronary deaths identified by community-based studies [25–27]. Finally, the study relied primarily on time-of-death data, which have not received the same criticism as have cause-of-death data, although a number of potential biases were considered and found not to account for the results.

There are a number of previous reports of the frequency of sudden coronary death during sleep that provide an unbiased estimate of the likelihood of its occurrence during the night. The review of these studies [12,15–20] presented in Table 3–2 indicates that only 12.3% of these deaths occurred during sleep, a number significantly below the 29% expected if sudden coronary death were randomly distributed over a 24 hour day with 7 hours of sleep. This finding provides independent support for a low frequency of sudden coronary death from 11 PM to 6 AM, which is a prominent feature of the morning increase observed in the present study.

In addition to the variation observed during the period from 9 PM to 9 AM, there is a marked decrease in the frequency of out-of-hospital sudden coronary death from 11 AM to 5 PM and a secondary peak from 5 to 7 PM. During these daytime hours, the reliability of ascertainment of the time of death and determination of the cause of death is likely to be constant.

Thus the data from the Massachusetts Death Certificate Study indicate that there is a prominent morning increase of sudden cardiac death. However, because of the limitations of the original source material (death certificates), it was considered desirable to utilize a more thoroughly studied population to confirm or refute the existence of a morning increase. We therefore turned to the database assembled by the Framingham Heart Study.

THE FRAMINGHAM SUDDEN CORONARY DEATH STUDY

Methods

Study population. The Framingham Sudden Death Study is based on mortality data that were collected in a standardized manner by the Framingham Heart Study for the past 38 years. The original cohort consisted of 5,209 residents of Framingham, Massachusetts, who were between 30 and 62 years of age in 1948 [28]. The Framingham Heart Study personnel learn of the death of a member of the study from the family, from an obituary notice, from monitoring of hospitalizations in the only hospital in Framingham, or, during an attempt to contact the subject for routine biennial examination. All data concerning the death, including autopsy reports if available, are supplied to the Mortality Review Committee of the Framingham Heart Study, which determines the underlying cause of death.

The analysis does not include deaths of patients who were hospitalized or bedridden, since their endogenous and exogenous activity rhythms were likely to have been altered, or deaths occurring within 1 month after a documented myocardial infarction, which were likely to be secondary to that event. Deaths of nursing home residents were included in the study unless there was evidence that the deceased was continuously confined to bed.

Identification of definite sudden cardiac deaths. Since its inception, the Framingham Heart Study has classified a death as a sudden cardiac death using the following definition [29]: "If a subject, apparently well, was observed to have died within a few minutes (operationally documented as under 1 hour) from onset of symptoms and if the cause of death could not reasonably be attributed on the basis of the full clinical information and the information concerning death to some potentially lethal disease other than coronary heart disease, this was called sudden death and was attributed to coronary heart disease." For the present study, deaths meeting this definition were considered *definite* sudden cardiac deaths.

Identification of possible sudden cardiac deaths. To permit the necessary inclusion of sudden cardiac deaths that occurred during the night (or at other times) but could not be termed definite because they were unwitnessed, the following definition was developed: Deaths that may have occurred within 1 hour of onset of symptoms, and in which there was no apparent noncardiac cause of death, were considered cases of *possible* sudden cardiac death. Possible sudden cardiac deaths were identified from a review of deaths originally classified as due to "coronary heart disease death not known to be sudden" or of "unknown cause." Cases for which inclusion in the present study was questionable were presented for arbitration to a study committee (D. Levy, J.E. Muller, M.B. Rocco), which was blinded to the time of day at which death occurred.

Determination of time of death. If conflicting data on time of death were encountered, the time was determined on the basis of the highest ranked of the following sources: First, interviews with witnesses of the death, or interviews with persons in close contact with the deceased, who could describe the circumstances surrounding the death; second, medical reports, including autopsy results; third, newspaper accounts of the death; fourth, death certificates. The times of unwitnessed deaths were estimated on the basis of the most precise information available. For purposes of analysis, the hourly probability of death was equally distributed over the interval during which the death was known to have occurred. In some cases, this period was the interval between the time the subject was last seen alive and the time the subject was found dead. In cases when the quarter of the day in which the death occurred could be determined but more precise timing was not possible, the probability of death was evenly distributed over the 6 hours of the quarter of the day. When the only information available about the nighttime interval was that the individual was found dead in bed, the probability of death was evenly distributed between midnight and 6 AM. If no estimate of time of death could be made, the probability of death was evenly distributed over 24 hours.

Statistical analysis

Assessment of the periodicity of sudden cardiac death. The distribution of sudden cardiac death was first tested for differences among the four 6 hour intervals of the day with a χ^2-test for goodness of fit. If this test showed significant differences, the period with the highest frequency was tested to evaluate its difference from the average of the other three periods. To quantify the periodic structure of the frequency distribution of sudden cardiac death, a double-harmonic regression model was fitted to the data. It contained sine and cosine functions in which the independent variable was the time of the day. As the time of day varied, this model generated a regression curve, which was compared with the observed hourly distribution of sudden cardiac death. Model goodness of fit was evaluated by t tests (two-tailed) on the estimated coefficients, an F test on the overall model, and R^2 and adjusted R^2 statistics [13]. A P value of less than 0.05 was considered significant.

Estimation of the time of occurrence of "primary" sudden cardiac death. To determine if the circadian variation of sudden cardiac death observed in the Framingham study simply reflects the circadian variation of myocardial infarction, a hypothetical analysis was performed based on two assumptions: first, that myocardial infarction causes approximately one-third of all cases of sudden cardiac death; second, that myocardial infarction in the morning is not more likely to have a fatal outcome than is myocardial infarction at other times of the day. One-third of all definite or possible sudden cardiac deaths assumed to be secondary to myocardial infarction were distributed in the previously observed circadian pattern of nonfatal myocardial infarction [5]. The estimated hourly number of these "secondary" sudden cardiac deaths was subtracted from the corresponding hourly number of all definite or possible sudden cardiac deaths, revealing the distribution of "primary" sudden cardiac death. The assumed percentage of "secondary" sudden cardiac death was then sequentially raised above 33% to determine the highest percentage of cases that could have been due to myocardial infarction and still leave a significant circadian variation for "primary" sudden cardiac death.

Results

Since its inception in 1948, a total of 2,458 (47%) of the 5,209 individuals originally enrolled in the Framingham Heart Study have died, and their causes of death have been recorded. The sudden death study identified 726 certain and 156 possible cardiac deaths. Among these, there were 264 definite sudden cardiac deaths (11% of total deaths) and 165 possible sudden cardiac deaths (7% of total deaths). The combined group of 429 definite or possible sudden cardiac death victims had a mean age of 69 ± 10.7 years. The gender distribution was 65% male and 35% female.

The primary source of information about time of death was an interview or a telephone discussion with a witness of the death or a close relative of the deceased in 43% of cases, a medical report in 34%, a newspaper account in 11%, and the death certificate in 12%. The precise time of death could be identified for 255 of the 429 (59%) individuals. For 82 individuals (19%), the quarter of the day in which death occurred was the most specific information that could be identified. The interval between the time a subject was last seen alive and the time he or she was found dead (unless found dead in bed) was the most precise timing that could be ascertained for 26 individuals (6%). In 42 subjects (10%), the only information available on time of death was the report that they were found dead in bed. No estimate of time of death could be made for 24 (6%) of individuals (one file was missing, three were unwitnessed deaths, and 20 were witnessed deaths whose file did not contain a report of time of death and whose time of death could not be ascertained retrospectively).

The known or estimated time of occurrence of definite sudden cardiac death exhibited a prominent morning increase ($P < 0.05$), with a low frequency during the night, as would be expected from the requirement that the deaths be witnessed (Fig. 3–4A). However, a morning increase remained when the known or estimated time of possible sudden cardiac death was added to that of definite sudden cardiac death (Fig. 3–4B). The hourly risk of sudden cardiac death was at least 70% greater between 7 and 9 AM than the average risk during the remaining 22 hours of the day. Significantly more sudden cardiac deaths occurred between 6 AM and noon than during the other quarters of the day ($P < 0.01$).

The morning increase of sudden cardiac death was similar for men and women and for the older and younger halves of the population. Sudden cardiac death was evenly distributed over the days of the week and over the

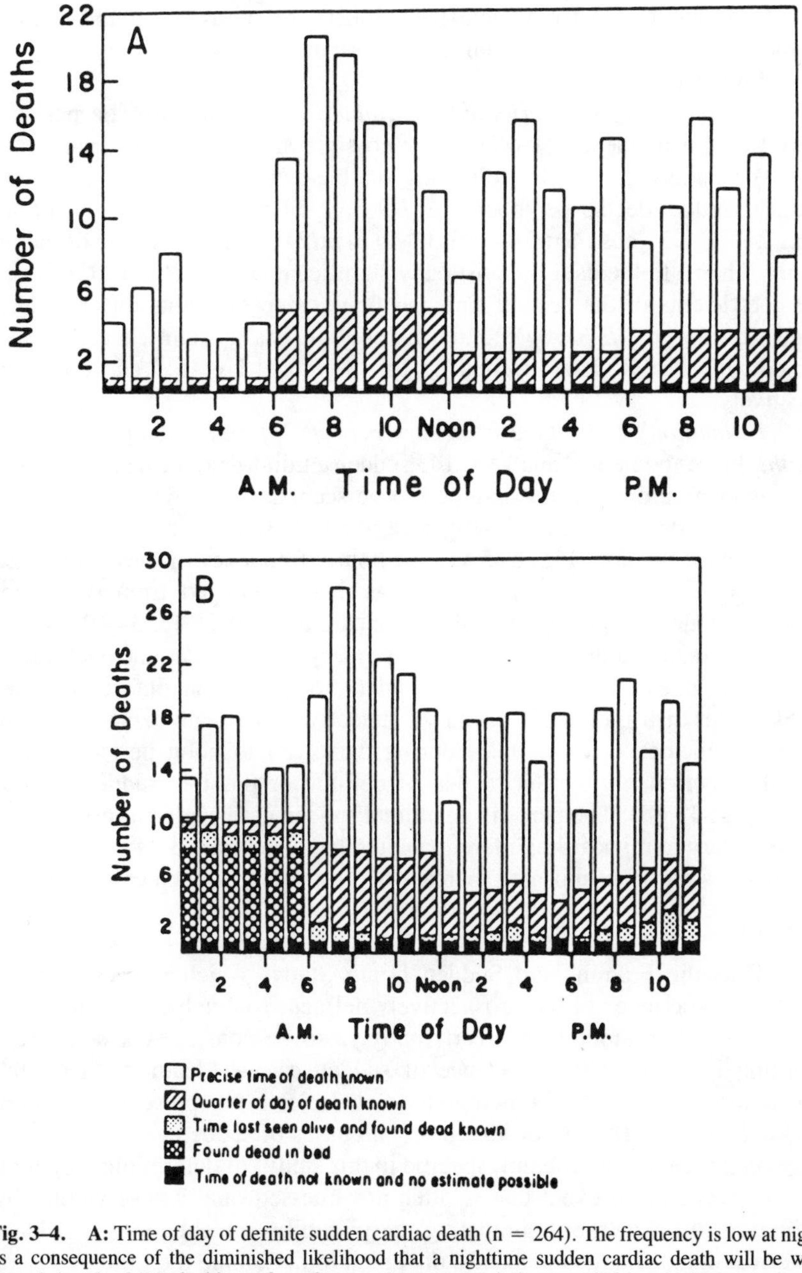

Fig. 3–4. **A:** Time of day of definite sudden cardiac death (n = 264). The frequency is low at night as a consequence of the diminished likelihood that a nighttime sudden cardiac death will be witnessed, but the fall in incidence from 9 AM to 1 PM occurs during a period in which observation is likely to be constant. **B:** Time of day of definite or possible sudden cardiac death (n = 429). The hourly risk of sudden cardiac death is approximately 70% higher from 7 to 9 AM compared to the average risk during the remaining 22 hours of the day.

months of the year. A fresh occlusive coronary thrombus was found in eight of the 24 cases (33%) for whom a postmortem report was available.

Statistical analysis

Assessment of the periodicity of sudden cardiac death. The periodic nature of the incidence of definite or possible sudden cardiac death (Fig. 3–4B) is indicated by the following double-harmonic regression model: sudden cardiac deaths per hour = $17.9 - 2.39 \cos(2\pi t/24) + 1.49 \sin(2\pi t/24) + 0.31 \cos(4\pi t/24) - 3.33 \sin(4\pi t/24)$, where t is time of day in hours. The fit to the data is statistically significant (F test, $P < 0.02$). Since the coefficients of the second sine and first cosine functions differ significantly from zero ($P < 0.05$), the distribution has a significant circadian periodicity. The R^2 and adjusted R^2 for the model are 46.9 and 35.8, respectively.

Estimation of the time of occurrence of "primary" sudden cardiac death. In a hypothetical analysis, 143 sudden cardiac deaths (the one-third of total sudden cardiac deaths assumed to be secondary to myocardial infarction) were distributed in the hourly pattern previously observed for nonfatal myocardial infarction (Fig. 3–5A). The hourly frequency of these presumed "secondary" sudden cardiac deaths was then subtracted from the corresponding hourly frequency of total sudden cardiac deaths (Fig. 3–4B), yielding the estimated hourly frequency of "primary" sudden cardiac death, i.e., those sudden cardiac deaths not secondary to myocardial infarction (Fig. 3–5B). This distribution of "primary" sudden cardiac death demonstrates an increased incidence ($P < 0.05$) during the 6 AM to noon period, with a circadian periodicity similar to that of definite or possible sudden cardiac death (Fig. 3–4B). The percentage of total sudden cardiac deaths assumed to be secondary to myocardial infarction could be raised from 33% to 40%, still yielding a significant morning increase of "primary" sudden cardiac death.

Discussion

Thus the Framingham Sudden Death Study, which is based on the mortality experience of the prospectively defined, routinely monitored population of the Framingham Heart Study, also demonstrates a significant morning increase in the incidence of sudden cardiac death, with a peak period from 7 to 9 AM. The two greatest obstacles to the present study were the well known difficulty of identifying all cases of sudden cardiac death in a population, and the problem, specific to this study, of determining the time of occurrence of an event that is often unwitnessed, and whose victim, by definition, dies, thereby eliminating the possibility of obtaining first hand historical data. The ideal database on which to determine the time of day of sudden cardiac death would consist of a large population followed for decades where a postmortem examination was performed for each death (to eliminate the need for assumptions about the cause of death) and in which some form of continuous surveillance would permit determination of the

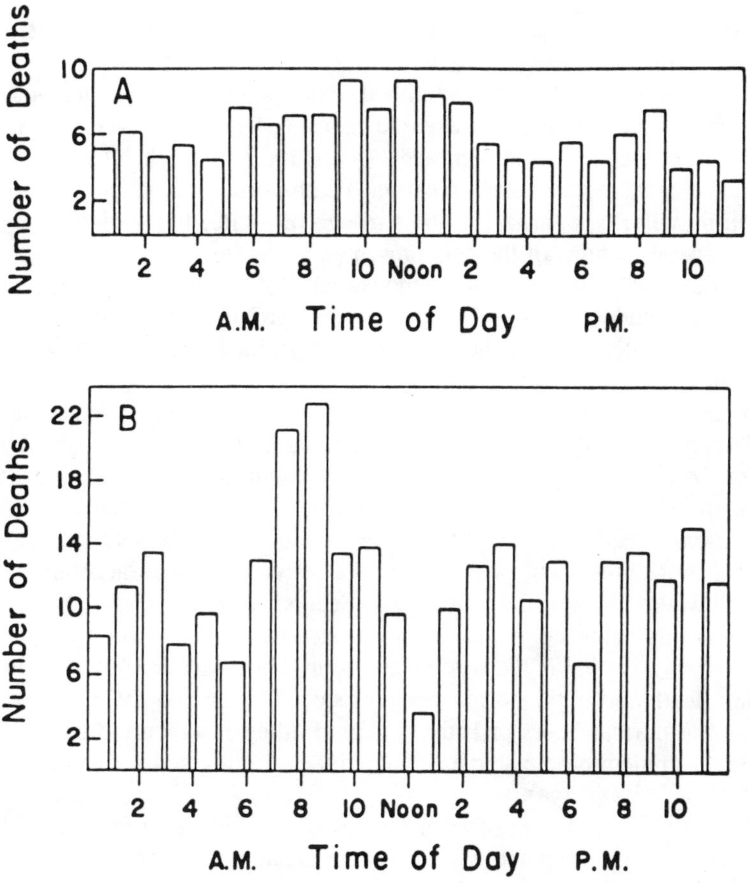

Fig. 3–5. **A:** Time of day of "secondary" sudden cardiac death assumed to be due to myocardial infarction (n = 143). On the basis of previous studies [7–21], which indicate that one-third or less of sudden cardiac deaths are due to acute occlusive coronary thrombosis, 143 deaths (one-third of deaths in B) are shown distributed in the previously observed circadian pattern of nonfatal myocardial infarction. **B:** Time of day of "primary" sudden cardiac death presumably not attributable to myocardial infarction (n = 286). The distribution is obtained by subtracting the hourly number of sudden cardiac deaths presumed to be secondary to myocardial infarction (A) from the corresponding hourly number of total definite or possible sudden cardiac deaths (Fig. 3–4B).

exact time of death (to eliminate the need for assumptions about the time of unwitnessed deaths). Since such a database does not exist and is unlikely to exist in the foreseeable future, we turned to the Framingham Heart Study as a close approximation to the ideal database for the present study. Commonly used estimates of the prevalence of sudden cardiac death are already based on data from the Framingham Heart Study [30,31].

The necessary assumptions about identification of cases of possible sudden cardiac death and their time of occurrence were then made in a manner most likely to diminish the possibility of detecting an increased frequency of sudden cardiac death in the period from 6 AM to noon. For instance, individuals found dead in bed, who might well have died at 7 or 8 AM, thereby augmenting an increased morning frequency, were considered to have died between midnight and 6 AM (Fig. 3–4B), thereby raising the estimated occurrence of sudden cardiac death during the hours of sleep, the period initially hypothesized to be a trough of a circadian variation.

Several features of the data presented in Figure 3–4A,B deserve comment. First, in addition to the demonstration of a morning increase in the incidence of sudden cardiac death, the figures provide upper and lower limits for its amplitude. The distribution of definite sudden cardiac death with time of death known (open bars in Fig. 3–4A) is an overestimate of the amplitude of the morning increase (unwitnessed deaths during the night and deaths for which the time of death is estimated are excluded), whereas the distribution of definite or possible sudden cardiac deaths with known or estimated time of death (Fig. 3–4B) is an underestimate, since it is partially based on ''worst-case'' assumptions. Furthermore, both figures would be likely to show a more prominent peak if the data were adjusted to account for the variable wake times of the individuals. Second, in Figure 3–4A,B, there is a decrease in incidence of sudden cardiac death from 9 AM to 1 PM, a period in which observation is likely to be constant. Third, the incidence of sudden cardiac death during the normal hours of sleep (11 PM to 6 AM) is lower than during the normal hours of activity. This finding is supported by previous results of epidemiologic studies of activity preceding sudden cardiac death [12,18].

There are a number of prior studies of time of death that support the conclusion of the both the Massachusetts Death Certificate Study and the Framingham Heart Study, although none feature their combination of size and specificity of diagnosis. In a summary report of 432,892 deaths from 49 separate studies, Smolensky et al. [32] reported a morning increase for total mortality with a peak at 6 AM. In a subgroup of 7,644 cases for whom death was reported to be due to a cardiovascular cause, there was a significant morning increase with a peak at 10 AM. Mitler et al. [33] demonstrated a morning increase for total mortality in a study of 4,619 deaths in New York State. The rhythm for total mortality was generated by a morning increase in ischemic heart disease mortality, which peaked at 8 AM. Finally, a study from the German Democratic Republic demonstrated a similar rhythm for out-of-hospital cardiac mortality [34].

It could be argued that the morning increase of sudden cardiac death reported in the present study is merely an expected result of the previously reported morning increase of nonfatal myocardial infarction [5] and the known relationship between myocardial infarction and sudden cardiac death. In our opinion, such a viewpoint would be an overinterpretation of the previously available studies about the myocardial infarction/sudden cardiac death relationship and an underestimate of the difficulties inherent in such studies. There are biologic barriers to confirmation of the diagnosis of myocardial infarction in individuals who die less than 1 hour after the onset of the event, since there is no time for myocardial enzymes to appear in plasma, and even direct observation of the myocardium provided by autopsy examination cannot reliably detect myocardial necrosis at such an early stage [35]. Of necessity, therefore, the autopsy studies focus on the incidence of an acute occlusive coronary thrombus, which has been found in 29% ± 8% of sudden cardiac death victims [36–45] (33% in the Framingham Study).

The other important source of information about the role of myocardial infarction in causing sudden cardiac death are findings in victims of cardiac arrest who are resuscitated [45–48]. However, in these studies, enzymatic or electrocardiographic evidence of myocardial infarction does not indicate whether infarction was the cause or the result of the cardiac arrest. Thus the reported 26% ± 12% and 39% ± 2% incidences of myocardial infarction (by electrocardiographic changes [45–48] or enzymatic changes [47–48], respectively) represent upper limits of the percent of cases in which myocardial infarction caused the cardiac arrest.

A statistical analysis based on the assumption that one-third of sudden cardiac deaths are caused by myocardial infarction indicated that there is a significant morning increase of "primary" sudden cardiac death. This is an important, conceptually new finding of the present study, since there have been few clues as to its cause, and, for resuscitated individuals, "primary" sudden cardiac death has been considered to have a worse prognosis than "secondary" sudden cardiac death [47,48].

The observation that sudden cardiac death is more likely to occur from 6 AM to noon is compatible with the two leading theories of causation of this disorder. First, it has been proposed that most cases of sudden cardiac death are a consequence of myocardial ischemia [49–51]. On the basis of the finding that coronary thrombi (intraluminal or intraintimal) could be identified in 95 of 100 cases of sudden cardiac death, the hypothesis has been advanced that sudden cardiac death results from ischemia secondary to platelet aggregates forming on an atherosclerotic coronary lesion [36]. This process could well be more likely to occur in the morning since it is a time of rising arterial pressure [52] (which may increase the likelihood of rupture of an atherosclerotic plaque, thereby exposing thrombogenic collagen [53]), increasing coronary artery tone [54], and increasing platelet aggregability [55]. Folts et al [56] developed an in vivo model supporting this theory. In this model, the induction of fixed partial coronary artery obstructions in dogs resulted in spontaneous cyclical reductions in coronary blood flow which were associated with the formation and distal embolization of platelet aggregates. Kowey et al. [49] observed that these changes were accompanied by reductions in the threshold for ventricular fibrillation. Second, it has been proposed that sudden cardiac death is frequently the result of a primary arrhythmic event [1,57,58]. Such a fatal arrhythmia might be more likely in the morning, since increased activity of the sympathetic nervous system, which is known to occur in the morning [59], may predispose to an arrythmia [60]. A retrospective analysis of the time of day of out-of-hospital sudden cardiac death in the NIH-sponsored Beta-Blocker Heart Attack Trial (BHAT) adds interest to the hypothesis that blockade of the morning surge in sympathetic activity may be beneficial [61]. This study found that propranolol therapy reduced the incidence of sudden cardiac death. However, the mechanism through which this beneficial effect was exerted was uncertain. Analysis of time of day of out-of-hospital sudden cardiac death in BHAT revealed that, in the placebo group, deaths were more frequent in the morning hours (from 2 AM to 2 PM) than during the remaining 12 hours of the day, indicating the presence of a morning increase similar to that observed in prior studies. However, in the group receiving propranolol, deaths during the morning period were 44% lower than in the placebo group. This suggestion that beta-blockade decreased the morning increase in sudden cardiac death needs to be confirmed in other randomized studies.

The primary value of the observation that sudden cardiac death is more likely to occur from 7 to 9 AM is not for the prevention of excess sudden cardiac deaths during that period but for the clue it may provide as to its mechanism. Further studies are needed to determine if this finding is present in other populations, to collect data regarding the timing and type of medications taken, and to determine activity immediately prior to death. The morning appears to be a time when "transient risk factors" proposed to precipitate sudden cardiac death [1] are likely to be prominent. Indeed, the clustering of sudden cardiac death cases in the morning hours strongly suggests that there are daily activities that "trigger" the onset of sudden cardiac death in vulnerable individuals. Studies of the physiologic changes occurring during the morning period of increased incidence of sudden cardiac death may provide additional evidence indicating the significance of one or another pathophysiologic triggering mechanism and may suggest possible means of prevention.

ACKNOWLEDGMENTS

We are grateful for the assistance of Ms. Kathleen Carney in the preparation of the manuscript.

REFERENCES

1. Lown B: Sudden cardiac death: the major challenge confronting contemporary cardiology. Am J Cardiology 43:313–328, 1979.
2. Kannel WB, Doyle JT, McNamara PM, Quickenton P, Gordon T: Precursors of sudden

cardiac death. Factors related to the incidence of sudden death. Circulation 51:606–613, 1975.
3. Spiekerman RE, Brandenburg JT, Achor RWP, Edwards JE: The spectrum of coronary heart disease in a community of 30,000. A clinicopathologic study. Circulation 25: 57–65, 1962.
4. Kuller L: Sudden and unexpected non-traumatic deaths in adults: A review of epidemiological and clinical studies. J Chronic Dis 19:1165–1192, 1966.
5. Muller JE, Stone PH, Turi ZG, et al.: Circadian variation in the frequency of onset of acute myocardial infarction. N Engl J Med 313:1315–1322, 1985.
6. Mattiolo G, Cioni G, Andreoli C: Time sequence of anginal pain. Clin Cardiol 9:165–169, 1986.
7. Rocco MB, Barry J, Campbell S, Nabel EG, Cook EF, Goldman L, Selwyn AP: Circadian variation of transient myocardial ischemia in patients with coronary artery disease. Circulation 75:395–400, 1987.
8. Robertson T, Marler J, Muller JE, et al.: Circadian variation in the frequency of onset of stroke. J Am Coll Cardiol 7 [Suppl A]:40A, 1986 (abstract).
9. Muller JE, Ludmer PL, Willich SN, Tofler GH, Aylmer G, Klangos I, Stone PH: Circadian variation in the frequency of sudden cardiac death. Circulation 75:131–138, 1987.
10. Willich SN, Levy D, Rocco MB, Tofler GH, Stone PH, Muller JE: Circadian variation in the incidence of sudden cardiac death in the Framingham Heart Study population. Am J Cardiol 60:801–806, 1987.
11. Manual of the International Statistical Classification of Diseases, Injuries, and Causes of Death: Based on the Recommendation of the Ninth Revision Conference, 1975, and adopted by the 29th World Health Assembly, WHO, Geneva, 1977.
12. Hinkle LE, Thaler HT: Clinical classification of cardiac deaths. Circulation 65:457–464, 1982.
13. Rosner BA: "Fundamentals of Biostatistics. 2nd Ed." Boston: Duxbury Press, 1986.
14. Brown BW Jr, Hollander M: "Statistics: A Biomedical Introduction." New York: John Wiley, 1977.
15. Bean WB: Infarction of the heart. A morphological and clinical appraisal of 300 cases. Part I. Predisposing and precipitating conditions. Am Heart J 14:684–702, 1937.
16. French AJ, Dock W: Fatal coronary arteriosclerosis in young soldiers. JAMA 124:1233–1237, 1944.
17. Moritz AR, Zamcheck N: Sudden and unexpected deaths of young soldiers. Diseases responsible for such deaths during World War II. Arch Pathol 42:459–494, 1946.
18. Myers A, Dewar HA: Circumstances attending 100 sudden deaths from coronary artery disease with coroner's necropsies. Br Heart J 37:1133–1143, 1975.
19. Baroldi G: Different types of myocardial necrosis in coronary heart disease. A pathologic review of their functional significance. Am Heart J 89:742–752, 1975.
20. Roelandt J, Klootwijk P, Lubsen J: Prodromal and lethal arrhythmias in 16 sudden death patients documented with long-term ambulatory electrocardiography. Circulation 68[Suppl III]:III-356, 1983 (abstract).
21. Kircher T, Nelson J, Burdo H: The autopsy as a measure of accuracy of the death certificate. N Engl J Med 313:1263–1269, 1985.
22. Lundberg GD, Voigt GE: Reliability of a presumptive diagnosis in sudden unexpected deaths in adults. JAMA 242:2328–2330, 1979.
23. Dobson AJ, Gibberd RW, Leeder SR: Death certification and coding for ischemic heart disease in Australia. Am J Epidemiol 117:397–405, 1983.
24. Glasser JH: The quality and utility of death certificate data. Am J Public Health 71: 231–237, 1981 (editorial).
25. Fraser GE: Sudden death in Auckland. Aust NZ J Med 8:490–499, 1978.

26. Madsen JK: Ischaemic heart disease and prodromes of sudden cardiac death. Is it possible to identify high-risk groups for sudden cardiac death? Br Heart J 54:27–32, 1985.
27. Kuller LH, Lilienfeld A, Fisher R: An epidemiological study of sudden and unexpected deaths in adults. Medicine 46:341–361, 1967.
28. Dawber TR, Meadors GF, Moore FE Jr: Epidemiological approaches to heart disease: The Framingham Study. Am J Public Health 41:279–286, 1951.
29. Shurtleff D: Some characteristics related to the incidence of cardiovascular disease and death: Framingham Study 18-year follow-up. In Kannel WB, Gordon T (eds): "The Framingham Study. Section 30." Washington, DC: U.S. GPO, 1974 (DHEW publication No. [NIH] 74-599).
30. Schatzkin A, Cupples LA, Heeren T, Morelock S, Kannel WB: Sudden death in the Framingham Heart Study. Am J Epidemiol 120:888–99, 1984.
31. Kannel WB, Doyle JT, McNamara PM, Quickenton P, Gordon T: Precursors of sudden coronary death. Factors related to the incidence of sudden death. Circulation 51:606–613, 1975.
32. Smolensky M, Halberg F, Sargent F: Chronobiology of the life sequence. In Itoh S, Ogata K, Yoshimura (eds). "Advances in Climatic Physiology." New York: Springer-Verlag, 1972, pp 281–318.
33. Mitler MM, Hadjukovic RM, Shafor R, Hahn PM, Kripke DF: When people die. Cause of death versus time of death. Am J Med 82:266–74, 1987.
34. Otto W, Hempel WE, Wagner CU, Best A: Some periodical and aperiodical variations of mortality from myocardial infarction in the German Democratic Republic. Z Gesamte Inn Med 37:756–763, 1982. (English Abstract)
35. Davies MJ: Pathological view of sudden cardiac death. Br Heart J 45:88–96, 1981.
36. Davies MJ, Thomas AC: Thrombosis and acute coronary-artery lesions in sudden cardiac ischemic death. N Engl J Med 310:1137–1140, 1984.
37. Kuller LH, Cooper M, Perper J, Fisher R: Myocardial infarction and sudden death in an urban community. Bull NY Acad Med 49:532–543, 1973.
38. Baba N, Bashe WJ Jr, Keller MD, Geer JC, Anthony JR: Pathology of atherosclerotic heart disease in sudden death. I. Organizing thrombus and acute coronary vessel lesions. Circulation 51/52[Suppl 3]:53–59, 1975.
39. Rissanen V, Romo M, Siltanen P: Prehospital sudden death from ischaemic heart disease—A postmortem study. Br Heart J 40:1025–1033, 1978.
40. Scott RG, Briggs RS: Pathological findings in pre-hospital deaths due to coronary atherosclerosis. Am J Cardiol 29:782–787, 1972.
41. Crawford T, Dexter D, Teare RD: Coronary artery pathology in sudden death from myocardial ischaemia. Lancet 1:181–185, 1961.
42. Lovegrove T, Thompson P: The role of acute myocardial infarction in sudden cardiac death. A statistician's nightmare. Am Heart J 96:711–713, 1978 (editorial).
43. Reichenbach DD, Moss NS, Meyer E: Pathology of the heart in sudden cardiac death. Am J Cardiol 39:865–872, 1977.
44. Goldstein S, Friedman L, Hutchinson R, Canner P, Romhilt D, Schlant R, Sobrino R, Verter J, Wasserman A, and the Aspirin Myocardial Infarction Study Research Group: Timing, mechanism and clinical setting of witnessed deaths in postmyocardial infarction patients. J Am Coll Cardiol 3:1111–1117, 1984.
45. Liberthson RR, Nagel EL, Hirschman JC, Nussenfeld SR, Blackbourne BD, Davis JH: Pathophysiologic observations in prehospital ventricular fibrillation and sudden cardiac death. Circulation 49:790–798, 1974.
46. Goldstein S, Landis JR, Leighton R, Ritter G, Vasu CM, Lantis A, Serokman R: Characteristics of the resuscitated out-of-hospital cardiac arrest victim with coronary heart disease. Circulation 64:977–984, 1981.

47. Baum RS, Alvarez H III, Cobb LA: Survival after resuscitation from out-of-hospital ventricular fibrillation. Circulation 50:1231–1235, 1974.
48. Schaffer WA, Cobb LA: Recurrent ventricular fibrillation and modes of death in survivors of out-of-hospital ventricular fibrillation. N Engl J Med 293:259–262, 1975.
49. Kowey PR, Verrier RL, Lown B, Handin RI: Influence of coronary platelet aggregation on ventricular electrical properties during partial coronary artery stenosis. Am J Cardiol 51:596–602, 1983.
50. Kubler W, Schomig A, Senges J: The conduction and cardiac sympathetic systems: metabolic aspects. J Am Coll Cardiol 5[Suppl]:157B–161B, 1985.
51. Fuster V, Steele PM, Chesebro JH: Role of platelets and thrombosis in coronary atherosclerotic disease and sudden death. J Am Coll Cardiol 5[Suppl]:175B–184B, 1985.
52. Millar-Craig MW, Bishop CN, Raftery EB: Circadian variation of blood pressure. Lancet 1:795–797, 1978.
53. Davies MJ, Thomas AC: Plague fissuring—The cause of acute myocardial infarction, sudden ischemic death, and crescendo angina. Br Heart J 53:363–373, 1985.
54. Willerson JT, Campbell WB, Winniford MD, Schmitz J, Apprill P, Firth BG, Ashton J, Smitherman T, Bush L, Buja LM: Conversion from chronic to acute coronary artery disease: speculation regarding mechanisms. Am J Cardiol 54:1349–1354, 1984 (editorial).
55. Tofler GH, Brezinski D, Schafer AI, Czeisler CA, Rutherford JD, Willich SN, Gleason RE, Williams GH, Muller JE: Concurrent morning increase in platelet aggregability and the risk of myocardial infarction and sudden cardiac death. N Engl J Med 316:1514–1518, 1987.
56. Folts JD, Crowell EB, Rower GG: Platelet aggregation in partially obstructed vessels and its elimination with aspirin. Circulation 54:365–370, 1976.
57. Skinner JE: Regulation of cardiac vulnerability by the cerebral defense system. J Am Coll Cardiol 5[Suppl]:88B–94B, 1985.
58. Eliot RS, Buell JC. Role of emotions and stress in the genesis of sudden death. J Am Coll Cardiol 5[Suppl 6]:95B–98B, 1985.
59. Turton MB, Deegan T: Circadian variations of plasma catecholamine cortisol, and immunoreactive insulin concentrations in supine subjects. Clin Chim Acta 55:389–397, 1974.
60. Corbalan R, Verrier R, Lown B: Psychological stress and ventricular arrhythmias during myocardial infarction in the conscious dog. Am J Cardiol 34:692–696, 1974.
61. Peters RW, Muller JE, Goldstein S, Byington R, Friedman IM: Propranolol and the circadian variation in the frequency of sudden cardiac death: The BHAT experience. Circulation 76[Suppl IV]:364, 1987 (abstract).

Chapter 4

Sudden Death in Noncoronary Heart Disease

Paul Kligfield, M.D.

Division of Cardiology, Department of Medicine, The New York Hospital—Cornell Medical Center, New York, New York 10021

INTRODUCTION

Death may occur as a predictable or as an unexpected event in patients with overt or occult cardiac and noncardiac disease, and it occasionally occurs, independent of trauma, in otherwise clinically normal subjects in whom no predisposing abnormalities can be found. With reference to cardiac performance, two major modes of death can be distinguished. The first is an abrupt cessation of effective circulation caused by arrhythmias, such as ventricular fibrillation, that may themselves be multifactorial in etiology. The second is a progressive deterioration in circulation to a level incapable of sustaining effective cellular perfusion, such as intrinsic pump failure, that occurs despite adequate electrical activity of the heart [1].

While it is widely appreciated that sudden death is a major consequence of ischemic heart disease, the prevalence and risk factors for arrhythmic death in noncoronary heart disease have been less well quantified. This discussion will examine sudden death in these subjects within a framework that relates complex arrhythmias to ventricular structure and function. Mitral valve prolapse will be used as a primary model for the estimation of sudden death incidence and prediction of risk in noncoronary heart disease according to this framework, with additional reference to related observations derived from patients with mitral regurgitation, dilated cardiomyopathy, and hypertrophic cardiomyopathy.

The Prevention of Sudden Cardiac Death, pages 43–81

TABLE 4–1. Cardiac Findings in Sudden Deaths

I. Ischemic heart disease
II. Nonischemic heart disease
  A. Valvular heart disease
    1. Mitral valve prolapse
    2. Mitral regurgitation
    3. Aortic stenosis
  B. Cardiomyopathy
    1. Idiopathic dilated cardiomyopathy
    2. Hypertrophic cardiomyopathy
    3. Alcohol cardiomyopathy
  C. Other cardiac findings
    1. Myocarditis
    2. Hypertensive heart disease
    3. Primary conduction tissue disease
    4. Primary malignant arrhythmia
    5. Arrhythmogenic dysplasia
    6. Sarcoidosis
    7. Congenital malformations and anomalies

SUDDEN DEATH: DEFINITIONS AND ETIOLOGIES

Sudden death will be considered to represent an abrupt arrhythmic event occurring in the setting of previously stable circulatory performance [1,2]. Evidence for a primary arrhythmic cause of death is found from several sources, including autopsy series of unexpected fatalities among clinically normal subjects and patients with disease [3–12], evaluation of subjects successfully resuscitated from out of hospital cardiac arrest [13–21], and ambulatory electrocardiographic recording coincident with unexpected death [22–26]. These observations demonstrate the most common underlying etiology of sudden death in the general population to be ischemic heart disease, found in 60–80% of cases. Although far smaller proportions of arrhythmic death are contributed by the various forms of cardiomyopathy, valvular heart disease, and hypertensive heart disease, as might be expected, the proportion of sudden death associated with noncoronary heart disease increases in younger subjects [6]. Major etiologies associated with sudden cardiac death are listed in Table 4–1.

Sudden death has been defined in alternate ways that, while clinically practical, often serve to obscure its pathophysiology. It is clear that definitions based on a discrete time period from the onset of symptoms, such as mortality within the first few hours of illness, cannot distinguish arrhythmic death from death caused by other factors. However, this distinction is itself further complicated by the obvious interdependence of potentially fatal arrhythmias with the metabolic, humoral, and hemodynamic consequences that accompany circulatory failure. Accordingly, the relationship between arrhythmias and ventricular function in the genesis of sudden death has been a central problem in the evaluation, prognosis, and treatment of various forms of heart disease.

Arrhythmias and Ventricular Function in Relation to Sudden Death

Several lines of evidence derived from the ischemic heart disease population, particularly in patients after myocardial infarction, suggest that complex arrhythmias and depressed ventricular function are independent and potentially synergistic risk factors for sudden death [27–40]. As an extreme, but theoretically important, example, Schulze et al. [35] found all cases of sudden death during a mean 7 month period after myocardial infarction to occur in patients who had both complex ventricular arrhythmias and reduced left ventricular ejection fraction at rest by radionuclide cineangiography. Sudden death did not occur in patients with preserved ventricular function, even in the presence of similarly complex rhythm disorders.

This framework can be extended to the noncoronary heart disease population, in which complex arrhythmias may or may not be present, and ventricular function may be normal and depressed. As has recently been summarized by Keefe et al. [15], several lines of investigation support the concept that sudden death results from an arrhythmic "trigger" acting on a vulnerable myocardial "substrate." Indeed, systolic ventricular dysfunction has emerged as a prognostically useful indicator of substrate vulnerability in many forms of noncoronary heart disease.

However, while hemodynamic profiles of patients resuscitated from out of hospital cardiac arrest reveal reduced cardiac index and ejection fraction in the majority, normal left ventricular function has been found in as many as one-third of this group [21]. It is therefore clear that other anatomic or physiologic substrates for sudden death, some of which may even be transient, remain to be characterized as predictors of mortality in some patients with overtly normal ventricular systolic function. Even with recognized limitations, however, stratification of sudden death risk according to ventricular function and the presence or absence of complex arrhythmias provides insights with clinical value.

In the case of mitral valve prolapse, most subjects have normal ventricular performance even when complex ventricular arrhythmias can be demonstrated by ambulatory electrocardiography, and risk of death is very low in this group. Depressed ventricular function in mitral prolapse may develop as a result of progressive mitral regurgitation, and complex arrhythmias are quite common in this relatively small group. As will be seen, risk of sudden death rises strikingly in these patients. Further, ventricular function emerges as an important determinant of arrhythmic mortality in patients with mitral regurgitation of all causes, and it will be demonstrated that risk of sudden death in these patients, even though most have complex arrhythmias, is markedly reduced when ventricular performance remains good.

Other observations support the prognostic usefulness of the framework relating arrhythmias to systolic performance. The independent risk of complex arrhythmias for sudden death in patients with uniformly poor ventricular function can be clearly demonstrated in the dilated cardiomyopathy population. On the other hand, it also remains clear that many resuscitated survivors of sudden death who have underlying mitral prolapse have entirely normal ventricular function and no mitral regurgitation. The risk of sudden death in other types of noncoronary heart disease, such as hypertrophic cardiomyopathy and primary electrical disorders, may be better assessed in other contexts.

Arrhythmias in Clinically Normal Subjects

Complex arrhythmias are often taken as an index of risk for sudden death within populations with known or suspected heart disease. For this purpose, ambulatory electrocardiography is commonly used to examine the prevalence of disorders of impulse formation and impulse conduction. However, the interpretation of arrhythmias in individuals and in groups of patients with ischemic heart disease, mitral valve prolapse, cardiomyopathy, and other specific types of heart disease must be related to the prevalence of rhythm findings in clinically normal populations. Appropriate control groups of age-matched normal subjects are required to separate arrhythmias that can be attributed to underlying disease from those that exist in the general population.

Data bearing on cardiac rhythm in apparently normal populations are available for newborn infants [41], healthy children [42], male medical students [43], young women [44], working adults [45–47], and active elderly people [48–50]. Several important trends and observations emerge from these studies. Most obvious is the extraordinarily high prevalence of potentially significant arrhythmias present in ambulatory subjects of all ages. Also apparent is a shift in the type of prevalent arrhythmia that accompanies aging. These data are summarized in Table 4–2.

Several important trends appear when the prevalence of arrhythmias is examined in relationship to age. Sinus pauses, various forms of sinus exit block, and marked sinus bradycardia with junctional escape rhythms are common in childhood and through young adulthood, but become very uncommon in middle and advanced age. Although far less common, moderately advanced sporadic atrioventricular node conduction delay also appears to decrease with aging in clinically normal subjects. On the other hand, disorders of impulse formation can be seen clearly to increase with age so that simple ventricular premature complexes, which are extraordinarily uncommon in children, are rather an expected finding in adults and are quite common in the elderly.

Since age is such an important factor in determining the prevalence of specific arrhythmias in apparently normal population, it is apparent that rhythm analysis of populations with specific diseases requires comparison

TABLE 4–2. Prevalence of Disorders of Impulse Formation and Conduction in Clinically Normal Populations, by Age (in Percent)

Population group and references	Sinus pauses, sinus block	Sinus bradycardia with AVJ escape	2° AVB	Any APCs	Any VPCs	VPC couplets	VT	Early cycle VPCs
Infants								
Southall et al. [41]	72	20	—	14	0	0	0	0
Children								
Southall et al. [42]	65	45	3	21	1	0	0	—
Young men								
Brodsky et al. [43]	50	22	6	56	50	2	2	6
Young women								
Sobotka et al. [44]	34	4	4	64	54	0	2	4
Working adults								
Clarke et al. [47]	—	10	2	—	73	13	2	2
Hinkle et al. [45]	1	—	1	76	62	—	3	—
Savage et al. [46]	—	—	—	89	68	15	—	—
Elderly								
Glasser et al. [48]	0	0	0	100	100	23	0	
Camm et al. [49]	0	4	1	37	69	6	6	
Kantelip et al. [50]	10	0	0	100	96	8	2	

AVJ, atrioventricular junctional; AVB, atrioventricular block; APCs, atrial premature complexes; VPCs, ventricular premature complexes; VT, ventricular tachycardia.

with age-matched controls. If this source of bias is not considered, it becomes easy to conclude that an arrhythmia is a feature of a specific disease rather than a characteristic of the population in which the disease occurs.

MITRAL VALVE PROLAPSE

The frequent occurrence of palpitation and arrhythmias were noted in early studies of mitral valve prolapse, which rapidly emerged as a combined auscultatory, electrocardiographic, and echocardiographic syndrome that unified previously unexplained symptoms and physical findings in large numbers of ambulatory subjects [51–55]. Occasional reports of sudden death in patients with mitral valve prolapse [54,56–58] have focused attention on the nature and treatment of associated arrhythmias, but at the same time it has also become well appreciated that mitral valve prolapse is most often a benign clinical finding with only a small incidence of complications [53,59].

Accordingly, mitral prolapse is an important model in which to examine the interaction of ventricular function and complex arrhythmias in noncoronary heart disease [60–63]. The high prevalence of mitral valve prolapse

TABLE 4–3. Prevalence of Arrhythmias in Adult Populations With Mitral Valve Prolapse, Detected by Ambulatory Electrocardiography

		Arrhythmia prevalence (%)			
Studies	N	APCs	PAT	VPCs	Complex VPCs
Kramer et al. [66]	63	81	32	63	43
Savage et al. [46]	61	90	24	89	56
De Maria et al. [64]	31	35	3	58	52
Campbell et al. [65]	20	—	10	80	50
Winkle et al. [67]	24	63	29	75	50

N, number of patients with mitral valve prolapse; APCs, atrial premature complexes; PAT, paroxysmal atrial tachycardia; VPCs, ventricular premature complexes (complex VPCs include VPC couplets and ventricular tachycardia with additional arrhythmias as defined in specific studies). Adapted from Kramer et al. [66] with permission of the publisher.

in the general population means that even a rare complication can affect large numbers of patients. While it is presumed that the basis for sudden death in mitral valve prolapse is arrhythmic, it is clear that the number of mitral valve prolapse patients with complex arrhythmias greatly exceeds the number who die suddenly [61,64–73].

In the large group of subjects with mitral prolapse who have normal ventricular function, it has been presumed, but not established, that complex arrhythmias that might be associated with sudden death are present prior to the fatal event. Thus, while some patients at potential jeopardy can be identified, the sensitivity and specificity of arrhythmias for identifying subjects at risk remains unknown. However, even with this uncertainty, it can be convincingly argued that the predictive value of complex arrhythmias for sudden death in the large majority of otherwise uncomplicated subjects with mitral prolapse is exceedingly low.

Prevalence of Arrhythmias in Mitral Valve Prolapse

The prevalence of various arrhythmias detected by ambulatory electrocardiography in patients with mitral valve prolapse is outlined in Table 4–3. With prolonged recording, generally for a period of 24 hours, atrial premature complexes have been found in 35–90%, atrial tachycardia in 3–32%, and ventricular premature complexes in 58–89% of mitral valve prolapse study groups. Complex ventricular arrhythmias have been reported in 43–56% of adult patients with mitral prolapse, but it must be appreciated that definitions of complexity have varied within these reports, often including frequent and multiform ventricular complexes [46,64] or multiform complexes alone [65,66], as well as repetitive ventricular arrhythmias such as ventricular couplets or ventricular tachycardia [67]. The reported prevalence of ventricular couplets has ranged from 6 to 50% and that for ventricular salvos or ventricular tachycardia from 5 to 21%.

However, patient selection has varied widely among these study populations, and this process can introduce significant interpretive bias in favor of arrhythmia complexity when highly symptomatic patients are concentrated in a study group [74]. Further, while prevalence data for arrhythmias in populations of patients with mitral value prolapse suggest that atrial and ventricular ectopy are common, these findings must be compared with rhythm abnormalities detected in clinically normal subjects and in appropriately selected controls [61–66]. As has been seen, both atrial and ventricular arrhythmias are highly prevalent in ambulatory adult subjects even in the absence of mitral valve prolapse [75] so that the excess prevalence of arrhythmias often attributed to mitral valve prolapse may be less than is indicated at first glance.

An excess prevalence of arrhythmias may also result when highly symptomatic subjects with mitral valve prolapse are compared with control populations that are uniquely free of symptoms. In contrast, the 28 control subjects studied by Kramer et al. [66] had prevalences of palpitation, chest pain, dyspnea, and dizziness comparable with those of 63 patients with mitral valve prolapse. Many of the control patients in this study were originally referred with a provisional diagnosis of mitral valve prolapse that was ultimately disproved by careful auscultatory and echocardiographic examination. Selection bias was avoided in the study of Savage et al. [46], in which 61 subjects with mitral valve prolapse and 179 randomly chosen controls were identified, independent of symptom status, as part of a systematic evaluation of offspring of the original cohort of the Framingham study.

In these reports, patients with mitral valve prolapse had modest trends toward more atrial couplets, a higher prevalence of brief supraventricular tachycardias, and a higher prevalence of multiform ventricular ectopy [46,66]. However, with similarly symptomatic controls or with randomly selected controls, no statistically significant excess prevalence of either atrial or ventricular arrhythmias could be demonstrated for patients with mitral valve prolapse (Figs. 4–1, 4–2). Both prolapse and control groups in the Framingham study had equal 15% prevalences of ventricular couplets or brief runs of ventricular tachycardia [46]. This does not exclude a modest excess prevalence of arrhythmia in the general mitral prolapse population, but it argues that, when present, this excess is not likely to be large. When the nearly identical increases in prevalence of paroxysmal atrial tachycardia associated with mitral valve prolapse in the Framingham and Cornell studies are combined, the difference does reach statistical significance (28% vs. 17%, $P < 0.02$).

Thus, when ambulatory populations of adult patients with mitral valve prolapse who do not have important mitral regurgitation are compared with comparably symptomatic, or comparably asymptomatic, control subjects, it

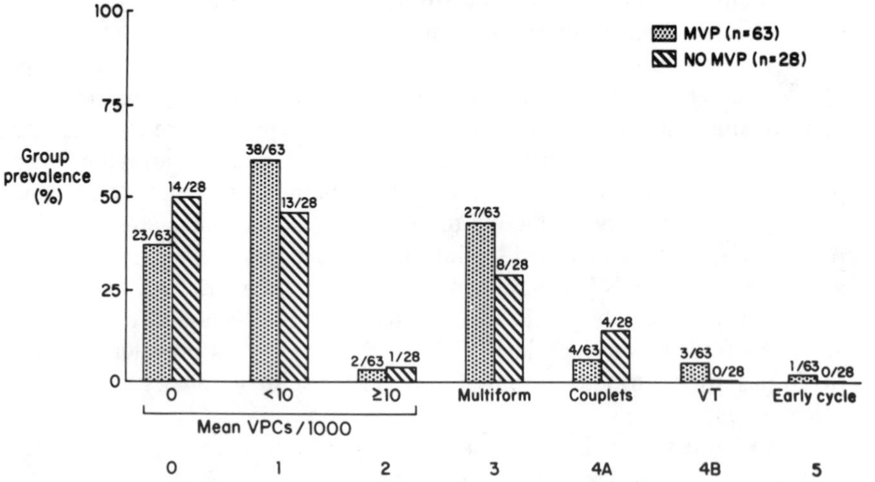

Fig. 4–1. Prevalence of ventricular arrhythmias in patients with mitral valve prolapse (MVP) without important mitral regurgitation and in similarly symptomatic, comparably aged control subjects. Arrhythmias are characterized according to mean frequency of ventricular premature complexes (VPCs) and according to group prevalence of multiform complexes, ventricular couplets, ventricular tachycardia (VT), and early-cycle forms. No significant differences are found between prolapse and control subjects. (Reproduced from Kramer et al. [66] with permission of the publisher.)

is difficult to demonstrate a higher prevalence of complex arrhythmias, other than atrial tachycardia, as an intrinsic feature of prolapse itself. The complexity of arrhythmias in mitral valve prolapse may be more strongly governed by demographic, structural, or functional factors that are independent of etiology, such as the development of significant mitral regurgitation. These findings do not address the potential association of complex arrhythmias with mortality in some subjects with mitral prolapse, but they do highlight the need to be cautious in equating the simple presence of arrhythmias alone with risk of sudden death.

Sudden Death and Malignant Arrhythmias in Mitral Valve Prolapse

Since rare cases of sudden death have been associated with mitral valve prolapse from its early recognition [53,54,56], it has become generally accepted that a small but important group of mitral valve prolapse subjects has complex arrhythmias that are potentially lethal [63]. Demonstration of mitral valve prolapse as the only autopsy finding in some cases of sudden death [76,77] is strong evidence for such an association, but at the same time this observation cannot be taken to prove mechanism or even to indicate cause and effect. A further link between arrhythmias and sudden death in mitral valve prolapse from recognition of mitral valve prolapse as the only abnormality in survivors of cardiac arrest [78] and in patients referred for man-

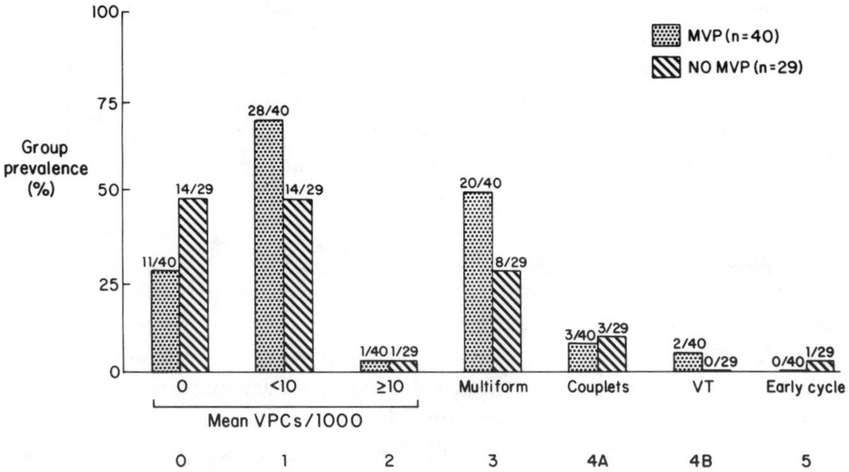

Fig. 4–2. Ventricular arrhythmias in asymptomatic and unmedicated subjects with mitral valve prolapse (MVP) and in asymptomatic controls. Prevalence of complex or repetitive forms is comparable in each group, similar to findings in larger numbers of randomly selected subjects and controls in the Framingham population [46]. VT, ventricular tachycardia; VPCs, ventricular premature complexes.

agement of refractory, symptomatic complex ventricular arrhythmias [57,79]. However, these observations do not mean that all patients with mitral valve prolapse who suffer sudden death have complex arrhythmias that could have been detected by routine monitoring. Sudden death in patients with mitral valve prolapse might also result from a unique or combined arrhythmogenic effect of transient autonomic, metabolic, or mechanical factors.

In previous reports, the incidence of sudden death during prospective follow-up of subjects with mitral valve prolapse has varied from 0 to as high as 0.5% yearly [59,80]. Unfortunately, these longitudinal data are derived from populations that may be quite heterogeneous as a result of different referral and selection patterns, and the usefulness and accuracy of these mortality figures may be complicated by inconstant reporting of associated findings such as mitral regurgitation and by lack of definitive autopsy documentation of mitral valve prolapse as the sole cause of death in older patients [81]. Even with limitations, some approximation of the relative risk and incidence of sudden death in subjects with mitral valve prolapse can be formulated from available observations. However, it must be appreciated that these estimates are based on data of uncertain general applicability and may therefore be subject to considerable error.

One can begin with the important observations of Davies et al. [77], derived from sudden deaths in a general population in England. Among forensic necropsies that were specifically and carefully screened for evidence of mitral valve prolapse, 13 cases of unexpected death associated with mitral prolapse were found during a 5 year period. Over two-thirds of these autopsy cases had evidence of significant mitral regurgitation caused by ruptured chordae, which is consistent with emerging evidence for the importance of mitral regurgitation as a potential substrate for sudden death in mitral valve prolapse [61,62]. In only four of the cases examined by Davies et al. were no important structural changes related to mitral regurgitation noted. The small proportion of deaths in which mitral regurgitation was absent suggests that mortality may vary considerably among subgroups of prolapse subjects with and without this finding.

Although no clear estimate of the proportion of sudden deaths accounted for by patients with mitral valve prolapse was presented by Davies et al. [77], it was noted that approximately 250 cases of sudden death caused by ischemic heart disease are generally encountered annually in the screened population. This suggests that on a yearly basis 10 sudden deaths might be expected among patients with mitral valve prolapse for every 1,000 ischemic sudden deaths. In the United States, where 400,000 sudden deaths from ischemic heart disease are estimated to occur annually [20], a similar proportion of sudden deaths caused by mitral valve prolapse would be 4,000 each year. Based on the findings data of Davies et al., about 2,700 of these deaths would likely be associated with hemodynamically important mitral regurgitation while approximately 1,300 deaths per year with no cardiac cause other than mitral valve prolapse might be predicted among the adult mitral valve prolapse population without important mitral regurgitation.

Sudden Death in Mitral Valve Prolapse Without Mitral Regurgitation

With an estimated 4% prevalence [82,83] of echocardiographically documented mitral valve prolapse among adults in the United States, approximately 7 million of the 180 million adults in this country are affected. Taking the yearly mortality of 1,300 people derived above for subjects without important mitral regurgitation, the annual risk of sudden death attributable to mitral valve prolapse alone can be estimated to be 1.9 per 10,000 subjects (approximately 0.02% per year). As will be shown, the estimated annual risk for subjects in whom hemodynamically significant mitral regurgitation has developed is markedly higher.

While the total number of deaths is high, the likelihood of sudden death for individuals with mitral prolapse who do not have mitral regurgitation is therefore quite small. This prolapse-related risk is lower than the annual risk of sudden death from all causes, which is 22 per 10,000 in the adult U.S. population [20]. Indeed, this risk is also lower than the 7 per 10,000 annual risk for sudden death found in subjects aged 45–54 without antecedent clinical evidence of coronary disease in the combined Albany-Framingham study [84]. As a result, sudden death in patients with mitral valve prolapse who do not have mitral regurgitation or coronary disease is sufficiently uncommon to be rarely encountered in any unselected study population, in accord with the emphasis previously placed on the generally benign prognosis of patients with this condition [53,59]. It might be argued from this analysis that sudden death in mitral valve prolapse patients without mitral regurgitation may be independent of mitral valve prolapse itself, and this possibility requires further study.

On the other hand, other observations argue strongly in favor of increased risk of sudden death in mitral valve prolapse, independent of important mitral regurgitation. Detection of mitral valve prolapse in a significant proportion of survivors of potentially fatal arrhythmia [57,78,79], and higher estimates of the incidence of sudden death in mitral valve prolapse [80] suggest that a true association of hemodynamically uncomplicated mitral valve prolapse and sudden death may exist. For example, Wei et al. [79] found 10 patients with mitral valve prolapse and a similar number with no detectable heart disease among 60 consecutive patients referred for management of refractory complex ventricular arrhythmias. In a larger series, J.C. Somberg and colleagues (personal communication) found 15 patients with mitral valve prolapse and 72 patients with no other detectable cardiac abnormality among more than 900 patients referred for electrophysiologic study after successful resuscitation from cardiac arrest or with sustained ventricular tachycardia.

If no selection bias governed referral to these study groups, the proportions of patients with mitral valve prolapse and without detectable disease, taken together with a 4% population prevalence of mitral valve prolapse, suggest that symptomatic refractory ventricular arrhythmias might be from 4 to 20 times more common among the mitral valve prolapse population. But it must be emphasized that this is likely to be an overestimate of relative risk, since clinically normal subjects would be less likely to have been referred for intensive evaluation than patients with mitral valve prolapse, and it is also uncertain how many of these patients were indeed at risk of sudden death.

Mitral valve prolapse populations with an increased risk of sudden death have been reported in the literature. Nishimura et al. [80] found six cases of sudden death among 237 minimally symptomatic mitral valve prolapse patients followed for an average of 6 years, suggesting an annual mortality of approximately 40 per 10,000. This is twice the incidence of sudden death expected in the general adult population [20]. All patients with sudden death in the report by Nishimura et al. had echocardiographic evidence of mitral leaflet redundancy (thickening), which was found in 41% of their patients and might represent an important discriminator between subjects with high and low risk. Sudden death was reported not to be independently associated with severe mitral regurgitation or with echocardiographic findings expected in patients with underlying moderate mitral regurgitation.

However, two-thirds of the cases of sudden death occurred in men over the age of 55, and it might be argued that in the absence of autopsy confirmation, occult ischemic disease might explain these deaths [84].

Risk of Arrhythmias for Sudden Death in Uncomplicated Mitral Prolapse

Because the number of subjects with mitral prolapse who do not have important mitral regurgitation is large in relation to estimated incidence of sudden death, and because complex arrhythmias are relatively common in this large population, the predictive value of complex arrhythmias alone for subsequent mortality can be shown to be quite low. Based on a 50% prevalence of multiform or repetitive ventricular arrhythmias in these subjects (Table 4–3), with an estimated 1,300 cases of sudden death among the 7 million affected adults in the United States, the predictive value of complex arrhythmias detected in any individual for mortality during the subsequent year can be calculated to be only about 0.04% (approximately 1 in 2,500). If only repetitive ventricular arrhythmias, including ventricular couplets or ventricular tachycardia found in 8–15% of these subjects [46,61,62] are considered risk factors, the predictive value still remains poor at about 0.12–0.23% per year (approximately 1 in 400–800).

These estimates assume, without evidence, that these specific forms of complex arrhythmias are indeed present prior to death in the mitral prolapse population at risk. If this is not reliably true, the predictive value of arrhythmias alone for sudden death among subjects with uncomplicated mitral prolapse may be considerably lower than suggested. Indeed, Nishimura et al. [80] reported antecedent complex ventricular arrhythmias in only three of six patients who died suddenly during a prospective study of the natural history of mitral valve prolapse. This suggests that in addition to low specificity and extremely poor predictive value for sudden death, complex ventricular arrhythmias detected by routine ambulatory monitoring may also suffer from low sensitivity for subsequent sudden death in the general mitral valve prolapse population. In approaching treatment of arrhythmias in patients with mitral valve prolapse who are otherwise asymptomatic and free of additional risk factors, this problem becomes an important consideration.

As a corollary of these estimates, it is apparent that complex arrhythmias in subjects with mitral prolapse, in the absence of mitral regurgitation, are of benign, short-term prognostic significance in well over 99% of cases. Clearly, additional descriptors of subsequent mortality, beyond arrhythmias alone, are needed to concentrate risk of sudden death in this large group.

Additional Risk Factors for Sudden Death in Mitral Valve Prolapse

Several clinical findings in addition to complex ventricular arrhythmias and important mitral regurgitation have been associated with sudden death in mitral valve prolapse (Table 4–4). Unfortunately, no single finding or com-

TABLE 4–4. Potential Risk Factors for Sudden Death in Mitral Valve Prolapse

Complex or repetitive ventricular arrhythmias
Mitral regurgitation
Prolonged QT interval
Inferolateral repolarization abnormalities
Redundant or thickened mitral leaflets
History of syncope, presyncope, palpitations
Age and sex

bination of findings has proven to be a consistent predictor of sudden death when potential risk factors in available reports are compared.

Risk stratification is further complicated by a paucity of prospective evidence concerning detection of suspected risk factors prior to sudden death. Thus, while it is clear that the mechanism of sudden death may be arrhythmic, detection of complex arrhythmias in mitral valve prolapse patients who have survived cardiac arrest does not demonstrate that complex arrhythmias regularly precede sudden death in less highly selected patients. Alternatively, it is possible that arrhythmic mortality in patients with mitral valve prolapse results from a cluster of additional pathophysiologic circumstances that might not be present during routine monitoring of rhythm prior to the fatal event.

Prolongation of the QT interval has been related to arrhythmias and to sudden death in patients with mitral valve prolapse [53,54,56,79,85,86], but this association has been inconstant. The relationship of the congenital long QT interval syndromes to autonomic dysfunction and to sudden death has been well reviewed by Schwartz et al. [87], and the effect of catecholamines on the QT interval has been examined by Abildskov [88]. It remains speculative whether these findings, together with observed catecholamine-sensitive automaticity and triggered activity in abnormal mitral valve tissue [89], provide a contributory mechanism for arrhythmogenesis in mitral valve prolapse.

In contrast, Levy and Savage [90] have found rate-corrected QT prolongation in only 8% of 240 randomly selected mitral valve prolapse offspring of the original Framingham cohort and in a similar proportion of unaffected subjects. This suggests that QT prolongation is not importantly concentrated in patients with mitral valve prolapse but does not exclude the possibility that abnormalities of repolarization may be prognostic indicators for arrhythmic death. Further, QT prolongation has been found in only a modest proportion of mitral valve prolapse patients who have died suddenly or who have demonstrated potentially fatal arrhythmias. Wei et al. [79] observed QT prolongation unrelated to drug effect in 5 of 10 patients with mitral valve prolapse referred for the management of refractory ventricular arrhythmias. But among nine survivors of cardiac arrest with underlying mitral valve prolapse examined by Boudoulas et al. [78] only one had QT prolongation, and prolongation of the QT interval was present in none of seven cases with available electrocardiograms among the 14 postmortem studies of mitral valve prolapse sudden death reviewed by Chesler et al. [76].

In addition to intrinsic QT prolongation, nonspecific repolarization changes have been associated with potentially malignant arrhythmias in mitral valve prolapse [58], and a thread linking serious arrhythmias to possible electrolyte and drug effects on the duration of repolarization has emerged. It is important to note that survivors of cardiac arrest with mitral valve prolapse reported by Winkle et al. [57] were often patients in whom diuretic therapy had produced potentially significant prolongation of repolarization caused by hypokalemia or other electrolyte abnormality, at times in the presence of simultaneous quinidine and digitalis administration. Thus, the possible proarrhythmic interactions of these drugs precludes entirely attributing these malignant arrhythmias to the presence of mitral valve prolapse. Indeed, Salmela et al. [91] have reported fatal ventricular fibrillation in a patient with mitral valve prolapse shortly after initiation of digoxin therapy, and aggravation and provocation of arrhythmias by antiarrhythmic drugs has become an increasingly recognized phenomenon [92].

The role of electrophysiologic assessment of ventricular arrhythmias in mitral valve prolapse has been controversial [93–96]. Although highly symptomatic patients with mitral valve prolapse may be inducible in the laboratory, it must be noted that inducibility in patients with mitral valve prolapse may be dissociated from prognostic and therapeutic utility [94,95]. The available data suggest that mitral valve prolapse patients without syncope or presyncope who are not inducible by the triple extrastimulus technique have a benign short-term natural history despite associated complex ventricular arrhythmias detected by ambulatory electrocardiography. Of course, this is consistent with the extremely low incidence of sudden death in asymptomatic patients with prolapse. This does not mean that electrophysiologic study might not be sensitive for the identification of asymptomatic patients at higher risk of arrhythmic death, but even if it were, because of the very low incidence of sudden death its predictive value is likely to be low. Thus many asymptomatic patients would have to be studied to detect one case at actual risk of sudden death. On the other hand, electrophysiologic guidance of drug therapy may provide benefit for some highly symptomatic patients with inducible sustained tachycardias or in those patients with sustained ventricular tachycardia who have nonsustained inducible rhythms [60,94].

Arrhythmogenesis in Uncomplicated Mitral Valve Prolapse

Extranodal accessory pathways have been found in up to 25% of symptomatic patients with mitral valve prolapse [97,98], which is likely a significant overestimate of the prevalence of bypass tracts in the general prolapse population. Levy and Savage [90] found no cases of Wolff-Parkinson-White

(WPW) conduction among 296 subjects with mitral valve prolapse who were identified by echocardiographic study in Framingham. However, the occasional occurrence of pre-excitation in patients with mitral valve prolapse has potentially important implications for arrhythmogenesis and drug therapy, since acceleration of conduction in anomalous pathways, particularly in the setting of paroxysmal atrial flutter or atrial fibrillation, is a recognized danger. Fortunately, only a minority of patients studied by Josephson et al. [97] had anterograde conduction down the anomalous pathway.

Wit and Cranefield [89] have observed triggered activity resulting from slow response potentials in simian mitral valve fibers, while endocardial friction lesions with scarring [76] and interstitial fibrosis with intramyocyte degenerative changes [99] also have been suggested as sources of arrhythmogenesis in patients with mitral valve prolapse. It is possible that duration of mitral valve prolapse in some older subjects, when combined with additional factors such as ventricular mass or blood pressure in the higher normal range, may facilitate arrhythmias according to these mechanisms, and these hypotheses require further testing.

MITRAL REGURGITATION

Complex ventricular arrhythmias are often found in patients with mitral regurgitation, and mortality may be high in unoperated patients with mitral regurgitation who have depressed right or left ventricular ejection fractions at rest [100,101]. Ventricular tachycardia has been associated with progression to severe mitral regurgitation in patients with mitral valve prolapse [102], and repetitive ventricular arrhythmias have been correlated with subsequent mortality in mitral regurgitation of diverse etiologies [101]. Death in patients with important mitral regurgitation might result either from severe hemodynamic failure or from a sudden arrhythmic event [1].

However, until recently the importance of arrhythmic death in mitral regurgitation has been supported by few previous observations beyond recognized mortality in medically treated patients [101,103] and arrhythmia-related postoperative mortality in patients undergoing mitral valve replacement [104]. Certainly, recognition of primary valvular disease among a small subset of survivors of cardiac arrest [20,21,105] suggests that arrhythmias in mitral regurgitation are not necessarily benign. Recent evidence argues that complex arrhythmias and sudden death among patients with nonischemic mitral regurgitation, with and without mitral prolapse, may be more common than is currently appreciated.

Because complex arrhythmias are so prevalent in mitral regurgitation, and because ventricular function may range from good to poor in these patients, this nonischemic disease provides a useful model in which to examine the interaction of ventricular performance with arrhythmias in the genesis of sudden death [62]. While mortality is observed to be exceedingly

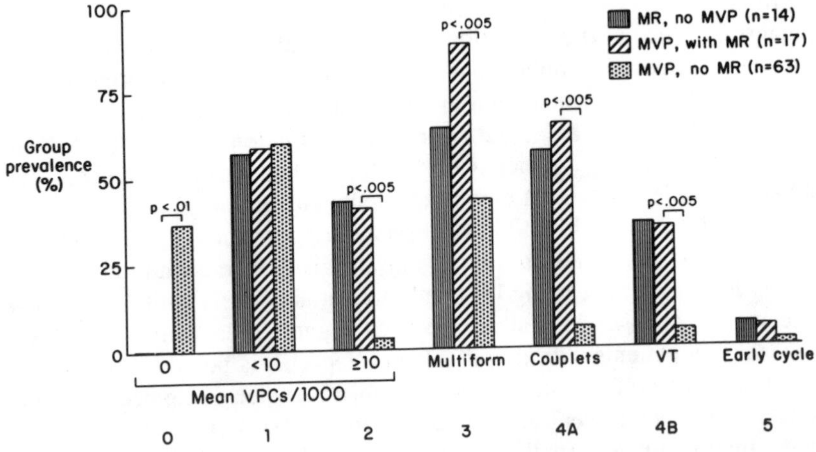

Fig. 4–3. Prevalence of ventricular arrhythmias (VT) in patients with mitral regurgitation (MR) with and without underlying mitral valve prolapse (MVP) and in patients with mitral prolapse without mitral regurgitation. Complex arrhythmias are common in mitral regurgitation, independent of etiology. VPC, ventricular premature complexes. (Reproduced from Kligfield et al. [100] with permission of the publisher.)

high in patients with depressed ejection fractions, nearly all of whom have complex ventricular arrhythmias, sudden death appears to be markedly lower when similarly complex complex arrhythmias exist in the setting of preserved ventricular function.

Arrhythmias in Nonischemic Mitral Regurgitation

The frequency and complexity of arrhythmias detected by ambulatory electrocardiography in 31 patients with hemodynamically severe mitral regurgitation of diverse etiology [100] are shown in Figure 4–3, in contrast to arrhythmias found in subjects with mitral prolapse but no regurgitation. In this population, mitral regurgitation was related to underlying mitral valve prolapse in 17, to rheumatic heart disease in four, to ruptured chordae in three, to healed infective endocarditis in one, and to unknown etiology in six. None of the patients had clinical evidence of ischemic heart disease, additional aortic valve disease, or mitral stenosis.

Frequent and complex atrial and ventricular arrhythmias were highly prevalent in this group. Sustained atrial fibrillation was present in 23% of the group, and among the patients in sinus rhythm, atrial premature complexes more frequent than 10 per 1,000 beats occurred in 17%, atrial couplets occurred in 54%, and brief bursts of atrial tachycardia occurred in 50%. All patients had ventricular premature complexes, and these were more frequent than 10 per 1,000 beats in 42% of the group. Multiform ventricular premature complexes were present in 77%, while 61% had repetitive ventricular arrhythmias, including ventricular couplets alone in 39% and ventricular couplets along with additional ventricular salvos or nonsustained ventricular tachycardia in 29%.

Arrhythmias in this group were more clearly associated with the presence of important mitral regurgitation than with the underlying etiology. When patients were separated according to mitral prolapse and nonprolapse causes of regurgitation, arrhythmia frequency and prevalence of complex forms were comparable in each subset (Fig. 4–2). These subsets were also similar with respect to age, sex, functional class, left atrial and left ventricular dimensions, and left ventricular ejection fractions [100]. Thus, despite differences in etiology, arrhythmias appear to be quite similar in patients with mitral regurgitation of comparable hemodynamic compromise.

Effect of Mitral Regurgitation on Arrhythmias in Mitral Prolapse

The development of significant mitral regurgitation is an infrequent but well-established complication of mitral valve prolapse. Indeed, because mitral valve prolapse is very common, it is now emerging as the most common cause of hemodynamically important mitral regurgitation [83,100]. The prevalence of ventricular arrhythmias in patients with mitral valve prolapse, with and without clinical evidence of hemodynamically important mitral regurgitation, is summarized from the data of Kligfield et al. [100] in Table 4–5.

All mitral prolapse patients with important mitral regurgitation had ventricular ectopy, and over 40% had very frequent ventricular premature complexes. In contrast, frequent ventricular premature complexes were present in only 3% of mitral valve prolapse patients without mitral regurgitation. Further, mitral valve prolapse patients with mitral regurgitation had a markedly increased prevalence of multiform ventricular premature complexes, ventricular couplets, and ventricular tachycardia, with peak Lown grades of 4A or 4B in nearly two-thirds of this subset.

Similarly, atrial arrhythmias were also more frequent and more complex in mitral valve prolapse patients who had mitral regurgitation [100]. Complex atrial arrhythmias might be related to sudden death in mitral valve prolapse if the anomalous bypass tracts found in some groups of symptomatic mitral valve prolapse patients [97,98] predisposed to unstable, rapid ventricular response rates during atrial flutter or atrial fibrillation. All patients with mitral regurgitation had supraventricular premature complexes, nearly one-third were in sustained atrial fibrillation, and one-fourth of the patients in sinus rhythm had very frequent atrial premature complexes. In contrast, none of the patients with mitral valve prolapse without mitral regurgitation had frequent atrial premature complexes or atrial fibrillation. Patients with mitral regurgitation were also more likely to have atrial couplets and episodes of

TABLE 4–5. Prevalence of Ventricular Arrhythmias in Mitral Valve Prolapse With and Without Mitral Regurgitation[a]

	MVP subgroups		
	MVP without MR (%; n = 63)	MVP with MR (%; n = 17)	*P*
VPC Frequency			
No VPCs	37 (23/63)	0 (0/17)	<0.01
Mean >10/1,000	3 (2/63)	41 (7/17)	<0.005
VPC complexity			
Multiform VPCs	43 (27/63)	88 (15/17)	<0.005
VPC couplets	6 (4/63)	65 (11/17)	<0.005
VPC salvos/VT	5 (3/63)	35 (6/17)	<0.005
Peak lown grade			
0–2	58 (36/63)	6 (1/17)	<0.001
3	33 (21/63)	24 (4/17)	ns
4A	3 (2/63)	35 (6/17)	<0.005
4B	5 (3/63)	29 (5/17)	<0.005
5	2 (1/63)	6 (1/17)	ns

[a]MR, mitral regurgitation; MVP, mitral valve prolapse; VPC, ventricular premature complex; VT, ventricular tachycardia. Adapted from Kligfield et al. [100] with permission of the publisher.

brief supraventricular tachycardia, but these differences did not reach statistical significance.

Thus mitral valve prolapse patients with important mitral regurgitation are far more likely to have frequent and complex atrial and ventricular arrhythmias than patients without mitral regurgitation. Since similar prevalences of complex arrhythmias occur in patients with comparable mitral regurgitation, whether the regurgitation is related to mitral valve prolapse [100], it would appear that these arrhythmias are more likely related to the presence of mitral regurgitation than to any direct structural or functional consequences of mitral valve prolapse itself. It is obvious from these findings that quantification of the proportion of patients with underlying mitral regurgitation is essential for accurate interpretation of both data on arrhythmia prevalence in mitral valve prolapse and data on the incidence of sudden death in patients with mitral valve prolapse in the general population.

Sudden Death in Mitral Valve Prolapse With Mitral Regurgitation

While the strength of association between sudden death and mitral valve prolapse in patients without mitral regurgitation is uncertain, sudden death does not appear to be a major risk among patients with mitral valve prolapse who have important mitral regurgitation. In the 12 cases of sudden death in mitral valve prolapse reviewed by Jeresaty [58], most of the patients who had undergone left ventriculography were noted to have mild to moderate mitral regurgitation.

However, it should be noted that among mitral valve prolapse survivors of potentially fatal arrhythmia, mitral regurgitation has not been commonly reported [57,78,79,20,105]. Two of seven patients reported by Winkle et al. [57] and at least one of 9 reported by Boudoulas et al. [78] had mitral regurgitation, but important mitral regurgitation was not noted by Wei et al. [79]. This might suggest that the proportion of mitral valve prolapse sudden death potentially associated with mitral regurgitation is less than that observed by Davies et al. [77]. But since these patients represent survivors of potential sudden death rather than fatalities, these findings may also be explained by a survival advantage for mitral valve prolapse patients in the presence of complex arrhythmias when mitral regurgitation is absent.

The magnitude of risk can be approximated from prevalence data for mitral regurgitation within the prolapse population combined with estimated yearly mortality in this group. Based on a 2% estimate of clinically significant mitral regurgitation, the 2,700 sudden deaths in mitral prolapse patients with mitral regurgitation estimated from the data of Davies et al. [77] would occur in a pool of approximately 144,000 adults, making annual mortality in this subgroup 188 per 10,000 (1.9%). Based on a 4% estimate for important mitral regurgitation among patients with mitral valve prolapse, annual mortality would be 94 per 10,000 (0.9%).

Thus, compared with the mitral valve prolapse population as a whole, the risk of sudden death may be as much as 50- to 100-fold more concentrated in mitral valve prolapse patients who have mitral regurgitation. This rather startling estimate is consistent with the high prevalence of complex ventricular arrhythmias in this group [100] and the high mortality found in patients with nonischemic mitral regurgitation who have poor ventricular function and complex ventricular arrhythmias [62,101], as will be demonstrated. Since a number of patients with primary valvular disease have been found in series of survivors of out of hospital cardiac arrest [20,105], these observations support an arrhythmic basis for sudden death in mitral valve prolapse patients with mitral regurgitation.

The magnitude of mitral regurgitation associated with increased risk has not yet been quantified. However, mitral valve prolapse patients with mitral regurgitation who had a high prevalence of complex arrhythmias in the report by Kligfield et al. [100] had pansystolic murmurs and large left atrial and left ventricular dimensions. In addition, the mortality in patients with mitral regurgitation reported by Hochreiter et al. [101] was strongly concentrated in those with reduced right and left ventricular ejection fractions at rest. These findings suggest that patients with mitral valve prolapse at greatest risk for sudden death have hemodynamically severe mitral regurgitation. Whether this risk develops discretely with hemodynamic compromise or is continuous with progressively important mitral regurgitation requires systematic evaluation.

Risk of Arrhythmias for Sudden Death in Mitral Prolapse With Regurgitation

These findings indicate that in patients with mitral valve prolapse who have associated significant mitral regurgitation, both the risk of sudden death and the prevalence of complex ventricular arrhythmias are increased with respect to the general prolapse population [60,62,100]. Based on the prevalences outlined above, complex or repetitive ventricular arrhythmias and important mitral regurgitation might occur together in under 2% of the prolapse population. Since patients with mitral regurgitation who have poor ventricular function have been found to have detectable complex arrhythmias prior to death [100,101], it is possible that the combination of arrhythmias and ventricular dysfunction may identify an even smaller subgroup of mitral valve prolapse patients at particularly high risk of sudden death. Indeed, if the proportion of patients with sudden death caused by mitral valve prolapse observed by Davies et al. [77] is generally applicable, it might be suggested that as many as two-thirds of the cases of sudden death caused by mitral valve prolapse may be concentrated within a detectable, high risk subgroup comprising only 2% or less of the entire prolapse population.

Based on an estimated 2,700 cases of sudden death yearly among the 168,000 prolapse patients with important mitral regurgitation who might be expected to have either ventricular couplets or ventricular tachycardia, the predictive value of these repetitive arrhythmias for yearly mortality in an affected individual can be calculated to be about 1.6% (approximately 1 in 60 each year). This is one order of magnitude greater than the predictive value of similarly repetitive ventricular arrhythmias in the general population of subjects with uncomplicated mitral prolapse, but still rather low to be of major clinical significance.

This estimate also assumes that these arrhythmias are present and detectable prior to death in prolapse patients with mitral regurgitation. Not enough data are present in the mitral prolapse population itself to assess this with confidence. However, recent data have emerged from a population of patients with mitral regurgitation of mixed etiology to suggest that complex ventricular arrhythmias are indeed reliably present prior to sudden death and are thus highly sensitive for subsequent arrhythmic mortality. Even so, the predictive value of complex arrhythmias for mortality in these patients is low. This results from the poor specificity of these arrhythmias for sudden death in mitral regurgitation, which of course is due to their extremely high prevalence in all subgroups of this population. On the other hand, this same finding makes mitral regurgitation a useful model for assessing the interaction of ventricular function with complex arrhythmias as a substrate for sudden death.

Arrhythmias and Ventricular Function in Mitral Regurgitation

From a prospective population of patients with valvular regurgitation, we followed 31 unoperated patients with pure, hemodynamically important mitral regurgitation annually for a mean period of 28 months [62]. Included were 16 men and 15 women, whose mean age was 49 years. Mitral regurgitation was related to mitral valve prolapse in 15 patients, to chronic rheumatic heart disease in six, to ruptured chordae with unknown primary disorder in one, to bacterial endocarditis with unknown primary disorder in two, to mitral anular calcification in three, and to undetermined etiology in four.

Characterization of arrhythmias was based on continuous ambulatory electrocardiographic recordings. Any frequency of single ventricular premature complexes was considered a simple ventricular arrhythmia, even when multiform ectopic morphology was present. Early-cycle ventricular premature complexes were not necessarily considered a complex arrhythmia in this population, and each patient having early-cycle forms was ranked according to the next highest grade that was present; in each case, ventricular couplets or salvos (three sequential ventricular premature complexes at a rate greater than 100/min) were also present. Repetitive ventricular arrhythmias (including ventricular couplets, salvos, and runs of ventricular tachycardia) were considered complex in these patients. Thus simple ventricular arrhythmias correspond to Lown grades 0–3, while complex (repetitive) ventricular arrhythmias correspond to Lown grades 4A and 4B.

Patients were separated into four groups based on resting right and left ventricular ejection fractions determined by radionuclide cineangiography at entry into the study and by the presence or absence of repetitive ventricular arrhythmias during serial ambulatory monitoring. Ventricular function was defined as depressed when either right ventricular ejection fraction at rest was $\leq$30% or left ventricular ejection fraction at rest was $\leq$45% on entry to the study. Patients with right ventricular ejection fraction at rest >30% and left ventricular ejection fraction at rest >45% were defined as having normal ventricular function. For the purpose of risk stratification, arrhythmias were considered simple when all available serial ambulatory electrocardiograms were free of ventricular couplets, salvos, or ventricular tachycardia. Arrhythmias were considered complex when these repetitive forms were present on any of the serial studies.

Defined in this way, there were eight patients with simple ventricular arrhythmias and normal ejection fraction, only one patient with simple ventricular arrhythmias and subnormal ejection fraction, 17 patients with complex (repetitive) ventricular arrhythmias and normal ejection fractions, and five patients with both complex ventricular arrhythmias and subnormal ejection fractions. No patient with simple arrhythmias was taking a type I antiarrhythmic drug. A type I drug was used in three of the patients with complex arrhythmias, including two patients who were also taking a beta-blocking agent. During longitudinal follow-up the only change in any potentially antiarrhythmic or proarrhythmic drug was institution of a type I agent in one patient with normal ventricular function, whose arrhythmias remained complex during serial study.

Mortality in Patients According to Ventricular Function and Arrhythmias

Classification of the type of death was based on the condition of the circulation as proposed by Hinkle and Thaler [1]. Accordingly, death was considered to be sudden when the patient was observed to collapse abruptly without prior deterioration of the circulation. Sudden death was inferred when the patient had been seen within several hours prior to death and was in stable condition with no symptoms of hemodynamic deterioration. Death occurring with progressive hypotension and shock was not considered sudden even when the clinical course was rapid.

Overall mortality in this population was strongly related to subnormal ejection fraction alone (67%, four of six), and less strongly related to complex arrhythmia alone (18%, four of 22, $P < 0.05$) because of the large number of patients with complex arrhythmia who had normal ventricular function. During the mean follow-up period of 27 months, mortality occurred in 80% (four of five) of patients with subnormal ejection fractions at entry who had repetitive ventricular forms during serial study, but in 0% (none of 26) of the remaining patients ($P < 0.001$). Of note, mortality in this high risk group was also significantly greater than the 0% mortality in the subgroup of 17 patients who had comparable repetitive ventricular arrhythmias but normal ejection fractions (Table 4–6).

Of the four deaths in this population, three were consistent with sudden death caused by arrhythmia and one occurred in a patient with worsening congestive heart failure. Sudden death was witnessed in two of these patients. The first was a 55-year-old physician with underlying mitral valve prolapse and mitral regurgitation, functionally class I according to New York Heart Association classification, who died instantaneously while playing tennis. Ambulatory studies had revealed salvos of ventricular premature complexes (three sequential ventricular complexes), borderline left ventricular ejection fraction, and depressed right ventricular ejection fraction. A second sudden death was witnessed in a 69-year-old woman with mitral regurgitation associated with calcification of the mitral anulus, who was functionally class III and had ventricular salvos together with depressed right and left ventricular ejection fractions. Arrhythmic death was inferred in a 33-year-old man with class III mitral regurgitation associated with remote, healed endocarditis caused by intravenous drug abuse, who was found dead in bed after being well at home the previous night. Previous studies had demonstrated ventricular couplets, and both right and left ventricular ejection fractions were depressed.

Thus, in unoperated patients with mitral regurgitation of mixed etiol-

TABLE 4–6. Mortality in Patients With Mitral Regurgitation, With and Without Mitral Valve Prolapse, According to Ventricular Function and Ventricular Arrhythmia[a]

	MR with MVP (n = 15)		MR with other etiology (n = 16)	
	Simple ventricular arrhythmias	Repetitive ventricular arrhythmias	Simple ventricular arrhythmias	Repetitive ventricular arrhythmias
Normal or not importantly depressed RVEF and LVEF	0/3	0/11	0/5	0/6
Importantly depressed RVEF or LVEF	0/0	1/1[b]	0/1	3/4[c]

[a]MR, mitral regurgitation; MVP, mitral valve prolapse; RVEF, right ventricular ejection fraction; LVEF, left ventricular ejection fraction.
[b]Witnessed sudden death.
[c]Sudden death (witnessed and inferred) in two of three deaths.
Reproduced from Kligfield et al. [62] with permission of the publisher.

ogy, 2 year mortality was exceedingly high when ventricular function was depressed, and complex arrhythmias were present in most of this group. While overall mortality in these patients was most strongly predicted by ventricular dysfunction alone, death in mitral regurgitation appears commonly to be sudden, and presumably arrhythmic in mechanism [1,2,62], when important ventricular dysfunction is associated with ventricular couplets, salvos, or ventricular tachycardia. In addition to a substrate of abnormal myocardial function, complex ventricular arrhythmias were found prior to death in all mitral regurgitation patients whose fatal events were not associated with progressive circulatory failure. This is consistent with previous observations that repetitive ventricular arrhythmias are associated with sudden death in patients with depressed ventricular function after recent myocardial infarction [35,40] and in patients with severe congestive cardiomyopathy [106].

These findings provide insight into the mechanism of death in unoperated patients with mitral regurgitation. The instantaneous witnessed deaths in two of our patients and the likely sudden death in one other strongly suggest that the ventricular arrhythmias are a significant cause of death in the high risk mitral regurgitation population defined by depressed ventricular performance. Although repetitive ventricular arrhythmias may not accurately predict sudden death in mitral regurgitation because of the large number of patients with these arrhythmias who survive, they appear to explain an important proportion of mortality in mitral regurgitation patients with ventricular dysfunction.

At the same time, mortality in mitral regurgitation appears to be quite low when the same repetitive ventricular arrhythmias occur in patients with preserved ventricular ejection fractions. This observation in nonischemic mitral regurgitation echoes findings in ischemic heart disease, most notably by Schulze et al. [35] in patients after myocardial infarction, that sudden death is relatively rare when complex or repetitive ventricular arrhythmias occur in the setting of well-preserved ventricular systolic function.

These findings do not address the effects of simple and complex arrhythmias on mortality in patients with comparably severe ventricular dysfunction. Only one patient with mitral regurgitation in this population had subnormal ventricular function that was associated with only simple ventricular arrhythmias during serial ambulatory monitoring; this patient was alive at the end of the follow-up period. The single patient in this subgroup precludes meaningful analysis of the potentially additive risk of complex arrhythmias to subnormal ventricular performance alone, but, as will be seen, patients with dilated cardiomyopathy provide a useful model for this distinction [106].

DILATED CARDIOMYOPATHY

Mortality is high in patients with dilated cardiomyopathy, and death is often sudden [107]. A recent study of 182 patients with severe heart failure secondary to ischemic and nonischemic disease revealed a 66% 1 year survival [108], and Fuster et al. [109] found similar results in 104 patients with idiopathic cardiomyopathy. Although survival in severe congestive heart failure caused by dilated cardiomyopathy has been related to the etiology of poor systolic function [108] and to ventricular performance itself [108–111], the prognostic value of coexistent arrhythmias on the natural history of this entity has been controversial [112–117].

Higher mortality in patients with congestive heart failure who have ventricular tachycardia were reported by Graboys et al. [118] and Follansbee et al. [119]. Meinertz et al. [113] described an independent association between the frequency of ventricular couplets and salvos and sudden death in patients with idiopathic dilated cardiomyopathy. The role of electropharmacologic testing in guiding drug therapy and predicting mortality in the nonischemic dilated cardiomyopathy population remains uncertain [120–122].

In contrast, Hamby [123] suggested that while complex ventricular arrhythmias are common in patients with nonischemic cardiomyopathy, prognosis was more closely related to the extent of failure than to arrhythmias. Further, von Olshausen et al. [117] found ambulatory monitoring to have little independent predictive value for arrhythmic or pump failure death in dilated cardiomyopathy. Huang et al. [124] found no correlation between the presence of ventricular tachycardia and short-term prognosis in idiopathic cardiomyopathy, but the unusually low 9% mortality during a mean follow-up period of 34 months in these patients suggests that this particular group may not be representative of the more typically aggressive forms of dilated cardiomyopathy.

Wilson et al. [112] reported that short-term survival in severe congestive heart failure was related to both functional status and the presence of five or more consecutive ventricular premature complexes, but suggested that functional class was the only independent predictor of mortality. Other studies suggest multifactorial contributions to mortality [125]. We examined the hypothesis that repetitive ventricular arrhythmias detected by ambulatory electrocardiography can stratify mortality risk in severe dilated cardiomyopathy and examined whether specific etiology, hemodynamic profile, and neurohumoral status influence the relation of arrhythmias to subsequent mortality.

Thirty-one patients with severe congestive heart failure caused by either ischemic or nonischemic dilated cardiomyopathy were examined [106]. All patients had been referred for vasodilator therapy because of poor clinical response to digitalis and diuretic drugs. Twenty-five were men and six were women, aged 34 to 78 years (mean, 56). The mean follow-up period was 14 months; the range was 2 to 25 months.

Patients were separated into ischemic and nonischemic etiologic subgroups. The diagnosis of ischemic dilated cardiomyopathy was made when there was documented previous myocardial infarction or by demonstration of occlusive coronary disease at cardiac catheterization. Nonischemic dilated cardiomyopathy was diagnosed when patients had no history of ischemia and no evidence was found for presumed idiopathic, postinfectious, postpartum, valvular, or alcoholic origin of ventricular dysfunction. Eleven patients underwent catheterization with coronary angiography, which confirmed the clinical diagnosis.

The overall mortality in this population was 45% (14 of 31) during the follow-up period. Survival was 51% as 12 months and 19% at 25 months. Based on available data from witnesses or clinical setting, 12 patients died suddenly, consistent with arrhythmic mortality, and two died in the setting of progressive circulatory failure.

Arrhythmias in Dilated Cardiomyopathy

A mean ventricular premature complex frequency of 10 or more per 1,000 beats occurred in 39% (12 of 31) of our patients, while multiform ventricular premature complexes were found in 87% (27 of 31). Repetitive ventricular complexes were common in this population (Fig. 4–4), independent of ischemic or nonischemic etiology, and arrhythmias were remarkably similar in prevalence and distribution to those found among patients with severe mitral regurgitation (compare with Fig. 4–2). Ventricular couplets were present in 65% (20 of 31), ventricular salvos or ventricular tachycardia in 39% (12 of 31), and early-cycle forms in 6% (2 of 31). According to peak

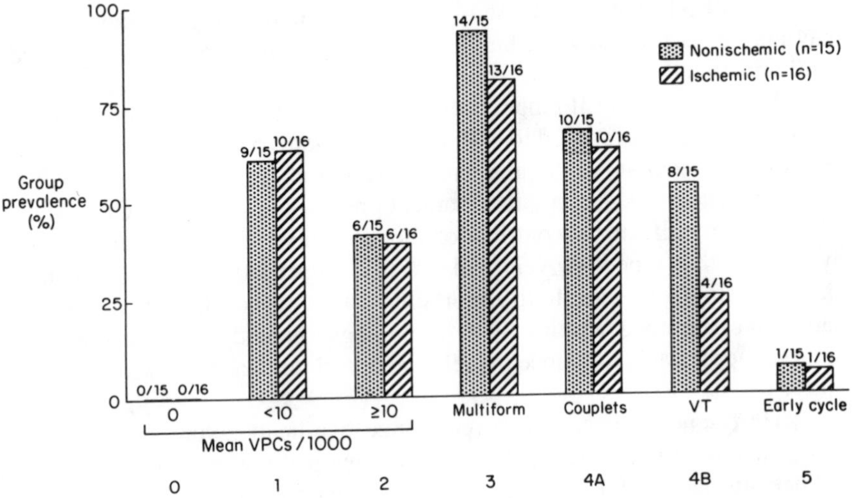

Fig. 4–4. Arrhythmias in patients with dilated cardiomyopathy of ischemic and nonischemic etiology according to frequency and complexity. Group prevalence of repetitive forms is high and nearly identical in distribution with arrhythmias found in severe mitral regurgitation (compare Fig. 4–3). VT, ventricular tachycardia; VPCs, ventricular premature complexes. (Reproduced from Holmes et al. [106] with permission of the publisher.)

ventricular arrhythmia grade, 71% (22 of 31) of all patients had Lown class 4 or 5 findings, including 29% (9 of 31) with ventricular couplets, 35% (11 of 31) with ventricular salvos or nonsustained ventricular tachycardia, and 6% (2 of 31) with early-cycle forms as the most advanced arrhythmia grade. These arrhythmias were considered complex for subgroup stratification, while any frequency of single ventricular premature complexes, even when multiform in morphology, were considered simple arrhythmias.

Sixteen patients had ischemic dilated cardiomyopathy, and 15 had nonischemic dilated cardiomyopathy. No significant frequency or complexity differences between subgroups were found with respect to nonmutually exclusive categories of ventricular arrhythmias or peak Lown grade. Sustained supraventricular arrhythmias (atrial fibrillation, flutter, and sustained atrial tachycardia) occurred in 25% (4 of 16) of patients with ischemic dilated cardiomyopathy and in 20% (3 of 15) of patients with ischemic dilated cardiomyopathy.

Complex Arrhythmias and Mortality in Dilated Cardiomyopathy

When patients were grouped according to complexity of ventricular arrhythmias, nine patients had peak Lown grades 1 to 2 arrhythmia (simple ventricular arrhythmia subgroup) and 22 patients had peak Lown grade 4 or 5 arrhythmia (complex ventricular arrhythmia subgroup). Striking mortality distinction was apparent with arrhythmia stratification (Fig. 4–5): Mortality

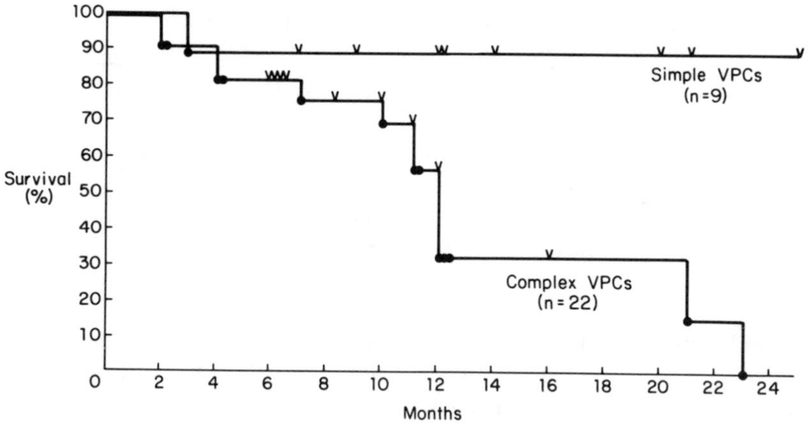

Fig. 4–5. Mortality in dilated cardiomyopathy, according to the presence or absence of complex ventricular arrhythmias. Sudden death was common and strongly associated with ventricular couplets or ventricular tachycardia. VPCs, ventricular premature complexes. (Reproduced from Holmes et al. [106] with permission of the publisher.)

was 11% (1 of 9) in the simple ventricular arrhythmia subgroup, but 59% (13 of 22) in the complex arrhythmia subgroup ($P < 0.025$ by log-rank test). Predictive value was similar for each form of complex ventricular arrhythmia. Specifically, mortality was 67% (6 of 9) in patients with ventricular couplets as their peak ventricular arrhythmia grade, 55% (6 of 11) for patients with ventricular tachycardia, and 50% (1 of 2) for those with early-cycle forms.

The increase in mortality among dilated cardiomyopathy patients with complex, rather than simple, ventricular arrhythmias, was not explained by important differences in clinical, functional, or neurohumoral findings in these subgroups [106]. Patients in each group were comparable with respect to age, sex, functional class, mean arterial pressure, cardiac index, systemic vascular resistance, norepinephrine level, and plasma renin activity. The only variable that differed significantly between simple and complex arrhythmia patients was mean pulmonary capillary wedge pressure, which was 14 mm Hg in the simple ventricular arrhythmia subgroup and 22 mm Hg in the complex ventricular arrhythmia subgroup.

However, analysis of survival distributions with respect to elevated pulmonary capillary wedge pressure (defined as greater than 18 mm Hg) revealed no significant excess in mortality associated with high filling pressures alone in these patients (Table 4–7). Among patients with simple ventricular premature complexes, the one patient who died had a pulmonary capillary wedge pressure greater than 18 mm Hg and a cardiac index of 1.00 liter/min/m^2, the lowest value of any patient in the study. In patients with complex ventricular arrhythmias, the mortality was the same in patients with

TABLE 4–7. Effect of Ventricular Arrhythmias and Pulmonary Wedge Pressure (PWP) on Mortality in Dilated Cardiomyopathy

	Percent ventricular arrhythmias	
	Simple	Complex
PWP ≤ 18 mm Hg	0 (0/6)	60 (3/5)
PWP > 18 Hg	33 (1/3)	59 (10/17)

Adapted from Holmes et al. [106] with permission of the publisher.

high and those with low wedge pressures (59% and 60%, respectively). Findings were also comparable when wedge pressure was partitioned at 16 mm Hg (61% vs. 50%) or at 20 mm Hg (60% and 57%). Similarly, the higher mortality associated with complex ventricular arrhythmias remained significant when patients were stratified for age and cardiac index.

Population profiles and hemodynamic and neurohumoral findings in the survivors and nonsurvivors were compared to determine if any characteristic other than ventricular arrhythmia complexity could identify patients most likely to die. No significant difference between survivors and nonsurvivors was found for age or sex. Mean cardiac index, mean arterial pressure, mean pulmonary capillary wedge pressure, and mean systemic vascular resistance were not significantly different in survivors and nonsurvivors. There were also no significant differences in utilization of antiarrhythmic medications, mean functional class rating, plasma renin activity, or plasma norepinephrine levels between survivors and nonsurvivors.

These observations suggest that repetitive arrhythmias may be an independent risk factor for sudden death in dilated cardiomyopathy in which a substrate of severe ventricular dysfunction is uniformly present. These findings are consistent with the observation that repetitive arrhythmias are detectable prior to sudden death in patients with mitral regurgitation who have poor ventricular function. However, it is apparent from the small, but important, group of patients with dilated cardiomyopathy who had only simple ventricular arrhythmias during ambulatory monitoring that repetitive arrhythmias associated with sudden death are not a necessarily inherent feature of severe heart failure. More important, severe failure alone, independent of repetitive arrhythmias, need not be a strong predictor of mortality. In this subset, sudden death was unlikely when ventricular dysfunction was present but complex arrhythmias were absent.

Survival distributions were also drawn to examine the effect of etiology on mortality in dilated cardiomyopathy subgroups with comparable arrhythmias. The 16 patients with ischemic dilated cardiomyopathy and 15 with nonischemic dilated cardiomyopathy were comparable by all hemodynamic, neurohumoral, and historical variables except for age. Patients with ischemic dilated cardiomyopathy were significantly older than those with nonischemic dilated cardiomyopathy (62 vs. 50 years, $P < 0.01$). The 1 year mortality was 44% in patients with nonischemic dilated cardiomyopathy and 54% in patients with ischemic dilated cardiomyopathy by Kaplan-Meier life-table analysis. Log-rank analysis of these survival distributions with stratification for increased age revealed no significant differences during the follow-up period.

The observation that prognosis is not markedly affected by etiology of dilated cardiomyopathy confirms similar findings of Wexler et al. [126]. However, Franciosa et al. [108] found a 23% 1 year mortality among patients with idiopathic dilated cardiomyopathy in contrast to a 46% mortality among patients with ischemic heart failure. Although mortality differences between etiologic subgroups might be explained if cardiac function were different, these patients were reportedly comparable by historical and hemodynamic variables. It is therefore relevant to note that ambulatory electrocardiograms were not evaluated in profiling this population, and differences in subgroup survival might actually reflect differences in ventricular arrhythmias in their subgroups rather than etiologic differences in natural history.

HYPERTROPHIC CARDIOMYOPATHY

It has long been recognized that patients with obstructive and nonobstructive forms of hypertrophic cardiomyopathy are at risk of sudden, presumably arrhythmic, death [127–129], with annual mortality approximating 3%. This mortality rate is similar to that found in patients with coronary artery disease, including patients discharged after myocardial infarction, and also is similar in order of magnitude to estimated mortality among medically treated patients with important mitral regurgitation [100,101], including those with underlying mitral valve prolapse [61]. From the data presented above, it can be seen that reported mortality in hypertrophic cardiomyopathy is approximately two orders of magnitude greater than that estimated among patients with uncomplicated mitral valve prolapse and one order of magnitude less that that observed in dilated cardiomyopathy.

Because systolic ventricular function in hypertrophic disease is generally good, assessment of risk for sudden death in the context of the general framework relating arrhythmia complexity to ventricular performance, which is of practical value in other forms of noncoronary heart disease, may not be appropriate in these patients. While it is possible that alternate clinically detectable substrates for arrhythmic death are important in hypertrophic disease, these have yet to be clarified. Thus, for example, Maron et al. [129] found no differences in ventricular septal thickness, left ventricular outflow gradient, or left ventricular end-diastolic pressure between patients with sudden death and comparably symptomatic survivors with hypertrophic cardiomyopathy. At the same time, complex arrhythmias are common and emerge as particularly strong correlates of mortality in these patients [130–136].

Hypertrophic cardiomyopathy provides a unique model of nonischemic disease in which repetitive arrhythmias have been shown to predict sudden death, and suppression of arrhythmias has been associated with improved survival.

Arrhythmias and Sudden Death in Hypertrophic Cardiomyopathy

The prevalence of repetitive ventricular arrhythmias, including ventricular couplets and ventricular tachycardia, in patients with hypertrophic cardiomyopathy studied by ambulatory electrocardiography has ranged from 23 to 39%, and ventricular tachycardia has been found in 19–26% of variously selected groups during cross-sectional study [130–135]. Of note, serial evaluation of 39 patients with hypertrophic cardiomyopathy who had no complex arrhythmias at entry by Frank et al. [136] revealed development of repetitive forms in 26% at 5 years and in 75% by 10 years, with ventricular tachycardia found in 40% of these patients by 10 years.

In a prospective study of 84 patients followed for a mean period of 3 years after initial ambulatory electrocardiography, Maron et al. [133] found a strong concentration of sudden death risk among those with ventricular tachycardia. There were six cases of arrhythmic death and one death associated with progressive heart failure during the follow-up period. In contrast to the 3% mortality among patients without ventricular tachycardia (2 of 66), subsequent short-term sudden death when brief bursts of even asymptomatic ventricular tachycardia were present was 24% (4 of 17). No differences in mortality were present when patients were separated according to other types of arrhythmia complexity. Similarly, McKenna et al. [134] found that five of seven episodes of sudden death during a comparable follow-up period in 86 patients occurred among the 24 patients with ventricular tachycardia during electrocardiographic monitoring. Thus the short-term risk of sudden death was 21% (5 of 24) in patients with ventricular tachycardia but only 3% (2 of 62) in patients without this finding.

Sudden death resulting from polymorphic ventricular tachycardia leading to ventricular fibrillation has been documented during ambulatory monitoring of a young patient with hypertrophic cardiomyopathy by Nicod et al. [127]. Taken together, these observations suggest that in patients with hypertrophic cardiomyopathy, risk of sudden death over several years following ambulatory recording may be concentrated by up to eightfold in the subset with ventricular tachycardia, which comprises approximately 20% of patients. It is important to recall the cumulative increase in ventricular tachycardia found during long-term serial evaluation by Frank et al. [136], which highlights the need for periodic assessment of these patients.

Most important, some evidence is available in the hypertrophic cardiomyopathy population that treatment of complex arrhythmias may alter the risk of sudden death. The effect of beta-blocking drugs on arrhythmia suppression in these patients has been controversial [129,131,132], but the observation by Maron et al. [129] that many patients with apparently adequate beta-blockade were included in their autopsy population suggests that these drugs may not prevent sudden death in hypertrophic cardiomyopathy. However, McKenna et al. [137,138] have demonstrated the frequent ability of amiodarone, but not verapamil, to eliminate ventricular tachycardia in a large proportion of these patients. Of note, amiodarone abolished ventricular tachycardia in each of 21 patients entered into longitudinal study beginning in 1978 [138], and, in contrast to their previous mortality experience in hypertrophic disease [134], none of these patients died during the subsequent 3 years.

SYNTHESIS

Taken together, these observations suggest that risk of sudden death in patients with noncoronary heart disease can be usefully stratified by noninvasive clinical evaluation. With particular reference to mitral valve prolapse, mortality can be demonstrated to be exceedingly low in subjects without important mitral regurgitation. Although complex arrhythmias in these subjects may be no more prevalent than in the general population, it remains to be clarified whether these arrhythmias, alone or in combination with other findings, might actually identify a subset of prolapse subjects at higher risk of sudden death. Because of the low mortality rate expected in this subset, study of large numbers of subjects will be required to address this problem, which will likely require a controlled, multicenter, prospective study for resolution.

In contrast, mortality is considerably higher in patients with mitral valve prolapse who have developed important mitral regurgitation, and complex arrhythmias are common in this group. With mitral regurgitation of diverse etiology as a model, it becomes apparent that sudden death is highly concentrated in the subgroup who have developed depressed systolic performance of either ventricle. In these patients, repetitive ventricular arrhythmias can be demonstrated prior to death. However, it is also apparent that similarly complex arrhythmias are not strongly predictive of sudden death in mitral regurgitation when ventricular function remains good.

Evidence for an independent risk of repetitive ventricular arrhythmias for sudden death, related to but independent of ventricular dysfunction itself, emerges from the dilated cardiomyopathy population. In this group, mortality appears to be importantly concentrated in those patients with ventricular couplets or ventricular tachycardia detected by ambulatory monitoring and is significantly lower, despite comparably poor ventricular function, when these arrhythmias are absent. The important role of ventricular arrhythmias in the genesis of sudden death, independent of systolic dysfunction but obviously related to otherwise abnormal myocardial substrate, is also found among patients with hypertrophic cardiomyopathy.

Additional descriptors of risk are needed to improve the predictive value of clinical assessment for sudden death in most forms of noncoronary heart disease. Whether other forms of noninvasive testing, such as signal-averaged electrocardiography, or more aggressive methods, such as electrophysiologic testing, can usefully concentrate risk in these patients remains to be clarified. Beyond more accurate prediction of risk, demonstration of effective therapeutic intervention remains an important challenge.

REFERENCES

1. Hinkle LE, Thaler HT: Clinical classification of cardiac deaths. Circulation 65:457–464, 1982.
2. Roberts WC: Sudden cardiac death: Definitions and causes [editorial]. Am J Cardiol 57:1410–1413, 1986.
3. Moritz AR, Zamcheck N: Sudden and unexpected deaths of young soldiers. Arch Pathol 42:459–494, 1946.
4. Bharati S, Lev M: Cardiac disease in sudden death. Arch Intern Med 144:1811–1812, 1984.
5. Maron BJ, Roberts WC, McAllister HA, Rosing DR, Epstein SE: Sudden death in young athletes. Circulation 62:218–229, 1980.
6. Raymond JR, van den Berg EK, Knapp MJ: Nontraumatic prehospital sudden death in young adults. Arch Intern Med 148:303–308, 1988.
7. Virmani R, Robinowitz M, McAllister HA Jr: Nontraumatic death in joggers. Am J Med 72:874–882, 1982.
8. Luke JL, Helpern M: Sudden unexpected death from natural causes in young adults. Arch Pathol 85:10–17, 1968.
9. Northcote RJ, Flannigan C, Ballanyne D: Sudden death and vigorous exercise—A study of 60 deaths associated with squash. Br Heart J 55:198–203, 1986.
10. Buxton AE: Sudden cardiac death—1986. Ann Intern Med 104:716–718, 1986.
11. Dungan WT, Garson A, Gillette PC: Arrhythmogenic right ventricular dysplasia: A cause of ventricular tachycardia in children with apparently normal hearts. Am Heart J 102: 745–750, 1981.
12. Clinton JE, McGill J, Irwin G, Peterson G, Lilja GP, Ruiz E: Cardiac arrest under age 40: Etiology and prognosis. Ann Emerg Med 13:1011–1015, 1984.
13. Vlay SC, Clayton HK, Weisfeldt ML, Reid PR: Anatomic substrate and clinical outcome in survivors of sudden cardiac death: A multivariate analysis. Cardiovasc Rev Rep 7:861–875, 1986.
14. Eldar M, Sauve MJ, Scheinman MM: Electrophysiologic testing and follow-up of patients with aborted sudden death. J Am Coll Cardiol 10:291–298, 1987.
15. Keefe DL, Schwartz J, Somberg JC: The substrate and the trigger: The role of myocardial vulnerability in sudden cardiac death. Am Heart J 113:218–225, 1987.
16. Schaffer WA, Cobb LA: Recurrent ventricular fibrillation and modes of death in survivors of out-of-hospital ventricular fibrillation. N Engl J Med 293:259–262, 1975.
17. Weaver MD, Cobb LA, Hallstrom AP: Ambulatory arrhythmias in resuscitated victims of cardiac arrest. Circulation 66:212–218, 1982.
18. Graboys TB, Lown B, Podrid PJ, DeSilva R: Long-term survival of patients with malignant ventricular arrhythmia treated with antiarrhythmic drugs. Am J Cardiol 50: 437–443, 1982.
19. Ptacin MJ, Tresch DD, Soin JS, Brooks HL: Evaluation of postresuscitation left ventricular global and segmental function by radionuclide ventriculography in sudden cor-

onary death survivors of prehospital cardiac arrest: Correlation to subsequent short-term prognosis. Am Heart J 100:54–56, 1982.
20. Ruskin JN, DiMarco JP, Garan H: Out-of-hospital cardiac arrest. Electrophysiologic observations and selection of long-term antiarrhythmic therapy. N Engl J Med 303: 607–613, 1980.
21. Meyerburg RJ, Conde CA, Sung RJ, Mayorga-Cortes A, Mallon SM, Sheps DS, Appel RA, Castellanos A: Clinical, electrophysiologic and hemodynamic profile of patients resuscitated from prehospital cardiac arrest. Am J Med 68:568–576, 1980.
22. Savage HR, Kissane JQ, Becher EL, Maddocks WQ, Murtaugh JR, Dizadji H: Analysis of ambulatory electrocardiogram in 14 patients who experienced sudden cardiac death during monitoring. Clin Cardiol 10:621–632, 1987.
23. Gradman AH, Bell PA, DeBusk RF: Sudden death during ambulatory monitoring: Clinical and electrocardiographic correlations: Report of a case. Circulation 55:210–211, 1977.
24. Hinkle LE, Argyros DC, Hayes JC, Robinson T, Alonso DR, Shipman SC, Edwards ME: Pathogenesis of an unexpected sudden death: Role of early cycle ventricular premature contractions. Am J Cardiol 39:873–879, 1977.
25. Denes P, Gabster A, Huang SK: Clinical, electrocardiographic and follow-up observations in patients having ventricular fibrillation during Holter monitoring: Role of quinidine therapy. Am J Cardiol 48:9–16, 1981.
26. Nikolic G, Bishop RL, Singh JB: Sudden death recorded during Holter monitoring. Circulation 66:218–225, 1982.
27. Chiang BN, Perlman LV, Ostrander LD, Epstein FH: Relationship of premature systoles to coronary heart disease and sudden death in the Tecumseh epidemiologic study. Ann Intern Med 70:1159–1166, 1969.
28. Chiang BN, Perlman LV, Fulton M, Ostrander LD, Epstein FH: Predisposing factors in sudden cardiac death in Tecumseh, Michigan: A prospective study. Circulation 41: 31–37, 1970.
29. Rodstein M, Wolloch L, Gubner RS: Mortality study of the significance of extrasystoles in an insured population. Circulation 44:617–625, 1971.
30. Desai DC, Hershberg PL, Alexander S: Clinical significance of ventricular premature beats in an outpatient population. Chest 64:564–569, 1973.
31. Moss AJ, Schnitzler R, Green R, Decamilla J: Ventricular arrhythmias 3 weeks after acute myocardial infarction. Ann Intern Med 75:837–841, 1971.
32. The Coronary Drug Project Research Group; prepared by Tominaga S, Blackburn H: Prognostic importance of premature beats following myocardial infarction: Experience in the Coronary Drug Project. J Am Med Assoc 223:1116–1124, 1973.
33. Kotler MN, Tabatznik B, Mower MM, Tominaga S: Prognostic significance of ventricular ectopic beats with respect to sudden death in the late postinfarction period. Circulation 47:959–966, 1973.
34. Moss AJ, DeCamill J, Mietlowski W, Greene WA, Goldstein S, Locksley R: Prognostic grading and significance of ventricular premature beats after recovery from myocardial infarction. Circulation 51/52:[Suppl III]204–210, 1975.
35. Schulze RA, Strauss HW, Pitt B: Sudden death in the year following myocardial infarction: Relation to ventricular premature contractions in the late hospital phase and left ventricular ejection fraction. Am J Med 62:192–199, 1977.
36. Vismara LA, Vera Z, Foerster JM, Amsterdam EA, Mason DT: Identification of sudden death risk factors in acute and chronic coronary artery disease. Am J Cardiol 39: 821–828, 1977.
37. Ruberman W, Weinblatt E, Goldberg JD, Frank CW, Shapiro S: Ventricular premature beats and mortality after myocardial infarction. N Engl J Med 14:750–757, 1977.
38. Bigger JT, Heller CA, Wenger TL, Weld FM: Risk stratification after acute myocardial infarction. Am J Cardiol 42:202–210, 1978.

39. Moss AJ, Davis HT, DeCamilla J, Bayer LW: Ventricular ectopic beats and their relation to sudden and nonsudden cardiac death after myocardial infarction. Circulation 60: 998–1003, 1979.
40. Ruberman W, Weinblatt E, Goldberg JD, Frank CW, Chaudhary BS, Shapiro S: Ventricular premature complexes and sudden death after myocardial infarction. Circulation 64:297–305, 1981.
41. Southall DP, Richards J, Mitchell P, Brown DJ, Hohnston PGB, Shinebourne EA: Study of cardiac rhythm in healthy newborn infants. Br Heart J 43:14–20, 1980.
42. Southall DP, Johnston F, Shinebourne EA, Johnston PGB: 24-Hour electrocardiographic study of heart rate and rhythm patterns in population of healthy children. Br Heart J 45:281–291, 1981.
43. Brodsky M, Wu D, Denes P, Kanakis C, Rosen KM: Arrhythmias documented by 24 hour continuous electrocardiographic monitoring in 50 male medical students without apparent heart disease. Am J Cardiol 39:390–395, 1977.
44. Sobotka PA, Mayer JH, Bauernfeind RA, Kanakis C, Rosen KM: Arrhythmias documented by 24-hour continuous ambulatory electrocardiographic monitoring in young women without apparent heart disease. Am Heart J 101:753–758, 1981.
45. Hinkle LE, Carver ST, Stevens M: The frequency of asymptomatic disturbances of cardiac rhythm and conduction in middle-aged men. Am J Cardiol 24:629–650, 1969.
46. Savage DD, Levy DL, Garrison RJ, Castelli WP, Kligfield P, Devereux RB, Anderson SJ, Kannel WB, Feinleib M: Mitral valve prolapse in the general population, part 3: Dysrhythmias. The Framingham study. Am Heart J 106:582–586, 1983.
47. Clarke JM, Shelton JR, Hamer J, Tayler S, Venning GR: The rhythm of the normal human heart. Lancet 508–512, 1976.
48. Glasser SP, Clark PI, Applebaum HJ: Occurrence of frequent complex arrhythmias detected by ambulatory monitoring: Findings in an apparently healthy symptomatic elderly population. Chest 75:565–568, 1979.
49. Camm AJ, Evans KE, Ward ED, Martin A: The rhythm of the heart in active elderly subjects. Am Heart J 99:598–603, 1980.
50. Kantelip J-P, Sage E, Duchene-Marullaz P: Findings on ambulatory electrocardiographic monitoring in subjects older than 80 years. Am J Cardiol 57:398–401, 1986.
51. Wooley CF: Where are the diseases of yesteryear? DaCosta's syndrome, soldiers heart, the effort syndrome, neurocirculatory asthenia—And the mitral valve prolapse syndrome [editorial]. Circulation 53:749–751, 1976.
52. Wooley CF: From irritable heart to mitral valve prolapse: The Osler connection. Am J Cardiol 53:870–874, 1984.
53. Devereux RB, Perloff JK, Reichek N, Josephson ME: Mitral valve prolapse. Circulation 54:3–14, 1976.
54. Hancock EW, Cohn K: The syndrome associated with midsystolic click and late systolic murmur. Am J Med 41:183–196, 1966.
55. Pocock WA, Barlow JB: Etiology and electrocardiographic features of the billowing posterior mitral leaflet syndrome. Am J Med 51:731–738, 1971.
56. Shappell SD, Marshall CE, Brown RE, Bruce TA: Sudden death and the familial occurrence of mid-systolic click, late systolic murmur syndrome. Circulation 48:1128–1134, 1973.
57. Winkle RA, Lopes MG, Popp RL, Hancock EW: Life-threatening arrhythmias in the mitral valve prolapse syndrome. Am J Med 60:961–967, 1976.
58. Jeresaty RM: Sudden death in the mitral valve prolapse-click syndrome [editorial]. Am J Cardiol 37:317–318, 1976.
59. Allen H, Harris A, Leatham A: Significance and prognosis of an isolated late systolic murmur. Br Heart J 36:525–532, 1974.

60. Kligfield P, Devereux RB: Arrhythmias in mitral valve prolapse. Clin Prog Electrophysiol Pacing 3:403–418, 1985.
61. Kligfield P, Levy D, Devereux RB, Savage DD: Arrhythmias and sudden death in mitral valve prolapse. Am Heart J 113:1298–1307, 1987.
62. Kligfield P, Hochreiter C, Niles N, Devereux RB, Borer JS: Relation of sudden death in pure mitral regurgitation, with and without mitral valve prolapse, to repetitive ventricular arrhythmias and right and left ventricular ejection fractions. Am J Cardiol 60: 397–399, 1987.
63. Alpert JS: Association between arrhythmias and mitral valve prolapse [editorial]. Arch Intern Med 144:2333–2334, 1984.
64. De Maria AN, Amsterdam EA, Vismara LA, Neumann A, Mason DT: Arrhythmias in the mitral valve prolapse syndrome: Prevalence, nature, and frequency. Ann Intern Med 84:656–660, 1976.
65. Campbell RWF, Godman MG, Fiddler GI, Marquis RM, Julian DG: Ventricular arrhythmias in syndrome of balloon deformity of mitral valve: Definition of possible high risk group. Br Heart J 38:1053–1057, 1976.
66. Kramer HM, Kligfield P, Devereux RB, Savage DD, Kramer-Fox R: Arrhythmias in mitral valve prolapse: Effect of selection bias. Arch Intern Med 144:2360–2364, 1984.
67. Winkle RA, Lopes MG, Fitzgerald JW, Goodman DJ, Schroeder JS, Harrison DC: Arrhythmias in patients with mitral valve prolapse. Circulation 52:73–81, 1975.
68. Swartz MH, Teichholz LE, Donoso E: Mitral valve prolapse: A review of associated arrhythmias. Am J Med 62:377–389, 1977.
69. Pocock WA, Barlow JB: Postexercise arrhythmias in the billowing posterior mitral leaflet syndrome. Am Heart J 80:740–745, 1970.
70. Gooch AS, Vicencio F, Maranhao V, Goldberg H: Arrhythmias and left ventricular asynergy in the prolapsing mitral leaflet syndrome. Am J Cardiol 29:611–620, 1972.
71. Sloman G, Wong M, Walker J: Arrhythmias on exercise in patients with abnormalities of the posterior leaflet of the mitral valve. Am Heart J 83:312–317, 1972.
72. Malcolm AD, Ahuja SP: The electrocardiographic response to exercise in 44 patients with mitral leaflet prolapse. Eur J Cardiol 8:359–370, 1978.
73. Webb Kavey R-E, Blackman MS, Sondheimer HM, Byrum CJ: Ventricular arrhythmias and mitral valve prolapse in childhood. J Pediatr 105:885–890, 1984.
74. Motulsky AG: Biased ascertainment and the natural history of diseases. N Engl J Med 298:1196–1197, 1978.
75. Kligfield P: Clinical applications of ambulatory electrocardiography. Cardiology 71: 69–99, 1984.
76. Chesler E, King RA, Edwards JE: The myxomatous mitral valve and sudden death. Circulation 67:632–639, 1983.
77. Davies MJ, Moore BP, Braimbridge MV: The floppy mitral valve: Study of incidence, pathology, and complications in surgical, necropsy, and forensic material. Br Heart J 40:468–481, 1978.
78. Boudoulas H, Schaal SF, Stang JM, Fontana ME, Kolibash AJ, Wooley CF: Mitral valve prolapse-sudden death with long term survival [abstract]. J Am Coll Cardiol 7:29A, 1986.
79. Wei JY, Bulkley BH, Schaeffer AH, Greene HL, Reid PR: Mitral-valve prolapse syndrome and recurrent ventricular tachyarrhythmias: A malignant variant refractory to conventional drug therapy. Ann Intern Med 89:6–9, 1978.
80. Nishimura RA, McGoon MD, Shub C, Miller FA, Ilstrup DM, Tajik AJ: Echocardiographically documented mitral-valve prolapse. N Engl J Med 313:1305–1309, 1985.
81. Barlow JB, Pocock WA: Mitral valve prolapse, the specific billowing mitral leaflet syndrome, or an insignificant non-ejection systolic click. Am Heart J 97:277–285, 1979.

82. Savage DD, Garrison RJ, Devereux RB, Castelli WP, Anderson SJ, Levy D, McNamara PM, Stokes J, Kannel WB, Feinleib M: Mitral valve prolapse in the general population. I. Epidemiologic features: The Framingham study. Am Heart J 106:571–578, 1983.
83. Devereux RB, Hawkins I, Kramer-Fox R, Lutas EM, Hammond IW, Spitzer MC, Hochreiter C, Roberts RB, Belkin RN, Kligfield P, Niles N, Alderman MH, Borer JS, Laragh JH: Complications of mitral valve prolapse: Disproportionate occurrence in men and older patients. Am J Med (in press), 1989.
84. Kannel WB, Doyle JT, McNamara PM, Quickenton P, Gordon T: Precursors of sudden coronary death: Factors related to the incidence of sudden death. Circulation 51:606–613, 1975.
85. Bekheit SG, Ali AA, Deglin SM, Jain AC: Analysis of QT interval in patients with idiopathic mitral valve prolapse. Chest 81:620–625, 1982.
86. Puddu PE, Pasternac A, Tubau JF, Krol R, Farley L, de Champlain J: QT interval prolongation and increased plasma catecholamine levels in patients with mitral valve prolapse. Am Heart J 105:422–428, 1983.
87. Schwartz PJ, Periti M, Malliani A: The long Q-T syndrome. Am Heart J 89:378–390, 1975.
88. Abildskov JA: Adrenergic effects on the QT interval of the electrocardiogram. Am Heart J 92:210–216, 1976.
89. Wit AL, Cranefield PF: Triggered activity in cardiac muscle fibers of the simian mitral valve. Circ Res 38:85–98, 1976.
90. Levy D, Savage D: Prevalence and clinical features of mitral valve prolapse. Am Heart J 113:1281–1290, 1987.
91. Salmela PI, Ikaheimo M, Juustila H: Fatal ventricular fibrillation after treatment with digoxin in a 27-year-old man with mitral leaflet prolapse syndrome. Br Heart J 46: 338–341, 1981.
92. Velebit V, Podrid P, Lown B, Cohen B, Graboys TB: Aggravation and provocation of ventricular arrhythmias by antiarrhythmic drugs. Circulation 65:886–893, 1982.
93. Engel TR, Meister SG, Frankl WS: Ventricular extrastimulation in the mitral valve prolapse syndrome. Evidence for ventricular reentry. J Electrocardiol 11:137–142, 1978.
94. Morady F, Shen E, Bhandari A, Schwartz A, Scheinman MM: Programmed ventricular stimulation in mitral valve prolapse: Analysis of 36 patients. Am J Cardiol 53:135–138, 1984.
95. Rosenthal ME, Hamer A, Gang ES, Oseran DS, Mandel WJ, Peter T: The yield of programmed ventricular stimulation in mitral valve prolapse patients with ventricular arrhythmias. Am Heart J 110:970–976, 1985.
96. Naccarelli GV, Prystowsky EN, Jackman WM, Heger JJ, Rahilly GT, Zipes DP: Role of electrophysiologic testing in managing patients who have ventricular tachycardia unrelated to coronary artery disease. Am J Cardiol 50:165–171, 1982.
97. Josephson ME, Horowitz LN, Kastor JA: Paroxysmal supraventricular tachycardia in patients with mitral valve prolapse. Circulation 57:111–115, 1977.
98. Ware JA, Magro SA, Luck JC, Mann DE, Nielsen AP, Rosen KM, Wyndham CRC: Conduction system abnormalities in symptomatic mitral valve prolapse: An electrophysiologic analysis of 60 patients. Am J Cardiol 53:1075–1078, 1984.
99. Mason JW, Kock FH, Billingham ME, Winkle RA: Cardiac biopsy evidence of a cardiomyopathy associated with symptomatic mitral valve prolapse. Am J Cardiol 42: 557–562, 1978.
100. Kligfield P, Hochreiter C, Kramer H, Devereux RB, Niles N, Kramer-Fox R, Borer JS: Complex arrhythmias in mitral regurgitation with and without mitral valve prolapse: Contrast to arrhythmias in mitral valve prolapse without mitral regurgitation. Am J Cardiol 55:1545–1549, 1985.

101. Hochreiter C, Niles N, Devereux RB, Kligfield P, Borer JS: Mitral regurgitation: Relationship of noninvasive descriptors of right and left ventricular performance to clinical and hemodynamic findings and to prognosis in medically and surgically treated patients. Circulation 73:900–912, 1986.
102. Duren DR, Becker AE, Durning AJ: Long-term follow-up of idiopathic mitral valve prolapse in 300 patients: A prespective study. J Am Coll Cardiol 11:42–47, 1988.
103. Rapaport E: Natural history of aortic and mitral valve disease. Am J Cardiol 35:221–227, 1975.
104. Phillips HR, Levine FH, Carter JE, Boucher CA, Osbakken MD, Okada RD, Akins CW, Daggett WM, Buckley MJ, Pohost GM: Mitral valve replacement for isolated mitral regurgitation: Analysis of clinical course and late postoperative left ventricular ejection fraction. Am J Cardiol 48:647–654, 1981.
105. Myerburg RJ, Conde CA, Sung RJ, Mayorgo-Cortes A, Mallon SM, Sheps DS, Appel RA, Castellanos A: Clinical, electrophysiologic and hemodynamic profile of patients resuscitated from prehospital cardiac arrest. Am J Med 68:568–576, 1980.
106. Holmes JR, Kubo SH, Cody RJ, Kligfield P: Arrhythmias in ischemic and nonischemic dilated cardiomyopathy: Prediction of mortality by ambulatory electrocardiography. Am J Cardiol 55:146–151, 1985.
107. Anderson KP, Freedman RA, Mason JW: Sudden death in idiopathic dilated cardiomyopathy. Ann Intern Med 107:104–106, 1987.
108. Franciosa JA, Wilen M, Ziesche S, Cohn JN: Survival in men with severe chronic left ventricular failure due to either coronary heart disease or idiopathic dilated cardiomyopathy. Am J Cardiol 51:831–836, 1983.
109. Fuster V, Gersh B, Giuliani G, Tajik A, Brandenburg R, Frye R: The natural history of idiopathic dilated cardiomyopathy. Am J Cardiol 48:525–531, 1981.
110. Feild BJ, Baxley WA, Russell RO, Hood WP, Holt JH, Dowling JT, Rackley CE: Left ventricular function and hypertrophy in cardiomyopathy with depressed ejection fraction. Circulation 47:1022–1031, 1973.
111. Johnson RA, Palacios I: Dilated cardiomyopathy of the adult. N Engl J Med 307: 1051–1058, 1119–1126, 1982.
112. Wilson JR, Schwartz JS, Sutton MSJ, Ferraro N, Horowitz LN, Relchek N, Josephson ME: Prognosis in severe heart failure: Relation to hemodynamic measurements and ventricular ectopic activity. J Am Coll Cardiol 2:403–410, 1983.
113. Meinertz T, Hofmann T, Kasper W, Treese N, Bechtold H, Stlenen U, Pop T, Leitner E, Andersen D, Meyer J: Significance of ventricular arrhythmias in idiopathic dilated cardiomyopathy. Am J Cardiol 53:902–907, 1984.
114. Huang SK, Messer JV, Denes P: Significance of ventricular tachycardia in idiopathic dilated cardiomyopathy: Observations in 35 patients. Am J Cardiol 51:507–512, 1983.
115. Ikegawa T, Chino M, Hasegawa H, Usuba F, Suzuki S, Ookura M, Nishikawa K: Prognostic significance of 24-hour ambulatory electrocardiographic monitoring in patients with dilative cardiomyopathy: A prospective study. Clin Cardiol 10:78–82, 1987.
116. Bigger JT Jr: Why patients with congestive heart failure die: Arrhythmias and sudden cardiac death. Circulation 75[Suppl IV]:IV-28, 1987.
117. von Olshausen K, Stienen U, Math D, Schwarz F, Kubler W, Meyer J: Long-term prognostic significance of ventricular arrhythmias in idiopathic dilated cardiomyopathy. Am J Cardiol 61:146–151, 1988.
118. Graboys TB, Lown B, Podrid PJ, DeSilva R: Long-term survival of patients with malignant ventricular arrhythmia treated with antiarrhythmic drugs. Am J Cardiol 50: 437–443, 1982.
119. Follansbee WP, Michelson EL, Morganroth J: Nonsustained ventricular tachycardia in

ambulatory patients: Characteristics and associations with sudden cardiac death. Ann Intern Med 92:741–747, 1980.

120. Meinertz T, Treese N, Kasper W, Geibel A, Hofmann T, Zehender M, Bohn D, Pop T, Just H: Determinants of prognosis in idiopathic dilated cardiomyopathy as determined by programmed electrical stimulation. Am J Cardiol 56:337–341, 1985.
121. Liem LB, Swerdlow CD: Value of electropharmacologic testing in idiopathic dilated cardiomyopathy and sustained ventricular tachyarrhythmias. Am J Cardiol 62:611–616, 1988.
122. Poll DS, Marchlinski FE, Buxton AE, Doherty JU, Waxman HL, Josephson ME: Sustained ventricular tachycardia in patients with idiopathic dilated cardiomyopathy: Electrophysiologic testing and lack of response to antiarrhythmic drug therapy. Circulation 70:451–456, 1984.
123. Hamby RI: Primary myocardial disease: A prospective clinical and hemodynamic evaluation in 100 patients. Medicine 49:55–78, 1970.
124. Huang SK, Messer JV, Denes P: Significance of ventricular tachycardia in idiopathic dilated cardiomyopathy: Observations in 35 patients. Am J Cardiol 51:507–511, 1983.
125. Unverferth DV, Magorien RD, Moeschberger ML, Baker PB, Fetters JK, Leier CV: Factors influencing the one-year mortality of dilated cardiomyopathy. Am J Cardiol 54:147–152, 1984.
126. Wexler IF, Boucher CA, Dinsmore RE, Johnson RA: Primary cardiomyopathy and cardiomyopathy syndrome due to coronary artery disease: A comparison of natural history [abstract]. Circulation 54[Suppl II]:II-79, 1976.
127. Nicod P, Polikar R, Peterson KL: Hypertrophic cardiomyopathy and sudden death. N Engl J Med 318:1255–1257, 1988.
128. Maron BJ, Roberts WC, Edwards JE, McAllister HA Jr, Foley DD, Epstein SE: Sudden death in patients with hypertrophic cardiomyopathy: Characterization of 26 patients without functional limitation. Am J Cardiol 41:803–810, 1978.
129. Maron BJ, Roberts WC, Epstein S: Sudden death in hypertrophic cardiomyopathy: A profile of 78 patients. Circulation 65:1388–1394, 1982.
130. Savage DD, Seides SF, Maron BJ, Myers DJ, Epstein S: Prevalence of arrhythmias during 24-hour electrocardiographic monitoring and exercise testing in patients with obstructive and nonobstructive hypertrophic cardiomyopathy. Circulation 59:866–875, 1979.
131. McKenna WJ, Chetty S, Oakley CM, Goodwin JF: Arrhythmia in hypertrophic cardiomyopathy: Exercise and 48 hour ambulatory electrocardiographic assessment with and without betaadrenergic blocking therapy. Am J Cardiol 45:1–5, 1980.
132. Canedo MI, Frank MJ, Abdulla AM: Rhythm disturbances in hypertrophic cardiomyopathy: Prevalence, relation to symptoms and management. Am J Cardiol 45:848–855, 1980.
133. Maron BJ, Savage DD, Wolfson JK, Epstein SE: Prognostic significance of 24 hour ambulatory electrocardiographic monitoring in patients with hypertrophic cardiomyopathy: A prospective study. Am J Cardiol 48:252–257, 1981.
134. McKenna WJ, England D, Doi YL, Deanfield JE, Oakley C, Goodwin JF: Arrhythmia in hypertrophic cardiomyopathy. I: Influence on prognosis. Br Heart J 46:168–172, 1981.
135. Bjarnason I, Hardarson T, Jonsson S: Cardiac arrhythmias in hypertrophic cardiomyopathy. Br Heart J 48:198–203, 1982.
136. Frank MJ, Watkins LO, Prisant LM, Stefadouros MA, Abdulla AM: Potentially lethal arrhythmias and their management in hypertrophic cardiomyopathy. Am J Cardiol 53: 1608–1613, 1984.
137. McKenna WJ, Harris L, Perez G, Krikler DM, Oakley C, Goodwin JF: Arrhythmia in

hypertrophic cardiomyopathy. II: Comparison of amiodarone and verapamil in treatment. Br Heart J 46:173–178, 1981.
138. McKenna WJ, Oakley CM, Krikler DM, Goodwin JF: Improved survival with amiodarone in patients with hypertrophic cardiomyopathy and ventricular tachycardia. Br Heart J 53:412–416, 1985.

Chapter 5

Risk Stratification for the Prevention of Sudden Cardiac Death by Noninvasive Methods

Michael Sanders, M.D., and John B. Kostis, M.D.

Division of Cardiovascular Diseases and Hypertension, UMDNJ—Robert Wood Johnson Medical School, New Brunswick, New Jersey 08903-0019

RISK STRATIFICATION: EXERCISE STRESS ELECTROCARDIOGRAPHY

Most cases of sudden death can be linked to a cardiac origin [1]. While certain anatomical catastrophes such as cardiac rupture or massive pulmonary embolism can result in sudden death, the preponderance of cases are known to follow ventricular fibrillation or sustained ventricular tachycardia [2,3]. Supraventricular tachycardia (except WPW with rapid atrial fibrillation) and profound bradyarrhythmia usually do not produce total cardiovascular collapse resulting in the syndrome of sudden cardiac death.

Ventricular tachyarrhythmia resulting in sudden death has become a well-recognized feature in the natural history of ischemic heart disease [3]. While other cardiac abnormalities have been associated with sudden arrhythmic death, (e.g. mitral valve prolapse (MVP) [4], IHSS [5], cardiomyopathy [6]), most cases involve atherosclerotic coronary artery obstruction with or without prior myocardial infarction. Ischemia by itself can produce an increase in myocellular automaticity and changes in refractory periods and conduction velocities and a decrease in fibrillatory threshold; ischemia plus

The Prevention of Sudden Cardiac Death, pages 83–107

myocardial fibrosis can result in dispersion of local refractoriness and conduction producing longitudinal dissociation, all of which serve as the underlying strata of reentry.

Pathologic examination studies of sudden death victims have underscored the importance of coronary artery disease. The majority of sudden death victims have severe triple vessel disease [7]. Nevertheless, recent myocardial infarction can be identified in only 5%, although 59% had old myocardial fibrosis and evidence of prior healed infarctions [8]. Rather, most pathologic studies find evidence of acute myocardial ischemia in 80–90% of subjects [9,10]. Transient cardiac ischemic and progressive myocardial fibrosis are the two parallel processes whose courses determine the prognosis of patients with coronary artery disease.

Exercise Stress Test

As atherosclerosis gradually or suddenly (plaque rupture) diminishes coronary artery lumen size, transient increases in oxygen demand and/or vasomotor tone (spasm) become more likely to cause ischemia. While the angiographic severity and distribution of coronary lesions have been shown to prognosticate myocardial infarction [11], the moment-to-moment relationship of oxygen supply and demand dictates the occurrence of each ischemic event [12].

Premature ventricular contractions are usually benign in the absence of underlying cardiac disease [13]. The progressive myocardial fibrosis of ischemic heart disease can produce the pathopysiologic substratum for sustained, lethal arrhythmias. Ischemia can be viewed as the "trigger" and the increased susceptibility of chronic myocardial fibrosis as the "powder" for the "explosion" of ventricular fibrillation and sudden death. In a study of over 1,000 survivors of out-of-hospital sudden death, 80% of those tested demonstrated objective evidence of myocardial ischemia, although only 10% had ever complained of exercise-induced angina (silent ischemia) [14,15].

The prevention of sudden cardiac death requires the identification of both risk factors: ischemia and susceptibility to sustained ventricular tachyarrhythmia. Exercise stress testing (EST) has been advocated for many years as the logical prognosticator of sudden death, since this one test can evoke both factors [16].

Ischemic ST Segment Response

ST segment depression has experimentally [17] and clinically [16,18] been found to be the primary electrocardiographic marker of myocardial ischemia. Electrocardiography during exercise was suggested as a test for coronary heart disease almost five decades ago [16]. In 1967 Robb and Markes [14] reported on an up to 15 year follow-up of 2,224 male applicants for life insurance who underwent exercise stress testing where a marked relationship between incidence of cardiac ischemia–ST segment depression and mortality was seen.

Many years of experience have led cardiologists to conclude that the risk stratification value of ischemic ST segment changes on EST is a function of the population in which it is applied [18–21]. Ellestad and Wan [22] evaluated 8,000 routine ESTs and reported an up to 8 year follow-up on 2,700 subjects with strongly positive (>2 mm) responses. The annual death rate among positive responders was 13.2% compared with only 1.1% for subjects without abnormal EKG changes. In another population of 1,472 patients with catheterization-documented coronary disease, McNeer et al. [23] found a 13% difference in the 2 year survival between positive and negative responders.

However, in applying EST to a large population of asymptomatic men, Bruce et al. [24] were able to find no additional predictive value in persons without conventional coronary risk factors. Nevertheless, as the single test for coronary risk, Giagnoni et al. [25] found that at 6 years after an ischemic EST response the relative risk of a significant coronary event was 5.55 in asymptomatic normotensive persons compared with control subjects. At the other extreme, applying EST to patients known to have severe coronary heart disease, a high risk subgroup was identified by Weiner et al. [26] on the basis of an ischemic EST response and poor exercise tolerance from the large Coronary Artery Surgery Study (CASS). The additional predictive value of developing chest pain during EST was reported recently by Falcone et al. [27]. They found no significant difference in survival in patients with ST segment depresssion during EST who developed angina versus those who did not: a syndrome that has come to be known as "silent ischemia."

Ventricular Ectopic Activity

The ability of EST to evoke ventricular ectopic activity (VEA) has been suggested as an independent predictor of sudden cardiac death. Chiang et al. [28] reported the findings of the large Tecumseh Community Health Study in which ventricular premature beats (VPBs) were associated with a greater death rate in persons with coronary heart disease. Kosowsky et al. [29] reported an improved ability to obtain evidence of incidence as well as seriousness of VEA by EST over ambulatory monitoring. Grayboys et al. [30] found EST to be additive to Holter monitoring for exposing VEA in patients with recurrent ventricular fibrillation or tachycardia.

The predictive value for sudden cardiac death of one or more VPBs during EST in patients suspected of having coronary disease was significantly greater in a study by Califf et al. [31] of 1,448 patients. In a similar report from the USSR, Ivanova and coworkers [32] found a fourfold increase in sudden death in patients with VEA on EST. They found that VEA on Holter monitoring was too sensitive to be a specific predictor for sudden death in their cohort of patients.

A study by Califf et al. [33] of 1,293 consecutive coronary artery disease patients undergoing EST within 6 weeks of cardiac catheterization demonstrated that even patients with "simple" VEA have a higher prevalence of significant coronary artery disease and an increased risk of sudden death; "complex" VEA carried an even worse prognosis against survival. However, in applying EST to a group of 280 persons without a diagnosis of coronary disease, Nair et al. [34] did not find VEA to be a predictor of subsequent coronary events in a 4 year follow-up.

Therefore, as with EST-induced ischemia, VEA's predictive power appears to depend on the patient group being studied. For example, Lampert et al. [35] recently reported a 63% sudden death rate in 161 patients with a documented history of ventricular fibrillation or sustained tachycardia. They identified VEA on EST as a major marker for these fatal outcomes. They furthermore reported that therapy that was successful in reducing EST-induced VEA also lowered the incidence of sudden death.

EST Following Acute Myocardial Infarction

Death during acute myocardial infarction (AMI) caused by ventricular fibrillation [3] was effectively addressed by the modern coronary care unit [36]. However, the 8–9% death rate in the first year among survivors of AMI has been a persistent problem plaguing contemporary cardiologists. Early postinfarction EST has been suggested as a means for identifying those patients at high risk for sudden death.

An ischemic response to a graded EST was reported by Sami et al. [37] in all of their MI survivors who subsequently died within 2 years. Theroux et al. [38] performed limited EST on 210 AMI patients 1 day before hospital discharge. They found a difference in first year mortality from 27% in patients with an ischemic EST to only 2.1% for negative responders. There was also a difference in sudden death of 10% versus 0.7% between patients with positive and negative responses to exercise. Starling et al. [39] followed 130 AMI survivors who had predischarge EST and found that ST segment deviation in conjunction with an inadequate blood pressure response during exercise best predicted those patients who would succumb to sudden death. Davidson and DeBusk [40] reported similar results but added angina as a predictive marker for subsequent coronary events. DeBusk et al. [41] found an ischemic response to exercise superior to exercise-induced VPBs in prognosticating a patient's outcome. In a report from Findland, Kentola and Repo [42] found that T wave changes following exercise added predictive power to ST segment shifts for sudden death in AMI survivors and postulated an enhanced sympathoadrenal activity as responsible. The induction of VEA during early post-AMI EST has also been extensively evaluated.

As early as 1973, Ericsson and coworkers [43] in Sweden found a positive association between an increased mortality and exercise-induced VPBs in 100 AMI survivors. This observation was later confirmed by

Granath et al. [44] in a large study of 205 patients. Weld et al. [45] found that while VPBs during EST 2 weeks following hospital discharge for AMI correlated with subsequent mortality, ST changes or angina during EST did not. Henry et al. [46] reported similar results demonstrating a 20% 2 year mortality rate for AMI survivors with EST-induced VEA compared with an 8% death rate among patients without this finding. They also failed to find a relationship between subsequent sudden death and ischemic ST changes, angina, or poor blood pressure response during EST.

Direction of Therapy by EST

Several large multicenter trials have documented improved survival in many subsets of patients with coronary artery disease who undergo coronary bypass surgery [47–49]. Similar trials are currently investigating the relative efficacy of PTCA. The decision to recommend CABG and PTCA is based on coronary arteriographic information concerning coronary anatomy and left ventricular function. However, many physicians find it difficult to apply these data across the board to all their patients regardless of functional activity or symptoms [50]. The extreme example—the asymptomatic patient—was recently evaluated utilizing the large CASS experience. Weiner et al. [51,52] demonstrated the efficacy of painless ischemia unmasked by EST in decision making. They were able to identify subgroups of "silent ischemia" patients whose survival was improved by surgery. Those patients with silent myocardial ischemia who had three-vessel disease had a 7 year survival of 90% when treated surgically compared with 37% with medical management.

Following AMI, uncertainty persists concerning the necessity of suppression of VEA [53]. Current pharmacologic therapy is complicated by frequent serious side effects (organ toxicity as well as proarrhythmia), is expensive, and has not been documented to alter survival. Until the results of current long-term multicenter trials on post-AMI arrhythmia suppression are available, practitioners need direction in patient selection and monitoring with antiarrhythmia drugs. EST was shown by Lampert et al. [35] to be a useful tool in managing these AMI survivors. The selection of patients for coronary arteriography, CABG, PTCA, and antiarrhythmic drugs can start with EST.

RISK STRATIFICATION: AMBULATORY ELECTROCARDIOGRAPHY

In the last section, the use of EST for sudden death risk stratification was described, i.e., its clinical usefulness in identifying those patients who have a greater than ordinary chance of suddenly dying from heart disease was explored. This accentuated risk of sudden cardiac death was found to be related to two exercise-provocable factors: ischemia and ventricular ectopic activity. The prognostic power of these two markers has also been investigated using a somewhat different electrocardiographic approach, the Holter Monitor, or ambulatory electrocardiography (AMB ECG). This approach has the advantages of sampling both a longer period (24 hours) as well as a patient's more normal or representative level of physical and emotional activity.

Ischemic ST Segment Response

While ST segment depression is a well-accepted marker for cardiac ischemia during exercise, up to 80% of ischemic episodes documented by AMB ECG do not correspond to chest pain or other symptoms, i.e., silent ischemia. Despite the correspondence of AMB ECG ST changes to other evidence of myocardial ischemia such as hypoperfusion during radionuclide studies, clinical studies demonstrating a direct relationship between the presence of silent ischemia diagnosed by AMB EKG and the risk of sudden death are not yet available. In addition, there is large day-to-day variability of ischemia detected by this method even when position and autonomic artifact are eliminated. Whether this difference between EST and AMB ECG is simply related to the intensity of myocardial oxygen demand or other factors is not known. Moreover, it is interesting to note anecdotal reports of lethal arrhythmias discovered fortuitously on Holter records being preceded by ST segment shifts.

Ventricular Ectopic Activity

Most of the data accumulated over the past several years on the use of AMB ECG to predict sudden death pertains to ventricular arrhythmia. VEA is well known to occur in normal subjects as well as in patients with a great variety of cardiac and extracardiac disorders. Its relationship to the prognosis of patients with MVP and other noncoronary causes of sudden cardiac death has been described in detail in Chapter 4 (Kligfield, this volume). In this section, we will explore the relationship of VEA as studied by AMB ECG to the risk of sudden cardiac death in both 1) subjects free of heart disease and 2) patients with coronary artery disease.

VEA in Normal Subjects

VEA has been recorded in persons free of heart disease by many investigators [54–61]. When recordings of adequate duration (e.g., 1 to several days) are performed, VEA can be found in the great majority of persons without heart disease. Ordinarily in such individuals, ventricular ectopy is of low frequency and complexity. A relationship between the duration of the recording and probability of detecting ventricular ectopic activity is obvious (Table 5–1).

Thus Lamb, studying normal Air Force recruits with 12 lead electrocardiograms, detected VPBs in less than 1% of his subjects, while longer

TABLE 5–1. Prevalence of Ventricular Premature Complexes in Normal Persons[a]

Studies	Population	Age range (years)	No. subjects	Screening method	Prevalence of VEA (%)
Averill et al.	Airmen	16–50	67,375	ECG	0.8
Hiss and Lamb	Airmen	16–50	122,043	ECG	0.6
Chiang et al.	Tecumseh (MI) population	>30	3,624	ECG	5
Hinkle et al.	Telephone workers	55–60	301	6 hour AE	62
Brodsky et al.	Male medical students	23–27	50	24 hour AE	50
Sobotka et al.	Female medical personnel	23–27	50	24 hour AE	50
Fleg and Kennedy	Healthy individuals	60–85	98	24 hour AE	80
Kostis et al.	Patients with normal coronary arteries	16–68	100	24 hour AE	39

[a]AE, ambulatory electrocardiogram; ECG, electrocardiogram; VEA, ventricular ectopic activity.

recordings, using 24 hour monitors, identify VEA in up to 40–50% of the subjects. In addition, VEA becomes more frequent and more complex with advancing age even in subjects without cardiac disease. In most of the studies in which AMB ECG was performed to detect arrhythmias, the patients were classified as normals by the absence of clinical evidence of cardiac disease on history and physical examination and on noninvasive testing of variable content. This, especially in the older age groups, did not exclude the possibility that the patients had silent coronary artery disease.

Our group at UMDNJ—Robert Wood Johnson Medical School performed AMB ECG on 100 normal subjects who were free of heart disease as evidenced by extensive noninvasive and invasive testing, including resting and exercise electrocardiography, chest X-ray, physical examination, echocardiography, right and left heart catheterization, and coronary arteriography [54]. Patients who had even minor abnormalities were excluded. Twenty-four hour AMB ECG detected cardiac arrhythmias in 40 of the 100 subjects. In the 40 normal subjects, however, the actual frequency of cardiac arrhythmia was quite low, with only four subjects having greater than 100 VPBs per 24 hours. Also, even in the absence of detectable heart disease, there was an increase in the prevalence and frequency of VEA with age. Importantly, repetitive forms were not recorded in this population with angiographically documented normal left ventricular anatomy and function. However, the number of patients over age 60 years was small, and a larger study of older normal subjects might identify repetitive forms in such individuals.

A somewhat different observation was reported by Kennedy and his associates [55], who reported on a small cohort of persons free from significant heart disease using similar noninvasive and invasive testing in whom VEA of significant frequency and complexity was recorded. In a longitudinal follow-up, these subjects' prognoses were no different from those of the general population, yielding the important clinical conclusion that even frequent and complex VEA in normal persons does not appear to increase the risk of sudden death [62]. Normal subjects may have sustained or even incessant ventricular tachycardia without a negative impact on their survival [63].

Most population studies confirm this prognostic impact of VEA on future mortality, including sudden death; however, in most studies mortality was usually limited to patients with additional evidence suggesting cardiac disease such as hypertension, pulmonary disease, or other ECG abnormalities. Only one study of clinically normal subjects, MRFIT participants, found an increase of sudden death (but not of nonsudden death) in those with VPBs [64]. Therefore, there appears to be an association between VEA and the risk of sudden death in the general population. This apparent relationship may at least partially be explained by the fact that arrhythmia itself may be a nonlethal marker of certain cardiac disorders and not the direct cause of death. This impression is strengthened by the finding in apparently normal persons of a relationship between the traditional risk factors for coronary disease (age, blood pressure, male gender, smoking) and the frequency and complexity of VEA [65]. In the general population a bimodal distribution according to VPB frequencys has been observed, implying two subgroups: one with a low frequency of VEA and one with a higher frequency [9,10,65]. Persons belonging to the high VEA subgroup may suffer from cardiovascular or other disease that is the cause of both the arrhythmia and the sudden cardiac death. The preferential association of VEA with sudden rather than nonsudden death, on the other hand, implies an (additional) causal mechanism.

Patients with frequent VEA but without structural heart disease who have suffered sudden death or were resuscitated from ventricular fibrillation have also been reported. While in some of these patients activation of the central nervous system had occurred, the majority were being treated with the classical antiarrhythmic agents. Thus it is not known whether the lethal arrhythmia was spontaneous or was a proarrhythmic effect of the antiarrhythmic drug. Thus, although in persons without cardiac disease VEA may rarely be associated with sudden death, it is reasonable to conclude 1) that subjects free of heart disease frequently have ventricular ectopy of low frequency and complexity, 2) that VEA increases with advancing age even in the absence of heart disease, and 3) that this arrhythmia may possibly be associated with a relative increase of risk of sudden cardiac death although in absolute terms the risk is quite small.

VEA in Patients With Coronary Artery Disease

Unlike VEA in normal persons, and unlike the finding of ST segment changes on AMB ECG, a direct relationship between VEA and the risk of sudden cardiac death has been reported by many investigators in patients with coronary heart disease [66–86]. Both prospective and retrospective studies have found an association between VEA and both sudden and nonsudden cardiac mortality.

Myocardial Infarction

A great deal of data on myocardial infarction pertain to studies of patients who survived the acute (1–3 week) phase. In this subset of coronary patients, VEA may be recorded on either early or late AMB ECG. Following myocardial infarction, arrhythmias may occur either as a result of the ischemia during the acute event or as a result of the chronic anatomic and physiologic changes attendant to the muscle death and scar formation. This difference may explain why there is only a weak relationship between those arrhythmias seen acutely after myocardial infarction and long-term mortality, while a stronger association exists between arrhythmias recorded several weeks after the acute infarction (during healing and scarring) and the subsequent risk of sudden death [66,73,74,83,87].

The ventricular ectopy of the acute ischemic event is usually transitory, related to the temporary alterations in the electrophysiologic substrate (cation fluxes, automaticity, local conduction, and refractoriness). If this disturbance results in ventricular fibrillation in the acute setting, there is no particularly high risk for recurrence after the initial ischemic episode has subsided. On the other hand, arrhythmias related to the chronic changes subsequent to cell death, fibrosis, and the architectural restructuring of the ventricle from scar contraction, expansion and compensatory hypertrophy define a subgroup for future development of serious and even fatal arrhythmias.

Patients studied by AMB ECG several weeks into the recuperative period following an AMI show a much higher frequency, prevalence, and complexity of VEA than does the normal population. Twenty-four hour Holter recordings during this period consistently demonstrate ventricular arrhythmia in over 80–90% of the patients. Approximately 20–40% demonstrate repetitive forms and 10–15% have more than 10 VPBs per hour. A small subgroup of these patients have more than 30 VPBs per hour [66,88,89].

The largest database of AMB ECG in acute myocardial infarction survivors comes from the Beta Blocker Heart Attack Trial (BHAT). Over 3,000 patients had a 24 hour AMB ECG at entry into the study before being randomized to receive either propranolol or placebo. A follow-up study of an average of 25 months after the acute infarction reported that 13% of this patient group had more than 10 VPBs per average hour and that 19.9% had repetitive forms. Although the mean hourly VPB count was 13.5, a large percentage of subjects had a very low VPB frequency, with a median count of only 0.298 VPBs per hour.

Determinants of VEA in Coronary Artery Disease

As suggested in the above section, the seriousness of coronary artery disease is associated with the extent of myocardial involvement that is in turn related to the frequency and complexity of VEA as demonstrated by AMB ECG. Age is also a major predictor of VEA in AMI survivors as it is in normal and apparently normal subjects and can be shown to be independent of disease severity [9,10,65].

Left ventricular dysfunction is a major determinant of VEA in myocardial infarction survivors even independently of its association with the extent of coronary artery disease [66,90]. The direct relationship between VEA and left ventricular dysfunction has been reported in both invasive and noninvasive studies. Higher grades of VEA have been observed in patients with both 1) clinical evidence of congestive heart failure and 2) past myocardial infarction. A relationship between VEA and objective measurements of left ventricular function, such as left ventricular end diastolic pressure, and ventriculographically measured regional hypokinesis has been convincingly demonstrated. Patients with greater depression in their global ejection fraction also tend to demonstrate more pronounced VEA, although this has not been uniformly observed.

Finally, the extent of coronary artery disease that is usually related to left ventricular function has also been found to be an independent predictor of VEA, suggesting a possible alternate pathway whereby coronary disease may mediate arrhythmia as well as an explanation for the relationship of VEA to mortality, especially nonsudden death mortality after accounting for LV dysfunction [90].

Other potential factors that might influence VEA following AMI have been looked for. However, a relationship of VEA to electrolyte imbalance, serum potassium level, infarction site, and the presence of angina has not been observed.

Relationship of VEA to Mortality

The observed associations of left ventricular dysfunction with risk of future mortality and also with VEA suggests that a link between ventricular ectopy and cardiac death should exist. In fact, this relationship has been reported in many prospective and retrospective studies using both simple 12 lead ECGs, such as in the Coronary Drug Project, and AMB ECG [66,90]. These studies have demonstrated this link both with sudden and nonsudden cardiac death. Earlier studies using small numbers of patients had suggested that sudden death risk required both factors (left ventricular dysfunction and complex ventricular ectopy), while either factor alone did not independently worsen prognosis. However, recent larger studies have determined that ecotpy worsens progressively even in the absence of left ventricular dysfunction [66,90,91].

The empiric relationship of left ventricular dysfunction, VEA, and sudden death still raises the question of whether VEA is not simply a marker of serious coronary artery disease manifested by left ventricular dysfunction or other risk factors rather than an independent predictor of risk. Most available data do support a relationship between VEA and the risk of sudden death that is at least partially independent of other factors and by inference is probably causally related to it.

Evidence for this position comes from several different types of analysis. For example, the early studies of Ruberman found that the presence of complex VEA increased the sudden death risk approximately twofold in patients both with and without congestive heart failure. Therefore, the inference was drawn that there was an independent relationship between these two cardiac abnormalities [91]. Such analyses do not consider the possibility that patients with congestive heart failure and arrhythmias may have a more serious degree of cardiac decompensation, and this may result in both the higher mortality and the greater degree of ventricular ectopy. This, however, is not born out in other studies such as MILIS and Bigger's in which left ventricular function was studied in detail using ejection fraction. In these studies ventricular ectopy worsened prognosis in both the high and low left ventricular dysfunction strata [90].

A third type of evidence of the independent relationship between VEA and sudden death derives from multivariate statistical analyses [66]. In several of these examinations, VEA determined by AMB ECG remained an independent predictor of sudden death after accounting for other variables associated with increased risk such as the degree of left ventricular dysfunction measured both invasively and noninvasively, the extent of ischemia, electrocardiographic abnormalities, and other factors.

A small number of studies, however, have not confirmed this independent relationship between VEA and sudden or nonsudden death, although a univariate relationship is almost always seen [92–94]. These studies are small and consequently have a low statistical power to detect a modest effect. Other factors that could be masking a real relationship in these studies include differences in severity of myocardial infarction, time from infarction, and other methodological differences in study design.

Relationship of VEA to Mortality in Subsets of Myocardial Infarction Survivors

Survivors of myocardial infarction have variable prognosis according to certain baseline characteristics describing the severity of the index infarction as well as other factors. Many stratification schemata utilizing a variety of clinical and laboratory indices including both invasive and noninvasive modalities have been proposed [95–105]. In most studies, the stratification factors considered to be important have been age; variables related to the degree of left ventricular damage subsequent to the infarction (e.g., left ventricular ejection fraction, cardiomegaly, clinical signs of heart failure, and the number of previous infarctions); measures of myocardial ischemia (e.g., positive EST, resting ECG abnormalities, and coronary arteriographic findings); and metabolic factors (e.g., electrolytes and coagulation parameters). The traditional risk factors for coronary artery disease such as smoking, hyperlipidemia, and hypertension also play a role especially in the later years of follow-up. Based on such criteria, patients who have survived an acute myocardial infarction may be stratified for risk of sudden death from the lowest to the highest risk strata. As would be predicted, sudden death mortality is concentrated in the highest risk strata. This has created the impression that VEA found during AMB ECG worsens prognosis only in the highest risk strata. However, this is only partially true. In several studies including the large BHAT, AMB ECG has found an increased risk of sudden cardiac death in both low and high risk strata with similar risk ratios in both groups [66,90]. In these important studies, the risk ratio was actually higher for the low risk patients than for the high risk patients. On the other hand, from the point of view of absolute rather than relative risk, the increment of risk imposed by VEA is greatest in the high risk subset. This was clearly seen in the BHAT in which patients were easily stratified according to the presence or absence of three readily obtainable clinical criteria: 1) more than one myocardial infarction, 2) cardiomegaly by chest X-ray, and 3) ST segment depression on the resting ECG. This stratification alone allowed identification of four subgroups according to the number of these criteria present. The rate of sudden death during the first 25 months following infarction was only 1.7 per 100 patients for the lowest risk category (no risk factors present). However, for patients who had one, two, or three of these predictive factors, the sudden death rate increased to 5.7, 8.8, and 22.6 per 100 over the same 25 month period [66].

In this study, the presence of VEA (defined as 10 or more VPBs per hour, or pairs of VPBs or ventricular tachycardia, or multiform VPBs during the 24 hour AMB ECG recording) increased the relative risk for sudden death from 2.06 times for the high risk to 4.26 times in the lowest risk subgroup. On the other hand, the absolute increment in risk was greatest in the high risk category (from 14.3% in those with high risk and no VEA to 29.4% in those high risk patients with VEA, an increase of about 15%); while in the low risk category, although the risk ratio was 4.26, the absolute increment in sudden death mortality was only 2.5%, i.e., an increase from 0.8% in low risk patients without VEA to 3.3% in those who had VEA. In most studies the relationship between VEA and risk is not affected by infarction site or depth (anterior vs. inferior, Q vs. non-Q).

Selection of Appropriate Arrhythmia Definition

Since the majority of AMI survivors have some degree of VEA, if this finding is to be considered in their prognostic stratification and therapeutic decisions it is important to consider the impact of different definitions of arrhythmia [66]. When dichotomous categorical definitions of arrhythmia are used, it is surprising to note that for those patients who do versus those who do not have a given arrhythmia definition the odds ratios of dying are quite similar among the various definitions selected, varying between 2 and 3. This holds when either total mortality or sudden death mortality is considered and whether the placebo or propranolol group is being studied (Table 5–2).

Both frequency and complexity of the VEA have been proposed as important predictors of sudden death mortality in these patients. It appears that both have prognostic importance. Thus the chance of suffering atherosclerotic sudden death within the 25 month study period following myocardial infarction was 2.3% in patients having no VPBs per 24 hours, with an odds ratio of 2.26. This separation is quite similar using a different arrhythmia cut-off frequency such as 10 VPBs per hour. Patients having 10 or more VPBs per hour had a 9% probability of sudden death, while those having nine or less VPBs per hour had 4.0 probability of sudden death, with an odds ratio of 2.38. Even the presence of repetitive forms acted similarly, with sudden death risk of 8.0 versus 3.8%, with an odds ratio of 2.18. Combining definitions of arrhythmias did not change the odds ratios; no definition of arrhythmia was intrinsically superior in discriminating survivorship.

A different approach to the relationship between mortality and the definition of arrhythmia is to compare the sensitivity and the specificity of each of the different definitions in predicting sudden death (Table 5–3). Analyzed this way, the presence of one or more VPBs per 24 hours was highly sensitive for predetermining victims of atherosclerotic sudden death (92.1%). This means that 92.1% of those who suffered sudden death had at least one VPB per 24 hours. On the other hand, the specificity of this definition, i.e., the percent of patients who did not suffer sudden death who also did not have arrhythmia by this definition, is rather low (16.2%). In other words, 83.8% of those who did not die suddenly did have this arrhythmia. Therefore, this rather lenient definition of arrhythmia has a very high sensitivity and low specificity.

This kind of reciprocal relationship between the sensitivity and specificity of the different definitions of arrhythmia in identifying sudden death victims has been observed as expected. Thus patients with 10 or more VPBs per hour and repetitive forms and multiform VPBs were only infrequently seen in this cohort (7%). This very stringent definition had very low sensitivity, since it identified only 15.8% of the patients who were to die suddenly during follow-up. On the other hand, its specificity was quite good, with 93.6% of those who did not die suddenly not having VEA by this definition.

TABLE 5–2. Total Mortality, Atherosclerotic Sudden Death, Atherosclerotic Nonsudden Death, and Seven Definitions of Ventricular Ectopic Activity

		Total mortality			Atherosclerotic sudden death (<1 hour)			Atherosclerotic nonsudden death		
	Total No. of patients	Death rate (%)	Odds ratio	Z of diff.	Death rate (%)	Odds ratio	Z of diff.	Death rate (%)	Odds ratio	Z of diff.
Overall	1,640	9.9	—	—	4.6	—	—	4.0	—	—
VPB >0/24 hours										
Yes	1,380	10.9			5.1			4.5		
No	260	5.0	2.32	2.90	2.3	2.25	1.95	1.5	3.01	2.22
VPB ≥10/hours										
Yes	211	19.9			9.0			8.1		
No	1,429	8.5	2.69	5.18	4.0	2.38	3.24	3.4	2.47	3.19
VPB pair or VT present										
Yes	327	16.5			8.0			6.7		
No	1,313	8.3	2.18	4.44	3.8	2.18	3.19	3.4	2.08	2.78
VPB ≥10 hours or VPB pair or VT)										
Yes	418	17.2			7.9			7.2		
No	1,222	7.4	2.59	5.77	3.5	2.35	3.67	2.9	2.55	3.80
Multiform present										
Yes	538	15.2			8.7			5.6		
No	1,102	7.4	2.27	5.02	2.6	3.54	5.52	3.3	1.75	2.23
VPB ≥10/hours and pair or VT and multiform complexes										
Yes	112	19.6			10.7			7.1		
No	1,528	9.2	2.40	3.56	4.2	2.75	3.17	3.8	1.95	1.74
VPB ≥10/hours or pair of VT or multiform complexes										
Yes	666	15.2			7.7			5.9		
No	974	6.4	2.63	5.85	2.6	3.15	4.82	2.8	2.18	3.12

VPB, ventricular premature beat; VT, ventricular tachycardia.

Thus the false positive rate was rather low (6.4%); i.e., only 6.4% of those who did not die suddenly had this arrhythmia [66].

This reciprocal relationship between sensitivity and specificity of different definitions of VEA has been displayed as a receiver operator characteristic curve (Fig. 5–1). This curve may be used to select the appropriate definition for a given therapeutic or research objective. When an intervention with low incidence of side effects is considered, a low specificity definition may be tolerated since treatment of many individuals who do not need the treatment (high false positive rate) would not result in unacceptable harm, while its high sensitivity would ensure that treatment would be received by most of those who did need it (high true positive rate). The opposite would be true for a toxic intervention where using a definition of high specificity

TABLE 5–3. Sensitivity and Specificity of Definitions of Arrhythmia in Predicting Sudden Death

Arrhythmia definition	No. of deaths (a)	No. with arrhythmia (b)	Sensitivity (c = b/a)	No. alive (d)	No. without arrhythmia (e)	Specificity (f = e/d)
Total mortality						
VPB >0/24 hours	163	150	0.920	1,477	247	0.167
VPB ≥10/hour	163	42	0.258	1,477	1,308	0.886
VPB pair or VT present	163	54	0.331	1,477	1,204	0.815
VPB ≥10/hour or VPB pair or VT	163	72	0.442	1,477	1,131	0.766
Multiform present	163	82	0.503	1,477	1,021	0.691
VPB ≥10/hour and pair or VT and multiform	163	22	0.135	1,477	1,387	0.939
VPB ≥10/hour or pair or VT or multiform	163	101	0.620	1,477	912	0.617
Atherosclerotic sudden death (<1 hour)						
VPB >0/24 hours	76	70	0.921	1,564	254	0.162
VPB ≥10/hour	76	19	0.250	1,564	1,372	0.877
VPB pair or VT present	76	26	0.342	1,564	1,263	0.808
VPB ≥10/hour or VPB pair or VT	76	33	0.434	1,564	1,179	0.754
Multiform present	76	47	0.618	1,564	1,073	0.686
VPB ≥10/hour and pair or VT and multiform	76	12	0.158	1,564	1,464	0.936
VPB ≥10/hour or pair or VT or multiform	76	51	0.671	1,564	949	0.607
Nonsudden atherosclerotic death						
VPB >0/24 hours	66	62	0.939	1,574	256	0.163
VPB ≥10/hour	66	17	0.258	1,574	1,380	0.877
VPB pair or VT present	66	22	0.333	1,574	1,269	0.806
VPB ≥10/hour or VPB pair or VT	66	30	0.455	1,574	1,186	0.753
Multiform present	66	30	0.455	1,574	1,066	0.677
VPB ≥10/hour and pair or VT and multiform	66	8	0.121	1,574	1,470	0.934
VPB ≥10/hour or pair or VT or multiform	66	39	0.591	1,574	947	0.602

would prevent its needless application (low false positive rate); however, its necessarily low sensitivity would result in treating only a small minority of those who really need treatment.

An approach to determine the appropriate definition of VEA for a specific clinical or research setting is demonstrated by the use of the infor-

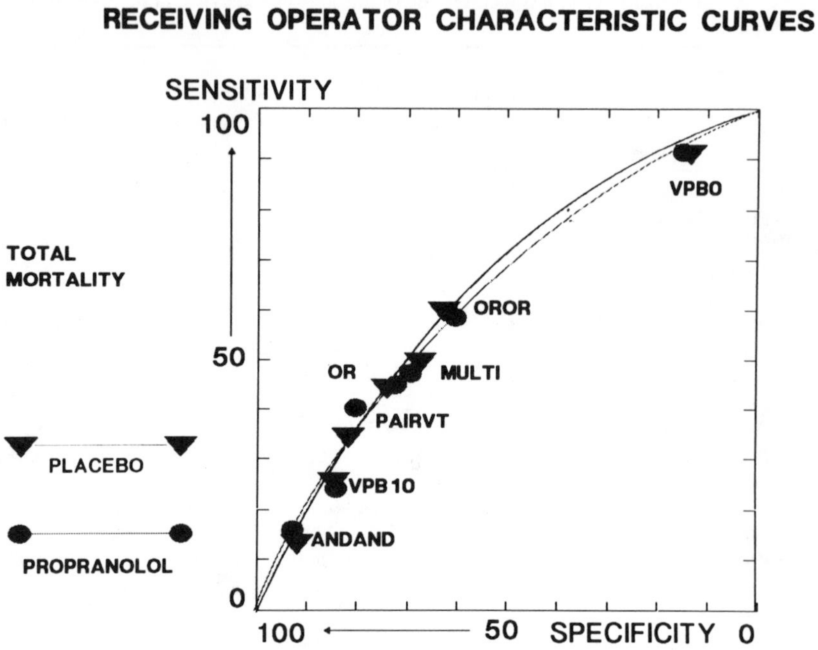

Fig. 5–1. Reciprocal relation between sensitivity and specificity of seven definitions of ventricular arrhythmias in predicting mortality rate of survivors of acute myocardial infarction. 1 = VPB > 0; 2 = VPB ≥ 10/h; 3 = VPB pair or VT; 4 = VPB ≥ 10/h; 5 = multiform complexes; 6 = VPB ≥ 10/h and VPB (pair or VT) and multiform complexes; 7 = VPB ≥ 10/h or VPB pair or VT or multiform complexes. VPB = ventricular premature beats; VT = ventricular tachycardia; triangles = placebo group; dots = propranolol group.

mation in Tables 5–2 and 5–3. For example, if a subset of patients with a high mortality is to be identified for treatment, persons with more than 10 VPBs per hour and multiform complexes and repetitive forms have a mortality rate approximately four times higher (19.6% in 25 months) than a person with no VPBs (5.0%). Treatment only of patients with this definition of VEA would afford a benefit to 13.4% of the patients likely to die and would therefore not benefit the majority at risk. Accordingly, it is important to consider not only the absolute risk of a given subset with a given definition of VEA but also the sensitivity of that definition in identifying patients who may die and its specificity in identifying patients not at risk (Fig. 5–1). By using this type of analysis, it becomes easier to tailor the definition of VEA to a proposed intervention.

The Influence of Beta-Blockers

Several large studies have shown an improved survival rate in patients who receive beta-blocking drugs during and after their myocardial infarction

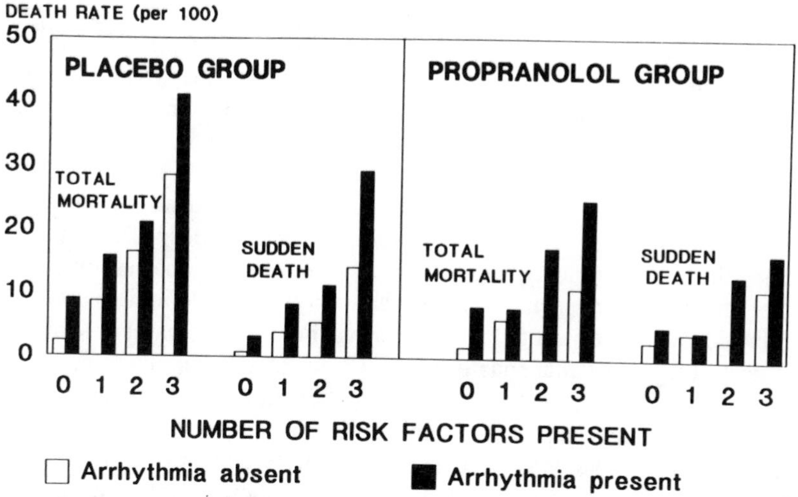

Fig. 5–2. Total mortality and sudden death mortality according to the number of risk factors (prior myocardial infarction, cardiothoracic ratio >0.5, ST depression on resting electrocardiogram) and the presence or absence of ventricular ectopic activity (ventricular premature complexes/hour ≥10 or [ventricular premature complexes pair or ventricular tachycardia event] or multiform) in the placebo or propranolol groups of the Beta-Blocker Heart Attack Trial.

and that this benefit persists for up to 2 or 3 years after the index event [106–108]. The exact mechanisms for this benefit have not yet been clearly elucidated, although an antiarrhythmic action has been suggested [109–111]. Several studies have shown that the increase in VEA during the weeks following myocardial infarction is blunted by beta-blockade. In addition, beta-blockers are known to have a direct antiarrhythmic potential, decreasing ventricular fibrillation threshold. Because of these common perceptions, many infarction survivors currently receive this class of drug.

The possible attenuation of the impact of VEA on myocardial infarction survival requires a more thorough examination. A review of the large BHAT database reveals that in infarction survivors who received propranolol, VEA was associated with sudden death by both multivariate and univariate analyses [112]. The relative risk of sudden death occurring in patients with or without VEA was similar in the propranolol and placebo groups, even slightly lower in the drug group (Fig. 5–2). In addition, the sensitivity and specificity for each definition of VEA in predicting mortality was similar in the two groups. Thus treatment with beta-blockers, at least with propranolol, does not diminish the predictive force of VEA in identifying patients prone to sudden death among survivors of acute myocardial infarction.

Association of VEA With Both Sudden and Nonsudden Coronary Death

The most likely pathophysiologic mechanism underlying the independent association between VEA and cardiac death is by the precipitation of ventricular fibrillation. Asymptomatic nonsustained ventricular ectopy may be a marker of "electrical instability" or a tendency of a patient's ventricular myocardium to fibrillate. From these considerations, one would expect the mortality risk ratios to be higher for sudden than for nonsudden coronary death.

In some studies, ventricular arrhythmias, especially repetitive forms, were found to be the best predictor for sudden cardiac death, whereas congestive heart failure was a stronger predictor of nonsudden death. In other studies this was not clearly evidenced. Factors that may be responsible for these varying results include 1) the variability in the definition of sudden cardiac death with respect to the time interval between the onset of symptoms and death (e.g., instantaneous death to 1 hour after symptoms); and 2) the allowable clinical circumstances of the fatal event (e.g., AMI, unwitnessed death, and during sleep; and 3) the differences in arrhythmia definition discussed in the previous section. The lack of preferential association of VEA with sudden rather than nonsudden cardiac death may imply the important conclusion that asymptomatic VEA is a marker of electrical instability that increases the risk of death in all patients with coronary artery disease regardless of the presence of clinically recognized ischemic events, including AMI. In addition, it is possible that the relationship between VEA and nonsudden death mortality may be mediated through the association of VEA with the extent of coronary artery disease [66,112].

Although VEA has been clearly shown to be associated with an increased mortality risk in survivors of AMI, and although it most probably contributes to the risk independently of other factors, there is no evidence to date that the treatment of this arrhythmia reduces the risk. Published studies of antiarrhythmic therapy in AMI have not proven a beneficial effect (Fig. 5–3). However, these studies were small (low statistical power), agents with low potency in suppressing VEA were used, single drugs in fixed doses were sometimes used, and AMB ECG was not always employed to define the risk and the efficacy of the treatment. A pilot study (CAPS) on this issue has been completed recently, and a large study on the protective effect of antiarrhythmic agents following myocardial infarction (CAST) is still in progress. Perplexing in this study is the fact that the two potent antiarrhythmic agents flecainide and encainide were associated with an increased mortality. This important trial is discussed in detail in Chapter 8 (Bigger, this volume).

CONCLUSIONS

Sudden cardiac death is the leading cause of death among 20–64-year-old men, occurring at the alarming rate of one victim every minute. The vast preponderance of these deaths is due to ventricular tachyarrhythmia in persons with coronary artery disease, even though 25% of victims have never experienced previous symptoms of their underlying disease.

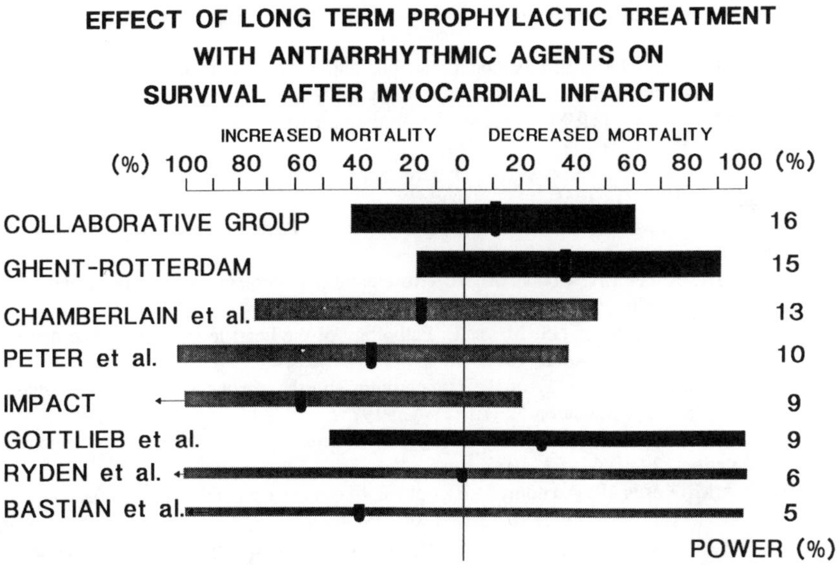

Fig. 5–3. The figure depicts the effect of antiarrhythmic therapy on total mortality, expressed as a percentage of placebo mortality. A decrease in mortality of a given percentage is depicted by a vertical line lying to the right of the zero line; an increase is shown by a line to the left of the zero line. The width of each bar around the vertical line corresponds to the 95% confidence intervals of each study. The height of each bar corresponds to the power of the study, i.e., the chance of proving a decrease in mortality by the intervention (in the case of these figures a 25% decrease), if such an effect were truly present. The numerical value of the power (percent) is listed on the right. Studies showing a beneficial trend are depicted by darker bars.

EST and AMB ECG have been proposed as logical tests for risk stratification, since they can induce or track signs of both coronary insufficiency and electrical instability. Extensive studies of large populations of persons have shown that both the ischemic ST segment response and/or VEA may identify individuals who both have coronary artery disease (symptomatic or silent) and may have an enhanced potential for lethal ventricular arrhythmia. A strong relationship has been firmly demonstrated between the increased risk of sudden cardiac death and EST and AMB ECG parameters in patients with known coronary heart disease, AMI survivors, and coronary surgery candidates. Once the potential for sudden death is identified, medical or surgical treatment of the underlying coronary heart disease may be more rationally tailored to reach the greatest benefit at the lowest risk.

REFERENCES

1. Burch GE, DePasquale NP: Sudden unexpected natural death. Am J Sci 249:86–89, 1965.
2. Savage DD, Castelli WP, Anderson SJ, Kannel WB: Sudden unexpected death during

ambulatory electrocardiographic monitoring. The Framingham study. Am J Med 74: 148–152, 1983.

3. Lown B, Kosowsky et al.: Pathogenesis, prevention and treatment of arrhythmias in myocardial infarction. Circulation 40 (II):261–267, 1969.
4. Broustet JP, Doward H, Mora: Exercise testing in arrhythmias of idiopathic mitral valve prolapse. Eur Heart J 8:37–42, 1987.
5. Nicod P, Polikar R, Peterson KL: Hypertrophic cardiomyopathy and sudden death. N England J Med 318:1255–1257, 1988.
6. Unverferth D, Magorien R, Moeschberger M, et al.: Factors influencing the one year mortality of dilated cardiomyopathy.
7. Perper JA, Kuller LH, Cooper M: Arteriosclerosis of coronary arteries in sudden expected death. Circulation 52 (II):27–33, 1975.
8. Reichenbach DD, Moss NS, Meyer E: Pathology of the heart in sudden cardiac death. Am J Cardiol 39:865–872, 1977.
9. Lie JT, Titus JL: Pathology of the myocardium and the conduction system in sudden coronary death. Circulation 52 (III):41–52, 1975.
10. Reichenbach DD, Moss NS: Myocardial wall necrosis and sudden death in humans. Circulation 52 (III):60–62, 1975.
11. Sanders M, Kostis JB: Anatomy versus physiology in the prognosis of coronary artery disease. J Am Coll Cardiol 10:1365–1366, 1987.
12. Sanders M: The physiology of chronic angina. In Haft JI, Bailey CP (eds): ''Advances in the Management of Clinical Heart Disease.'' Mount Kisco, NY: Futura Press, pp 183–220, 1975.
13. Kostis JB, McCrone K, Moreyra AE, et al.: Premature ventricular complexes in the absence of identifiable heart disease. Circulation 63:1351–1356, 1981.
14. Robb GP, Markes HH: Postexercise electrocardiogram in atherosclerotic heart disease. JAMA 200:918–926, 1967.
15. Sharma B, Wyeth RP: Six year survival of patients with and without painless myocardial ischemia and out-of-hospital ventricular fibrillation. Am J Cardiol 61:9F–12F, 1988.
16. Masters AM, Friedman R, Dadi S: The electrocardiogram after standard exercise as a functional test of the heart. Am Heart J 24:777–793, 1942.
17. Bayley RW, LaDue JS, York DJ: Electrocardiographic changes (local ventricular ischemia and injuries) produced in the dog by temporary occlusion of a coronary artery showing a new stage in the evolution of myocardial infarction. Am Heart J 27:164–172, 1944.
18. Allen WH, Aronow WS, Goodman P, Stinson P: Five year follow-up of maximal treadmill stress test in asymptomatic men and women. Circulation 62:522–527, 1986.
19. Bruce RA: Noninvasive clinical and exercise predictors of sudden cardiac death in men with coronary artery disease. Texas Med 77:55–59, 1981.
20. Ryan M, Lown B, Horn H: Comparison of ventricular ectopic activity during 24 hour monitoring and exercise testing in patients with coronary heart disease. N Engl J Med 292:7249–7253, 1975.
21. McHenry PL: Role of exercise testing in predicting sudden death. J Am Coll Cardiol 5:9B–12B, 1985.
22. Ellestad MH, Wan MKC: Predictive implications of stress testing. Follow-up of 2700 subjects after maximum treadmill stress testing. Circulation 51:363–369, 1975.
23. McNeer JF, Margolis JR, Lee KL, et al.: The role of the exercise test in the evaluation of patients for ischemic heart disease. Circulation 57:64–70, 1978.
24. Bruce RA, DeRowen TA, Hossack KF: Value of maximal exercise tests in risk assessment of primary coronary heart disease events in healthy men. Am J Cardiol 46: 371–378, 1980.

25. Giagnoni E, Secchi B, Wu SC, et al.: Prognostic value of exercise EKG testing in asymptomatic normotensive subjects. N Engl J Med 309:1985–1089, 1983.
26. Weiner DA, Ryan TJ, McCabe CH, et al.: Prognostic importance of a clinical profile and exercise test in medically treated patients with coronary artery disease. J Am Coll Cardiol 3:772–779, 1984.
27. Falcone C, deServi S, Poma E, et al.: Clinical significance of exercise induced silent myocardial ischemia in patients with coronary artery disease. J Am Coll Cardiol 9: 295–299, 1987.
28. Chiang BN, Perlman LV, Ostrander LD, Epstein FH: Relationship of premature systoles to coronary heart disease and sudden death in the Tecumseh Epidemiologic Study. Ann Intern Med 70:1159–1166, 1969.
29. Kowsowsky BD, Lown B, Whiting R, Guiney T: Occurrence of ventricular arrhythmias with exercise as compared to monitoring. Circulation 44:826–832, 1971.
30. Grayboys TB, DeSilva RA, Lown B: Ambulatory monitoring and exercise stress testing in the management of patients with malignant ventricular arrhythmia. Am J Cardiol 41:400, 1978.
31. Califf RM, McNeer F, Lee K, Rosati R: Prognostic implications of ventricular arrhythmias in treadmill exercise testing. Circulation 58(II):198, 1978.
32. Ivanova LA, Mazur NA, Smirnova TM, et al.: Electrocardiographic exercise testing and ambulatory monitoring to identify patients with ischemic heart disease at risk of sudden death. Am J Cardiol 45:1132–1138, 1980.
33. Califf RM, McKinnin RA, McNeer F, et al.: Prognostic value of ventricular arrhythmias associated with treadmill exercise testing in patients studied with cardiac catheterization for suspected ischemic heart disease. J Am Coll Cardiol 2:1061–1067, 1983.
34. Nair CK, Aronow WJ, Sketch MH, et al.: Diagnostic and prognostic significance of exercise induced premature ventricular complexes in men and women: A four year followup. J Am Coll Cardiol 1:1201–1206, 1983.
35. Lampert S, Lown B, Grayboys TB, et al.: Determinants of survival in patients with malignant ventricular arrhythmias associated with coronary artery disease. Am J Cardiol 61:791–797, 1988.
36. Killip T, Kimball JT: Treatment of myocardial infarction in a coronary care unit. Am J Cardiol 20:457–464, 1967.
37. Sami M, Kraemer H, DeBusk RF: The prognostic significance of serial exercise testing after myocardial infarction. Circulation 60:1230–1246, 1979.
38. Theroux P, Waters DD, Halphen C, et al.: Prognostic value of exercise testing soon after myocardial infarction. N Engl J Med 301:341–345, 1979.
39. Starling MR, Crawford MH, Kennedy GT, O'Rourke RA: Exercise testing early after myocardial infarction: Predictive value for subsequent unstable angina and death. Am J Cardiol 46:909–914, 1980.
40. Davidson DM, DeBusk RF: Prognostic value of a single exercise test 3 weeks after uncomplicated myocardial infarction. Circulation 61:236–242, 1980.
41. DeBusk RF, Davidson DM, Houston N, Fitzgerald J: Serial ambulatory electrocardiography and treadmill exercise testing after uncomplicated myocardial infarction. Am J Cardiol 45:547–554, 1980.
42. Kentola E, Repo UK: Sudden death after myocardial infarction and T wave changes in connection with exercise testing. Ann Clin Res 15:109–112, 1983.
43. Ericsson M, Granath A, Ohlsen P, et al.: Arrhythmias and symptoms during treadmill three weeks after myocardial infarction. Br Heart J 35:787–796, 1973.
44. Granath A, Sodermark J, Winge T, et al.: Early work load tests for evaluation of long term prognosis of acute myocardial infarction. Br Heart J 39:758–763, 1977.
45. Weld FM, Chu K, Bigger TJ, Rolnitzky MS: Risk stratification with low level exercise testing 2 weeks after acute myocardial infarction. Circulation 64:306–314, 1981.

46. Henry RL, Kennedy GT, Crawford MH: Prognostic value of exercise induced ventricular ectopic activity for mortality after acute myocardial infarction. Am J Cardiol 59:1251–1255, 1987.
47. Kaiser GC, Davis KB, Fisher LD, et al.: Survival following coronary artery bypass grafting in patients with severe angina pectoris (CASS): An observational study. J Thorac Cardiovasc Surg 89:513–523, 1925.
48. Veterans Administration Coronary Artery Bypass Surgery Cooperative Study Group: Seven year survival in Veterans Administration randomized trial of coronary bypass surgery for stable angina. N Engl J Med 311:1333–1339, 1984.
49. European Cooperative Surgery Study Group: Long term results of prospective randomized study of coronary artery bypass surgery in stable angina pectoris. Lancet 2:1173–1180, 1982.
50. Norris RM, Barnaby PF, Brandt PWT, et al.: Prognosis after recovering from first myocardial infarction: Determinants of reinfarction and sudden death. Am J Cardiol 53:408–413, 1984.
51. Weiner DA, Ryan TJ, McCabe CH, et al.: The role of exercise testing in identifying patients with improved survival after coronary artery bypass surgery. J Am Coll Cardiol 8:741–748, 1986.
52. Weiner DA, Ryan TJ, McCabe CH, et al.: Comparison of coronary artery bypass surgery and medical therapy in patients with exercise induced silent myocardial ischemia: A report from the Coronary Artery Surgery Study (CASS) Registry. J Am Coll Cardiol 12:595–599, 1988.
53. Surawicz B: Noninvasive assessment of ventricular arrhythmias in clinical practice: Prognostic implications. Can J Cardiol 2:285–294, 1986.
54. Kostis JB, McCrone K, Moreyra AE, Gotzoyannis S, Aglitz NM, Natarajan N, Kuo PT: Premature ventricular complexes in the absence of identifiable heart disease. Circulation 63(6):1351–1356, 1981.
55. Kennedy HL, Pescarmona JE, Bouchard RJ, Goldberg RJ: Coronary artery status of apparently healthy subjects with frequent and complex ventricular ectopy. Ann Intern Med 92:179, 1980.
56. Hinkle LE Jr, Carver ST, Stevens M: The frequency of asymptomatic disturbances of cardiac rhythm and conduction in middle-aged men. Am J Cardiol 24:629, 1969.
57. Hinkle LE, Carver ST, Argyros DC: The prognostic significance of ventricular premature contractions in healthy people and in people with coronary artery disease. Acta Cardiol [Suppl 18]:5, 1974.
58. Raftery EB, Cashman PMM: Long-term recording of the electrocardiogram in normal population. Postgrad Med J 52[Suppl 7]:32, 1976.
59. Brodsky M, Wu D, Denes P, Kanakis C, Rosen KM: Arrhythmias documented by 24-hour continuous electrocardiographic monitoring in 50 male medical students without apparent heart disease. Am J Cardiol 39:390, 1977.
60. Clarke JM, Shelton JR, Hamer J, Taylor S: The rhythm of the normal human heart. Lancet 2:508, 1976.
61. Glasser SP, Clark PT, Applebaum HJ: Occurrence of frequent complex arrhythmias detected by ambulatory monitoring. Chest 75:565, 1979.
62. Kennedy HL, Whitlock JA, Sprague MK, Kennedy LJ, Buckingham TA, Goldberg RJ: Long-term follow-up of asymptomatic healthy subjects with frequent and complex ventricular ectopy. N Engl J Med 312(4):193–197, 1985.
63. Lemery R, Burgada P, Paola DB, et al.: Nonischemic ventricular tachycardia. Clinical course and long-term follow-up in patients without clinically overt heart disease. Circulation 79:990–999, 1989.
64. Abdalla IS, Prineas RJ, Neaton JD, Jacobs DR, Crow RS Jr: Relation between ventric-

ular premature complexes and sudden cardiac death in apparently healthy men. Am J Cardiol 60(13):1036–1042, 1987.
65. Kostis JB, McCrone K, Moreyra AE, Hosler M, Cosgrove N, Kuo PT: The effect of age, blood pressure and gender on the incidence of premature ventricular contractions. Angiology 33(7):464–473, 1982.
66. Kostis JB, Byington R, Friedman LM, Goldstein S, Furberg C for the BHAT Study Group: Prognostic significance of ventricular ectopic activity in survivors of acute myocardial infarction. J Am Coll Cardiol 10:231–242, 1987.
67. Moss AJ, Schnitzler L, Green R, DeCamilla J: Ventricular arrhythmias 3 weeks after acute myocardial infarction. Ann Intern Med 75:837, 1971.
68. Tominaga S, Blackburn H: The coronary drug project research group: Prognostic importance of premature beats following myocardial infarction. JAMA 223:1116, 1973.
69. Kotler MN, Tabatznik B, Mower MM, Tominaga S: Prognostic significance of ventricular ectopic beats with respect to sudden death in the late postinfarction period. Circulation XLVII:959, 1973.
70. Moss AJ, DeCamilla J, Engstrom F, Hoffman W, Odoroff C, Davis H: The posthospital phase of myocardial infarction: Identification of patients with increased mortality risk. Circulation 49:460, 1974.
71. Schulze RA Jr, Rouleau J, Rigo P, Bowers S, Strauss HW, Pitt B: Ventricular arrhythmias in the late hospital phase of acute myocardial infarction: Relation of left ventricular function detected by gated cardiac blood pool scanning. Circulation 52:1006, 1975.
72. Vismara LA, Amsterdam EA, Mason DT: Relation of ventricular arrhythmias in the late hospital phase of acute myocardial infarction to sudden death after hospital discharge. Am J Med 59:6, 1975.
73. Moss AJ, DeCamilla J, Davis H, Bayer L: The early posthospital phase of myocardial infarction: Prognostic stratification. Circulation 54(1):58, 1976.
74. Rehnqvist N: Ventricular arrhythmias prior to discharge after acute myocardial infarction. Eur J Cardiol 4:63, 1976.
75. Luria MH, Knoke JD, Margolis RM, Hendricks FH, Kuplic JB: Acute myocardial infarction: Prognosis after recovery. Ann Intern Med 85:561, 1976.
76. Ruberman W, Weinblatt E, Frank CW, Goldberg JD, Shapiro S, Feldman CL: Prognostic value of one hour of ECG monitoring of men with coronary heart disease. J Chronic Dis 29:497, 1976.
77. Schulze RA Jr, Strauss HW, Pitt B: Sudden death in the year following myocardial infarction: Relation to ventricular premature contractions in the late hospital phase and left ventricular ejection fraction. Am J Med 62:192, 1977.
78. Vismara SA, Vera A, Foerster JM, Amsterdam IA, Mason DT: Identification of sudden death risk factors in acute and chronic coronary artery disease. Am J Cardiol 39:821, 1977.
79. Anderson KP, DeCamilla J, Moss AJ: Clinical significance of ventricular tachycardia (3 beats or longer) detected during ambulatory monitoring after myocardial infarction. Circulation 57(5):890, 1977.
80. Moss AJ, DeCamilla J, Davis H: Cardiac death in the first 6 months after myocardial infarction: Potential for mortality reduction in the early posthospital period. Am J Cardiol 39:816, 1977.
81. Rehnqvist N, Sjogren A: Ventricular arrhythmias prior to discharge and one year after acute myocardial infarction. Eur J Cardiol 5(5):425, 1977.
82. Ruberman W, Weinblatt E, Goldberg J, Frank CW, Shapiro S: Ventricular premature beats and mortality after myocardial infarction. N Engl J Med 297:750, 1977.
83. Bigger JT Jr, Heller CA, Wenger TL, Weld FM: Risk stratification after acute myocardial infarction. Am J Cardiol 42:202, 1978.

84. Rehnqvist N: Ventricular arrhythmias after an acute myocardial infarction. Eur J Cardiol 7:169, 1978.
85. Moss AJ, Davis HT, DeCamilla J, Bayer LW: Ventricular ectopic beats and their relation to sudden and nonsudden cardiac death after myocardial infarction. Circulation 60:998, 1980.
86. Luria MH, Knoke JD, Wachs JS, Luria MA: Survival after recovery from acute myocardial infarction: Two and five year prognostic indices. Am J Med 67:7, 1979.
87. DeSoyza N, Bennett FA, Murphy ML, et al.: The relationship of paroxysmal ventricular tachycardia complicating the acute phase and ventricular arrhythmia during the late hospital phase of myocardial infarction to long-term survival. Am J Med 64:377, 1978.
88. Bigger JT Jr, Weld FM, Rolnitzky LM: Prevalence, characteristics and significance of ventricular tachycardia (three or more complexes) detected with ambulatory electrocardiographic recording in the late hospital phase of acute myocardial infarction. Am J Cardiol 48:815, 1981.
89. Mukharji J, Rude RE, Poole WK, Gustafson N, Thomas LJ Jr, Strauss HW, Jaffe AS, Muller JE, Roberts R, Raabe DS, Croft CH, Passamani E, Braunwald E, Willerson JT: Risk factors for sudden death after acute myocardial infarction: Two-year follow-up. Am J Cardiol 54:31, 1984.
90. Bigger JT Jr, Fleiss JL, Kleiger R, Miller JP, Rolnitzky LM: The relationships among ventricular arrhythmias, left ventricular dysfunction, and mortality in the 2 years after myocardial infarction. Circulation 69:250, 1984.
91. Ruberman W, Weinblatt E, Goldberg JD, Frank CW, Chaudhary BS, Shapiro S: Ventricular premature complexes and sudden death after myocardial infarction. Circulation 64(2):297, 1981.
92. Califf RM, McKinnis RA, Burks JM, Lee KL, Harrell FE Jr, Behar VS, Pryor DB, Wagner GS, Rosati RA: Prognostic implications of ventricular arrhythmias during 24 hour ambulatory monitoring in patients undergoing cardiac catheterization for coronary artery disease. Am J Cardiol 50:23, 1982.
93. Taylor GJ, Humphries JO, Mellits ED, Pitt B, Schulze RA, Griffith LSC, Achuff SC: Predictors of clinical course, coronary anatomy and left ventricular function after recovery from acute myocardial infarction. Circulation 62:960, 1980.
94. Madsen EB, Gilpin E, Henning H, Ahnve S, LeWinter M, Ceretto, Joswig W, Collins D, Pitt W, Ross J Jr: Prediction of late mortality after myocardial infarction from variables measured at different times during hospitalization. Am J Cardiol 53:47, 1984.
95. Williams WL, Nair RC, Higginson LAJ, Baird MG, Allan K, Beanlands DS: Comparison of clinical and treadmill variables for the prediction of outcome after myocardial infarction. J Am Coll Cardiol 4:477, 1984.
96. Theroux P, Waters DD, Halphen C, Desbaisieux JC, Mizgala HF: Prognostic value of exercise testing soon after myocardial infarction. N Engl J Med 361:341, 1979.
97. Weld FM, Chu KL, Bigger JT Jr, Rolnitzky LM: Risk stratification with low-level exercise testing 2 weeks after acute myocardial infarction. Circulation 64:306, 1981.
98. DeBusk RF, Kraemer HC, Nash E: Stepwise risk stratification soon after acute myocardial infarction. Am J Cardiol 52:1161, 1983.
99. Rigo P, Bailey IK, Griffith LSC, Pitt B, Wagner HN, Becker LC: Stress thallium-201 myocardial scintigraphy for the detection of individual coronary arterial lesions in patients with and without previous myocardial infarction. Am J Cardiol 48:209, 1981.
100. Corbett JR, Dehmer GJ, Lewis SE, Woodward W, Henderson E, et al.: The prognostic value of submaximal exercise testing with radionuclide ventriculography before hospital discharge in patients with recent myocardial infarction. Circulation 64:535, 1981.
101. Greene HL, Reid PR, Schaeffer AH: The repetitive ventricular response in man: A predictor of sudden death. N Engl J Med 299:729, 1978.
102. Hamer A, Vohra J, Hunt D, Sloman G: Prediction of sudden death by electrophysiologic

studies in high risk patients surviving acute myocardial infarction. Am J Cardiol 50:223, 1982.

103. Richards DA, Cody DV, Denniss AR, Russell PA, Young AA, Uther JB: Ventricular electrical instability: A predictor of death after myocardial infarction. Am J Cardiol 51:75, 1983.
104. Norris RM, Caughey DE, Mercer CJ, Deeming LW, Scott PJ: Coronary prognostic index for predicting survival after recovery from acute myocardial infarction. Lancet 2:485, 1970.
105. Coronary Drug Project Research Group: Factors influencing long-term prognosis after recovery from myocardial infarction—Three-year findings of the coronary drug project. J Chronic Dis 27:267, 1974.
106. Beta-Blocker Heart Attack Trial Research Group: A randomized trial of propranolol in patients with acute myocardial infarction. JAMA 247:1707–1714, 1982.
107. Norwegian Multicenter Study Group: Timolol-induced reduction in mortality and reinfarction in patients surviving acute myocardial infarction. N Engl J Med 304:801–807, 1981.
108. Hjalmarson A, Elmfeldt D, Herlitz J, Holmberg S, Malek I, Nyberg G, Ryden L, Swedberg K, Vedin A, Waagstein F, Waldenstrom A, Waldenstrom J, Wedel H, Wilhemsen L, Wilhelmsson C: Effect on mortality of metroprolol in acute myocardial infarction: A double-blind randomized trial. Lancet 2:823–827, 1981.
109. Ryden L, Ariniego R, Arnman K, Herlitz J, Hjalmarson A, Holmberg S, Reyas C, Snodgard P, Svedberg K, Vedin A, Waagstein F, Waldenstrom A, Wilhelmsson C, Wedel H, Yamamoto M: A double-blind trial of metoprolol in acute myocardial infarction: Effects on ventricular tachyarrhythmias. N Engl J Med 308:614–618, 1983.
110. Olsson G, Rehnqvist N: Ventricular arrhythmias during the first year after acute myocardial infarction: Influence of long-term treatment with metoprolol. Circulation 69: 1129–1134, 1984.
111. Bigger JT Jr, Coromilas J: How do beta-blockers protect after myocardial infarction [editorial]? Ann Intern Med 101:256–258, 1984.
112. Kostis JB, Wilson AC, Sanders MR, Byington RP for the BHAT Study Group: Prognostic significance of ventricular ectopic activity in survivors of acute myocardial infarction who receive propranolol. Am J Cardiol 61:975–978, 1988.

Chapter 6

Risk Stratification for Sudden Death in Patients With Complex Ventricular Arrhythmias: Value of Electrophysiologic Testing and the Signal-Averaged Electrocardiogram

Nabil El-Sherif, M.D., and Gioia Turitto, M.D.

Cardiology Division, Department of Medicine, State University of New York Health Science Center, and Veterans Administration Medical Center, Brooklyn, New York 11203

INTRODUCTION

Sudden cardiac death is currently the major contributor to overall cardiovascular mortality in the modern world. It accounts for approximately 60% of all coronary heart disease fatalities occurring annually [1]. The need for a systematic approach that would identify the high risk patient, aid in initiating appropriate therapy, and prevent the occurrence of sudden cardiac death is paramount. It has been amply documented that patients with sustained ventricular tachyarrhythmias, including those resuscitated from cardiac arrest, have a high incidence of sudden cardiac death [2–6]. Those

The Prevention of Sudden Cardiac Death, pages 109–138

patients, however, represent only a small proportion of the total population with complex ventricular arrhythmias. The relationship of complex ventricular arrhythmias, short of sustained ventricular tachycardia (VT)/ventricular fibrillation (VF) to sudden cardiac "arrhythmic" death, however, remains controversial. A number of recent studies suggest that complex ventricular arrhythmias in the postinfarction patient are independent markers for risk of sudden cardiac arrest [7–9], but there is general agreement that their sensitivity and specificity are relatively low [10].

In the last several years many studies have investigated the role of programmed electrical stimulation (PES) as a means of classifying patients with complex ventricular arrhythmias into low and high risk groups for sudden cardiac death [11–37]. The present chapter reviews the role of PES and the recently introduced noninvasive technique of signal-averaged electrocardiogram (ECG) in risk stratification and management of patients with complex ventricular arrhythmias. Although complex ventricular arrhythmias are usually defined as frequent, multiform, and repetitive ventricular premature complexes (VPCs), the role of nonsustained VT (three or more consecutive VPCs and <30 seconds in duration at a rate of >100/min) is particularly emphasized. Nonsustained VT is thought to represent a strong marker for sudden cardiac death [10,38–40].

COMPLEX VENTRICULAR ARRHYTHMIAS AND SUDDEN DEATH IN THE PRESENCE OR ABSENCE OF ORGANIC HEART DISEASE AND/OR IMPAIRED VENTRICULAR FUNCTION

Complex ventricular arrhythmias are uncommon in the absence of organic heart disease, and their presence does not increase the risk of either cardiac death or sudden death [41]. A long-term follow-up (average, 6.5 years) of 73 asymptomatic subjects who had frequent and complex ventricular arrhythmias, including nonsustained VT, showed no increased risk of death compared with that of the healthy U.S. population [42].

The incidence of complex ventricular arrhythmias is higher in patients with heart disease. However, in the absence of impaired ventricular function, the arrhythmia does not seem to be associated with an increased incidence of sudden death. Of 92 patients with normal left ventricular ejection fraction studied after coronary artery bypass surgery, 57% had complex ventricular arrhythmias, including 21.5% who had nonsustained VT. The incidence of complications in patients with complex ventricular arrhythmias was not higher than that in those with no arrhythmias, and there were no cardiac or sudden deaths during an average follow-up period of 16 months [43]. In another series of 130 patients with chronic stable angina pectoris complex ventricular arrhythmias were not associated with an increased risk of sudden cardiac death [44].

In the presence of impaired left ventricular function, complex ventricular arrhythmias may be an independent risk for sudden cardiac death. This view is not without controversy [41]. In the first quantitative study of the relationship between impaired left ventricular function and complex ventricular arrhythmias after myocardial infarction cardiac death was strongly associated with a low left ventricular ejection fraction, and the independent role of the arrhythmia could not be established [45]. The interrelationships between impaired ventricular function, complex ventricular arrhythmias, and sudden cardiac death were systematically analyzed later in two groups of patients. These were patients with congestive heart failure, commonly the result of ischemic or idiopathic dilated cardiomyopathy, and patients who survived the early phase of myocardial infarction. Packer [46] summarized the results of seven studies comprising 891 patients with congestive heart failure. The incidence of nonsustained VT ranged from 39 to 60%. The total mortality rate averaged 37.4%, and the rate of sudden cardiac death averaged 14.3% per year. Surawicz [41] reviewed eight studies comprising 398 patients with congestive heart failure. The incidence of nonsustained VT ranged from 49 to 100% and averaged 65%, while the total mortality and sudden cardiac death rates averaged 42.4% and 21.4%, respectively, during a follow-up period of 18.5 months (range, 11 to 34 months). In a majority of the above studies, sudden cardiac death was unrelated to nonsustained VT. In one study nonsustained VT was present in 26 of 35 patients. Of those, 80% died within 2 years, and only one of the deaths was attributed to arrhythmias [47]. Other studies, however, found that complex ventricular arrhythmias were an independent risk factor for sudden cardiac death [48–50], although the correlation was not strong [41].

In survivors of myocardial infarction three studies addressed the interrelationships between impaired ventricular function, complex ventricular arrhythmias, and sudden cardiac death in a large series of patients [7–9]. All three studies suggested that complex ventricular arrhythmias constitute an independent risk factor for sudden cardiac death. The Multicenter Post-Infarction Research Group was a nine hospital natural history study of patients under age 70 years who had a proven myocardial infarction [7]. In 766 patients, 86 deaths occurred during a 3 year follow-up period. When multivariate survivorship techniques were used to evaluate the independent contribution of ventricular arrhythmias and impaired left ventricular function to postinfarction mortality, VPC frequency, VPC runs, and left ventricular ejection fraction were each independently associated with both total mortality and arrhythmia-specific mortality.

The Multicenter Investigation of the Limitation of Infarct Size (MILIS) study was a five hospital intervention study of the effect of hyaluronidase, propranolol, or both in patients under age 76 years who had acute myocardial infarction [8]. Five hundred thirty-three patients who survived 10 days after infarction were followed for a mean of 18 months. Frequent VPCs (>10/hour) and left ventricular ejection fraction <40% were independently significant markers of risk for subsequent sudden death believed to be the result of primary ventricular arrhythmia. The incidence of sudden death was 18% in patients with both left ventricular dysfunction and frequent VPCs, an 11-fold increase compared with patients in whom neither risk factors was present. Seventy-nine percent of all sudden deaths occurred within 7 months after the index infarction.

Maisel et al. [9] studied 191 survivors of non-Q wave myocardial infarction and 586 survivors of Q wave infarction. Complex ventricular arrhythmias at the time of hospital discharge were an important predictor of mortality only in patients with non-Q wave infarction. The 10% incidence of sudden cardiac death in this group was much higher than in patients with Q wave infarction as well as the incidence of sudden death reported in most other studies. It was postulated that this was caused by the presence of an unstable ischemic state in the patients.

Although recent multicenter studies have shown that complex ventricular arrhythmias are an independent risk factor for sudden cardiac death, especially in survivors of myocardial infarction, the corollary observation that suppression of those arrhythmias would reduce the incidence of sudden death has not yet been demonstrated. Of eight trials of antiarrhythmic agents conducted thus far and summarized by Furberg and May [51] in one, both the drug and the placebo produced the same result; in two, the drug improved the outcome, and in four, the drug worsened it. These studies suffered from the small numbers of enrolled patients and the exclusion of patients with severe ventricular arrhythmias. A large multicenter study that addresses some of the limitations of previous studies is currently underway, sponsored by the National Institutes of Health.

The Cardiac Arrhythmia Suppression Trial (CAST) [52] will determine if suppression of asymptomatic ventricular arrhythmias will reduce the incidence of sudden death in patients at moderate risk. This trial is being done at 27 sites in the United States, Canada, and Sweden. Four thousand four hundred patients with previous myocardial infarction, asymptomatic ventricular arrhythmias documented by ambulatory electrocardiography, and reduced left ventricular function will be enrolled over a 3 year period. Patients whose arrhythmias are suppressed by antiarrhythmic drugs will be randomly assigned to receive placebo or effective suppressive therapy during 2 to 5 years of follow-up, and the incidence of sudden death in the two groups will be compared. An advantage of this study is that the hypothesis is being tested using three different randomly assigned drugs, each of which can effectively suppress VPCs. Therefore, it is anticipated that the results of this study can be extrapolated to any safe drug that suppresses VPCs. Woosley [52] has argued that if the CAST study is successful, antiarrhythmic agents will join the β-receptor antagonist as medications indicated for prevention of sudden death. If not, two possibilities should be considered: either the concept that ventricular arrhythmias in this population progress to cause sudden death is invalid or these agents prevent sudden death in some patients and cause sudden death in others, cancelling any overall benefit. In a preliminary report from CAST, patients treated with encainide or flecainide were found to have a higher rate of death from arrhythmia than the patients assigned to placebo during an average of 10 months of follow-up [52a]. Because of these results, the part of the trial involving encainide and flecainide, but not moricizine, has been discontinued.

Even if the CAST study eventually shows that suppression of complex ventricular arrhythmias would decrease the incidence of sudden cardiac death in survivors of myocardial infarction, a risk stratification strategy other than the mere presence of complex ventricular arrhythmias on ambulatory monitoring would probably be required. This is because of the low sensitivity and specificity of Holter monitoring alone as a marker of sudden cardiac death in these patients. Because of its low sensitivity a number of patients with no complex ventricular arrhythmias but who still may be at risk for sudden cardiac death could be deprived of appropriate therapy. Further, the low specificity of this marker would lead to unnecessary chronic therapy in a large percentage of patients. This would be of relatively less concern if antiarrhythmic drugs (and/or other forms of antiarrhythmic therapy) are consistently effective, affordable, and without serious side effects. None of these premises is currently in sight. Because of this and similar arguments, the role of PES and more recently of the signal-averaged ECG in risk stratification and management of patients with complex ventricular arrhythmias has received considerable interest.

PROGRAMMED ELECTRICAL STIMULATION IN PATIENTS WITH COMPLEX VENTRICULAR ARRHYTHMIAS

Several studies have investigated the role of PES in identifying subsets of patients with complex ventricular arrhythmias at low and high risk for sudden cardiac death [11–37]. Patients in whom PES fails to induce sustained VT may have a low risk of sudden cardiac death. In those patients antiarrhythmic therapy may not be warranted. On the other hand, patients with inducible sustained VT may be at increased risk of sudden cardiac death. It is possible that antiarrhythmic therapy guided by the results of PES would decrease the risk of sudden death in this group.

Stimulation Protocols

The incidence and type of ventricular arrhythmias induced by PES depends on the stimulation protocol. Table 6–1 lists all studies of PES in patients with nonsustained VT in which details of the stimulation protocol were reported. The stimulation protocol varied with regard to the nature of the basic drive (sinus or ventricular paced rhythm), the cycle length of the basic paced drive, the current strength of the stimulus, the nature of the

TABLE 6–1. Techniques and Endpoints for Programmed Stimulation Studies in Patients With Spontaneous Nonsustained Ventricular Tachycardia[a,b]

Authors	Basic drive(s)	No. of extrastimuli	Burst pacing	Site(s) of stimulation		Drugs (isp)	Endpoints
				RV	LV		
Vandepol et al., 1980 [60]	SR; VP at ≥ 1 CL	2	Yes	≥ 1	≥ 1	No	Reproducible VT (≥ 3 RVR)
Naccarelli et al., 1982 [11]	SR; VP at CL = 600, 500, 400 msec	2	Yes	2 (apex, OT)	≥ 1 in some cases	No	VT
Livelli et al., 1982 [69]	AP; VP at CL = 600, 400 msec	2	Yes	2 (apex, OT)	No	No	Reproducible sustained VT (requiring intervention for termination)
Buxton et al., 1983 [13]	SR; VP at CL = 600–400 msec	2; 3 in some cases	Yes	2 (apex, OT)	≥ 1 in some cases	Yes	Reproducible VT resembling clinical VT
Gomes et al., 1984 [15]	SR; VP at CL = 600, 500 msec	2	Yes	2 (apex, OT)	No	No	Reproducible VT (≥ 5 RVR)
Veltri et al., 1985 [18]	VP at CL = 600, 500, 450 msec	2	Yes	2 (apex, OT)	2 in some cases	No	Sustained VT (≥ 30 seconds)
Spielman et al., 1985 [19]	SR; VP at CL = 600, 450 msec	3	No	2 (apex, OT)	No	No	Sustained VT (≥ 15 seconds); VF
Schoenfeld et al., 1985 [65]	SR, AP; VP at > 1 CL	2; 3 in some cases	Yes	1 (apex)	No	No	Reproducible sustained VT (> 100 complexes) or symptomatic nonsustained VT

Zheutlin et al., 1986 [21]	SR; VP at CL = 600, 500, 400 msec	2	Yes	≥ 1 (apex, OT in some cases)	No	No	Reproducible VT (> 6 RVR)
Breithardt et al., 1986 [22]	SR; VP at CL = 500, 430, 370, 330 msec	2 or 3	No	1 or 2 (apex, OT)	No	In some cases	VT
Poll et al., 1986 [24]	VP at CL = 600, 400 msec	3	Yes	2 (apex, OT)	No	No	Sustained VT (> 30 seconds)
Estes et al., 1986 [53]	SR; VP at ≥ 1 CL = 700–400 msec	2; 3 in some cases	Yes	≥ 1 (apex, OT in some cases)	No	No	VT (≥ 5 RVR); VF
Prystowsky et al., 1986 [54]	SR; VP at CL = 600, 500, 400 msec	2; 3 in some cases	Yes	2 (apex, OT)	In some cases	No	VT (≥ 3 RVR) resembling clinical VT
Buxton et al., 1987 [29]	VP at CL = 600, 400 msec	3	Yes	2 (apex, OT)	No	No	Reproducible sustained VT (> 30 seconds) resembling clinical VT
Sulpizi et al., 1987 [30]	VP at CL = 600–400 msec	2; 3 in some cases	No	1 (apex); ≥ 2 in some cases	In some cases	No	Reproducible sustained VT (> 15 complexes)
Zehender et al., 1987 [63]	SR; VP at CL = 600, 500, 430 msec	3	No	1 (apex)	No	No	Sustained monomorphic VT (≥ 30 seconds)
Turitto et al., 1988 [33]	SR; VP at CL = 600, 500, 400 msec	3	No	2 (apex, OT)	No	No	Sustained monomorphic VT (≥ 30 seconds); VF
Kharsa et al., 1988 [35]	VP at CL = 600, 500, 400 msec	3	No	2 (apex, OT)	No	No	Sustained monomorphic VT (≥ 30 sec); VF

[a]AP, atrial pacing; CL, cycle length; isp, isoproterenol; LV, left ventricle; OT, outflow tract; RVR, repetitive ventricular responses; RV, right ventricle; SR, sinus rhythm; VF, ventricular fibrillation; VP, ventricular pacing; VT, ventricular tachycardia.

[b]Listed, in chronological order, are only those full reports in which patients with nonsustained VT represented all, or a significant fraction, of the study population.

stimulating train (basic drive followed by one or more extrastimuli, burst pacing, and alternation of short and long cycle), the site of stimulation, the use of drugs such as isoproterenol to facilitate induction of VT, and, finally, what constitutes a specific endpoint for the stimulation protocol.

The introduction of a single ventricular extrastimulus during sinus rhythm rarely resulted in the induction of VT which most often required two or more extrastimuli in patients with spontaneous nonsustained VT. In the studies of Estes et al. [53] and Prystowsky et al. [54], approximately 20% of all episodes of VT (sustained or nonsustained) were induced by one to three extrastimuli delivered during sinus rhythm. Spielman et al. [19] reported that only 13% of all induced sustained VT was induced by triple extrastimuli during sinus rhythm. Extrastimuli applied during ventricular pacing were consistently more effective in inducing ventricular tachyarrhythmias. However, the optimal duration and cycle length of the pacing drive are not clearly established [55]. Based on results obtained both in patients with spontaneous sustained ventricular tachyarrhythmias [56,57] and in those with nonsustained VT [19], it seems advisable to use more than one pacing drive, with cycle lengths between 600 and 400 msec. In these studies, the yield of inducing sustained VT with up to three extrastimuli increased by approximately 20% with the use of a second pacing drive and by an additional 20% when a third drive was included in the protocol. In a study by Breithardt et al. [58] shortening the cycle length of the basic drive allowed induction of sustained VT by extrastimuli with longer coupling intervals. However, this finding was not reproduced by other groups [59].

The incidence of inducible ventricular tachyarrhythmias varied directly with the number of extrastimuli applied during basic ventricular pacing in patients with either spontaneous sustained or nonsustained VT. In patients with spontaneous sustained VT, the probability of inducing sustained monomorphic VT ranged from 22 to 33% (mean, 27%) with one extrastimulus, from 47 to 73% (mean, 66%) with two extrastimuli, and from 72 to 94% (mean, 88%) with the use of three extrastimuli [56,57,60–63]. Thus the introduction of a second and a third extrastimulus increased the sensitivity of the stimulation protocol for sustained monomorphic VT by an average of 45% and 23%, respectively. The same phenomenon was reported in patients with spontaneous nonsustained VT. Four studies [19,29,33,63] that utilized a similar stimulation protocol (three extrastimuli, one or two right ventricular pacing sites, and multiple basic drives) and similar endpoints (induction of sustained ventricular tachyarrhythmias) reported their data according to the number of extrastimuli required for induction. The fraction of patients who had sustained monomorphic VT induced by one extrastimulus was low (0–3%), rose substantially with two extrastimuli (9–24%), and showed further increase with three extrastimuli (21–39%). A similar trend was described for the induction of ventricular fibrillation (VF), which increased from 0% with one extrastimulus to 2–7% with two extrastimuli and 10–14% with three extrastimuli [19,33,63].

Burst pacing was used by several authors to induced ventricular tachyarrhythmias in patients with spontaneous nonsustained VT. The additional yield of this mode of stimulation above the use of two extrastimuli ranged from 3 [53,54] to 11% [60]. Similar results were reported in patients with spontaneous sustained VT [53,60,64,65]. However, burst pacing may have no advantage over the use of three extrastimuli [54]. Further, animal studies [66] have shown that the technique of burst pacing is highly dependent on the number of beats in the paced train and the cycle length of stimulation in a fashion that makes it very difficult to standardize or to reproduce in the clinical setting. A protocol employing an abrupt short–long sequence of the basic drive before the introduction of one or more extrastimuli was reported to initiate sustained VT in patients not otherwise inducible with conventional protocols [67]. However, when the efficacy of such a technique was compared with the use of triple extrastimuli, no significant difference was found [68].

Programmed stimulation is usually limited to right ventricular sites. In patients with spontaneous nonsustained VT, there was little advantage of stimulating a second right ventricular site (usually the outflow tract or the septum) after three extrastimuli applied at the right ventricular apex had failed to induce VT. In the studies by Turitto et al. [33] and Kharsa et al. [35], VT initiated at the outflow tract represented 0–4% of all induced sustained VT. Similarly, Zheutlin et al. [21], using up to two extrastimuli and VT lasting six or more complexes as the endpoint, found that only 3% of inductions occurred during stimulation at the outflow tract. However, Spielman et al. [19] reported that stimulation at the outflow tract was effective in 14% of patients and accounted for 53% of induced sustained VT.

Specificity of Induced Tachyarrhythmias

In patients with recurrent sustained monomorphic VT, the sensitivity of the technique of programmed stimulation is defined as the ability to reproduce the clinical arrhythmia. Such a definition is not applicable in patients with spontaneous nonsustained VT. In these patients programmed stimulation can induce nonsustained VT, sustained monomorphic or polymorphic VT, or VF. There is some evidence that the induction of sustained monomorphic VT rather than that of nonsustained VT or VF should be considered as the specific endpoint of PES in patients with spontaneous nonsustained VT. Nonsustained VT was as commonly induced in patients with as in those without heart disease (34% and 21%, respectively) [69–72]. Induced nonsustained VT was polymorphic in 80% of the cases [56,68,69,71]. Polymorphic nonsustained VT induced in patients without organic heart disease did not differ in their cycle length and mode of initiation from those elicited in postinfarction patients with spontaneous sustained ventricular tachyarrhythmias [72]. These data strongly suggest that the specificity of induced nonsustained VT is low. Although some authors tried to improve the specificity of induced nonsustained VT by comparing its QRS configuration [13] and/or cycle length [18,54] to the spontaneous arrhythmias, this approach is fraught with difficulties. Careful comparison between the QRS configuration of spontaneous and induced rhythms may be difficult to accomplish because of limitations on the number of simultaneously recorded ECG leads. It will be almost impossible to compare adequately the QRS configuration of polymorphic nonsustained VT. Further, there is usually little correlation between the cycle length of spontaneous and induced VT [19,74,75].

The induction of VF may be a nonspecific response to programmed stimulation in patients with nonsustained VT. Ventricular fibrillation was induced with comparable frequency in patients with spontaneous sustained ventricular tachyarrhythmias (3–13%) [63,70,73,76,77], survivors of myocardial infarction without documented sustained VT/VF (1–14%) [63, 78,79], and in patients with spontaneous nonsustained VT (0–15%) (see Table 6–2). The frequency of induced VF was related to the aggressiveness of the stimulation protocol [3,19,70,71].

On the other hand, sustained monomorphic VT could not be induced by PES in patients without organic heart disease; thus its specificity is close to 100% [69,70–72]. The arrhythmia was considered a marker for an electrophysiologic substrate of reentry [80] and may not be induced in the absence of such substrate. However, sustained monomorphic VT could be induced in patients with heart disease regardless of the presence of spontaneous sustained VT. Its prevalence was less than 3% in studies on a miscellaneous population [56,60,69,70,71,73], but it was much higher in patients with spontaneous nonsustained VT (see Table 6–2) and in survivors of myocardial infarction. In the latter setting, sustained monomorphic VT was inducible in 28–51% of patients with spontaneous nonsustained VT [33,63,81] as well as in 11–45% of those without documented arrhythmias [63,78,79,82].

In summary, the induction of sustained monomorphic VT in patients with spontaneous nonsustained runs could be interpreted as a demonstration of the ability of programmed stimulation to expose a fixed electrophysiologic abnormality. Such an abnormality may be implicated in the high risk of sudden cardiac death in these patients.

Results of Programmed Stimulation

Table 6–2 summarizes the results of PES in patients with complex ventricular arrhythmias and nonsustained VT in 25 studies published between 1980 and 1988. It includes an early study from our laboratory by Gomes et al. [15] and a more recent series by Turitto et al. [33].

Programmed electrical stimulation initiated sustained monomorphic VT in 20% of patients (range, 0–50%), VF in 5% (range, 0–15), and nonsustained VT in 32% (range, 10–64). Forty-three percent of patients

TABLE 6–2. Ventricular Tachyarrhythmias Induced by Programmed Stimulation in Patients With Spontaneous Nonsustained Ventricular Tachycardia and/or Complex Ventricular Ectopy[a]

Authors	No. of patients	S-VT (%)	VF (%)	ns-VT (%)	NI (%)	VT/VF (%)
Vandepol et al., 1980 [60]	29	0	0	62	38	
Naccarelli et al., 1982 [11]	44	0	0	34	66	
Livelli et al., 1982 [69]	18	11	—	44	44	
Swerdlow et al., 1982 [12][b]	41	22	7	32	39	
Buxton et al., 1983 [13][c]	83	8 mono 10 poly	0	24 mono 24 poly	49	
Gomes et al., 1984 [15]	73	11	7	10	73	
Miles et al., 1984 [17][b]	139	16	—	46	38	
Reddy and Jivrajka, 1984 [16][b]	52	—	—	—	73	27 (S-VT/VF)
Veltri et al., 1985 [18]	33	21	—	21	58	
Spielman et al., 1985 [19]	58	26 mono	14	3 mono 21 poly	36	
Schoenfeld et al., 1985 [65]	66	15	2	30 mono 14 poly	39	
Zheutlin et al., 1986 [21]	88	—	—	—	63	38
Breithardt et al., 1986 [22]	106	12	2	44	42	
Poll et al., 1986 [24]	20	10 mono 10 poly	10	20 mono 25 poly	25	
Estes et al., 1986 [53]	110	—	—	—	38	62
Prystowsky et al., 1986 [54]	104	15	—	49	36	
Miles et al., 1986 [26][b]	53	25 (mono S-VT and VF by ≤2 extra-stimuli)	15	36	25	
Batsford et al., 1986 [28][b]	81	21	—	44	35	
Klein and Machell, 1986 [27][b]	22	50 mono	0	—	50	
Buxton et al., 1987 [29]	62	39 mono 7	0	24	31	
Buxton et al., 1987 [81]	43	49 mono 2 poly	0	21 mono 5 poly	23	
Sulpizi et al., 1987 [30]	61	15 mono	0	28 mono 18 poly	39	
Zehender et al., 1987 [63][c]	50	32 mono 16	10	20 mono 44 poly	18	
Turitto et al., 1988 [33]	105	21 mono	13	8 mono 16 poly	43	
Kharsa et al., 1988 [35]	40	20 mono	5	10 mono 20 poly	45	

[a]Mono, monomorphic; NI, no induced arrhythmia; poly, polymorphic; VF, ventricular fibrillation; VT, ventricular tachycardia; ns, nonsustained; S, sustained; —, not reported. Refer to Table 6–1 for details on the stimulation protocols used in the reported studies.
[b]Abstract report.
[c]Study in which more than one induced arrhythmia was reported for some patients (total > 100%).

(range, 18–73) did not have any inducible arrhythmias. Induced nonsustained VT was monomorphic in 46% of cases and polymorphic in the remaining 54%. The difference in the results of the reported studies may be related, in part, to the use of different stimulation protocols and endpoints (see Table 6–1). The proportion of patients with induced sustained monomorphic VT was lower (11%) when a maximum of two extrastimuli and burst pacing were delivered and higher (29%) when three extrastimuli was used. The use of three extrastimuli was associated with a proportional, but not greater, increase in the induction of ventricular fibrillation. In studies by Turitto et al. [33] and Spielman et al. [19], VF accounted, respectively, for 31% and 44% of sustained tachyarrhythmias induced by two extrastimuli compared with 45 and 29% of those induced by three extrastimuli with no statistically significant differences.

The cycle length of induced sustained monomorphic VT was relatively short, ranging between 190 and 280 msec in most studies [18,19,22, 26,30,33,63,81]. These cycle lengths were shorter than those induced in patients with spontaneous sustained VT (285–370 msec) [56,58,59,61, 63,73,75,76]. This may be due, at least in part, to the fact that the induction of sustained monomorphic VT usually required more extrastimuli in patients without than in those with spontaneous sustained VT [63]. The cycle length of induced VT tended to shorten as the number of extrastimuli necessary for induction increased. This was demonstrated in patients with spontaneous nonsustained VT [20,21] as well as in those with sustained VT [56].

Noninvasive Predictors of the Results of Programmed Stimulation

Because only a fraction of patients with spontaneous nonsustained VT had inducible sustained monomorphic VT on PES, several noninvasive determinants of VT inducibility have been investigated as means to screen patients for the invasive electrophysiologic procedure (Table 6–3). The presence and type of heart disease, as well as other clinical variables, ECG characteristics of the spontaneous arrhythmia, and left ventricular function indices, have been investigated separately or in combination. More recently, the value of the signal-averaged ECG was also assessed.

Clinical variables. Induction of VT was more common in patients with than in those without heart disease [11,13,15,18,30,33,35,54]. In a majority of studies all patients with induced sustained VT [18,30,35] or induced nonsustained/sustained VT [15,18] had structural heart disease. In a few reports, the incidence of induced nonsustained/sustained VT in patients with apparently normal heart ranged from 12% [54] to 17% [13] to 40% [11]. Observed differences reach statistical significance when data from several reports are pooled together, even though this approach may not be entirely satisfactory because of the different design of individual studies. A total of 483 patients with heart disease and 112 subjects with apparently normal heart were subjected to PES in eight studies [11,13,15,18,30,33,35,54]. When

TABLE 6–3. Determinants of Ventricular Tachyarrhythmia Inducibility by Programmed Stimulation in Patients With Nonsustained Ventricular Tachycardia and/or Complex Ventricular Ectopy[a]

Variables	Buxton et al. [13,14], VT	Spielman et al. [19], S-VT/VF	Veltri et al. [18], VT	Sulpizi et al. [30]*, S-VT, m	Turitto et al., [33]*, S-VT, m	Gomes et al. [15], VT/VF	Zheutlin et al. [21], VT	Gradman et al. [84], VT	Schoenfeld et al. [65]*, VT/VF	Nalos et al. [83]*, S-VT, m
Age	—	No	—	—	No	—	No	—	No	Yes
Sex	—	No	—	—	No	—	No	—	Yes	No
Presence of HD	Yes	—	Yes	No	No	—	—	—	—	—
Ischemic HD	Yes	No	—	No	No	Yes	No	—	No	—
Prior MI	—	—	—	No	No	Yes	No	—	Yes	Yes
Syncope	No	No	—	No	Yes	—	—	—	Yes	Yes
VPCs/h	—	No	—	—	No	—	—	Yes	—	—
Couplets/24 h	—	—	—	—	No	—	—	Yes	—	—
Repetition index	—	—	—	—	No	—	—	Yes	—	—
VT runs/24 h	No	No	No	—	No	—	—	—	—	—
VT duration	No	No	No	—	No	—	—	—	—	—
VT rate	—	No	—	—	No	—	—	—	—	—
VT morphology	—	—	—	—	No	—	—	—	—	—
Ejection fraction	Yes	No	No	Yes	Yes	Yes	No	—	No	Yes
LV dyskinesia	Yes	Yes	—	—	No	—	—	—	No	Yes
Signal-averaged ECG	—	—	—	—	Yes	—	—	—	—	Yes

Study population included only patients with spontaneous nonsustained VT in the reports from Buxton et al., Spielman et al., Veltri et al., Sulpizi et al., Turitto et al.; patients with nonsustained VT and/or complex ventricular ectopy in the reports from Gomes et al. and Zheutlin et al.; patients with various clinical presentations (sustained VT, cardiac arrest, nonsustained VT, syncope) in the reports from Gradman et al., Schoenfeld et al., and Nalos et al.

[a]Each column heading lists the authors and the induced arrhythmia that was predicted by the variables analyzed in each study. Asterisks indicate studies in which multivariate methods to predict inducibility of the index arrhythmia were used. Univariate methods were utilized in the remaining studies. Yes, significant variable; No, variable not significantly related to inducibility; —, variable not studied; ECG, electrocardiogram; HD, heart disease; LV, left ventricle; MI, myocardial infarction; VF, ventricular fibrillation; VPCs, ventricular premature complexes; VT, ventricular tachycardia; S, sustained; m, monomorphic.

inducible nonsustained and sustained VT were considered together, they were significantly more frequent in patients with than in those without heart disease (48 vs. 30%, respectively, $P < 0.05$). When inducible sustained monomorphic VT was considered alone, the difference between its incidence in patients with or without organic heart disease (20 vs. 2%, respectively) became more statistically significant ($P < 0.01$). Organic heart disease was present in 86% of patients with induced nonsustained/sustained VT [11,13,15,18,54] and 98% of those with induced sustained VT [13,30,33,35].

The relationship between the type of heart disease and inducibility can be demonstrated by combining data from seven studies on a total of 315 patients with coronary artery disease and 152 patients with other types of organic heart disease, including 88 patients with idiopathic dilated cardiomyopathy [13,15,18,21,33,35,54]. Only induction of nonsustained/sustained VT was more frequent in the group with coronary artery disease compared with other groups (56 vs. 29%, $P < 0.0001$), while the induction of sustained VT occurred with similar frequency in the two groups (28 vs. 16%). When patients with coronary artery disease were compared with those with idiopathic cardiomyopathy, the frequency of induced nonsustained/sustained VT was still higher in the group with coronary artery disease (56 vs. 39%, $P < 0.05$), while the frequency of induced sustained VT was not statistically different in the two groups (28 vs. 16%).

A previous myocardial infarction was documented more often in patients with than in those without induced nonsustained/sustained VT in studies by Kharsa et al. [35] (88 vs. 44%, $P < 0.05$) and Gomes et al. [15] (85 vs. 43%, $P < 0.001$), while the difference was not statistically significant in the report from Zheutlin et al. [21] (73 vs. 53%). In a study by Sulpizi et al. [30], all patients with recent myocardial infarction (within 3 months of programmed stimulation) had inducible sustained or nonsustained VT, yielding a higher inducibility rate than in the remaining population (100 vs. 54%, $P < 0.007$). However, this variable was not considered to be independently related to VT inducibility by multivariate analysis. On the other hand, old myocardial infarction was a significant variable in multivariate models published by Schoenfeld et al. [65] ($P < 0.001$) and Nalos et al. [83] ($P < 0.0002$). The influence of the site of prior myocardial infarction on induction of sustained monomorphic VT was studied by Zehender et al. [63] in 106 postinfarction patients. In the group with spontaneous nonsustained VT or no documented VT, inducibility was 34% for inferior infarction compared with 65% for anterior infarction ($P < 0.05$).

Symptoms were significantly related to VT induction only in the series by Turitto et al. [33]. A history of syncope/presyncope was present in 50% of patients with and in 22% of those without induced sustained monomorphic VT ($P < 0.05$). Other investigators did not find any significant difference in the frequency of syncope between patients with or without inducible VT [13,19,30].

Electrocardiographic variables. In a study by Gradman et al. [84], three quantitative variables derived from 24 hour ambulatory ECG were found to be significantly related to the induction of VT by PES: a mean VPC frequency of ≥100/1,000 normal beats, a mean couplet frequency of ≥1/1,000 normal beats, and a repetition index value of ≥15/1,000 VPCs. The repetition index was defined as the ratio of the number of couplets to the total number of VPCs. These data are at variance with other studies in which ECG characteristics of the spontaneous arrhythmia did not predict VT inducibility [13,18,19,33].

Left ventricular function indices. Several studies found that patients with ejection fraction <40% had a greater frequency of induced VT compared with those with ejection fraction ≥0.40. This difference was significant in studies by Buxton et al. [14] (60 vs. 28%, $P < 0.03$), Gomes et al. [15] (85 vs. 38%, $P < 0.0006$), and Turitto et al. [33] (86 vs. 36%, $P < 0.0001$). Ejection fraction was a significant predictor of inducibility in multivariate analysis models reported by Turitto et al. [33] and Nalos et al. [83]. In a study by Sulpizi et al. [30], impairment of left ventricular function, defined as an ejection fraction lower than 0.35 or functional class III to IV with cardiomegaly on chest X-ray, was identified as the only variable independently related to the induction of sustained VT. On the other hand, the degree of left ventricular dysfunction was similar in patients with or without induced VT in reports from Zheutlin et al. [21], Veltri et al. [18], and Spielman et al. [19].

Besides left ventricular ejection fraction, the relationship between wall motion abnormalities and inducibility was considered in a number of studies. Spielman et al. [19] found that induced sustained VT/VF was more frequent in patients with at least one akinetic or dyskinetic left ventricular segment, as shown by radionuclide angiography, compared with those without such abnormalities (69 vs. 29%, $P < 0.01$). Buxton et al. [13] reported that among patients with coronary artery disease sustained VT was induced more often in the presence of left ventricular aneurysm than in its absence (69 vs. 20%, $P < 0.01$). However, this finding was not corroborated by subsequent studies from the same authors [29] or other groups [33].

The signal-averaged ECG. The signal-averaged ECG is recorded by amplifying, averaging, and filtering the signal recorded on the body surface by orthogonal leads [85]. The recording detects low amplitude cardiac electrical signals in the late QRS/ST segment that may represent delayed activation of abnormal myocardial tissue [86]. These signals are usually called *late potentials*. The signal-averaged ECG was initially found to predict accurately the results of PES in patients with spontaneous sustained VT [87–89]. The predictive value of the signal-averaged ECG for the induction of sustained VT was confirmed in a study by Nalos et al. [83] in patients with miscellaneous presenting arrhythmias and by Buxton et al. [81] in patients with spontaneous nonsustained VT after healing of myocardial infarction.

The first prospective study of the value of the signal-averaged ECG as a predictor of the results of programmed stimulation in patients with nonsustained VT using stepwise discriminant function analysis was published from our laboratory by Turitto et al. [33]. The study found that the signal-averaged ECG is the single most accurate screening test to predict the inducibility of sustained VT in patients with spontaneous nonsustained VT. A consecutive series of 105 patients with spontaneous nonsustained VT on 24 hour ambulatory ECG were studied. The study population consisted of 60 patients with coronary artery disease, 26 with idiopathic dilated cardiomyopathy, and 19 with no identifiable heart disease. Patients were divided into

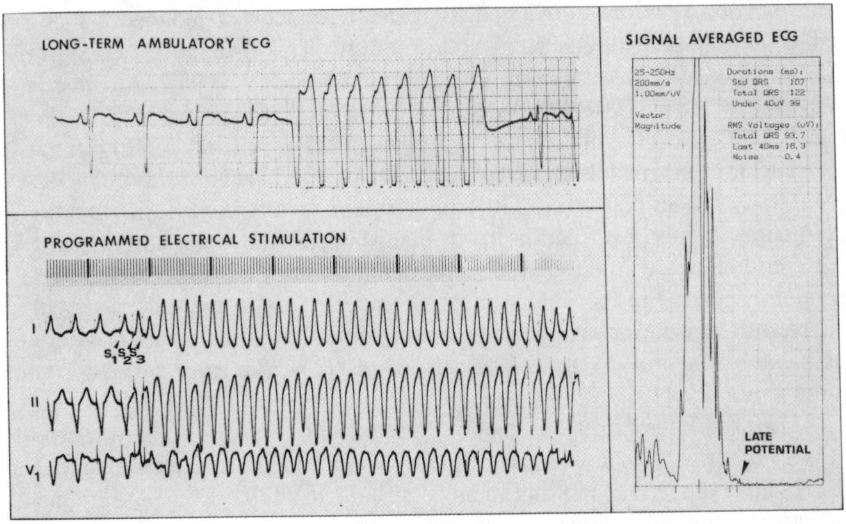

Fig. 6–1. Recordings of ambulatory ECG, programmed electrical stimulation and signal- averaged ECG from a 56-year-old man with coronary artery disease. A 24 hour ambulatory ECG showed frequent ventricular premature complexes and runs of nonsustained ventricular tachycardia. The signal-averaged ECG showed late potentials (the root mean square [RMS] voltage of the last 40 msec of the filtered QRS = 16.3 μV, and the duration of the low amplitude signal under 40 μV = 39 msec). Programmed electrical stimulation utilizing an $S_1S_2S_3$ protocol from the right ventricular apex induced a sustained monomorphic tachycardia.

three groups according to the results of programmed stimulation (three extrastimuli, two right ventricular sites): Group 1 included 22 patients with induced sustained monomorphic VT (Fig. 6–1); group 2, 14 patients with induced VF; and group 3, 69 patients without induced sustained ventricular tachyarrhythmias (Fig. 6–2).

Table 6–4 shows the characteristics of patients in the three groups. Group 1 patients showed a significantly higher frequency of syncope/presyncope, left ventricular ejection fraction <0.40, and late potentials on the signal-averaged ECG compared with group 3. Late potentials were defined as low amplitude signals in the terminal part of the QRS with duration ≥38 msec and root mean square voltage ≤25 μV. The etiology of underlying heart disease, the ECG characteristics of the spontaneous arrhythmia (number, duration, and cycle length of nonsustained VT runs), and the prevalence of left ventricular wall motion abnormalities were not significantly different in groups 1 and 3. On the other hand, when patients with induced VF (group 2) were compared with patients without induced sustained VT/VF (group 3), none of the variables showed significant differences. Further analysis of group 3 patients revealed no significant differences in clinical and ECG variables, left ventricular function indices, and the signal-averaged ECG between patients in whom monomorphic nonsustained VT,

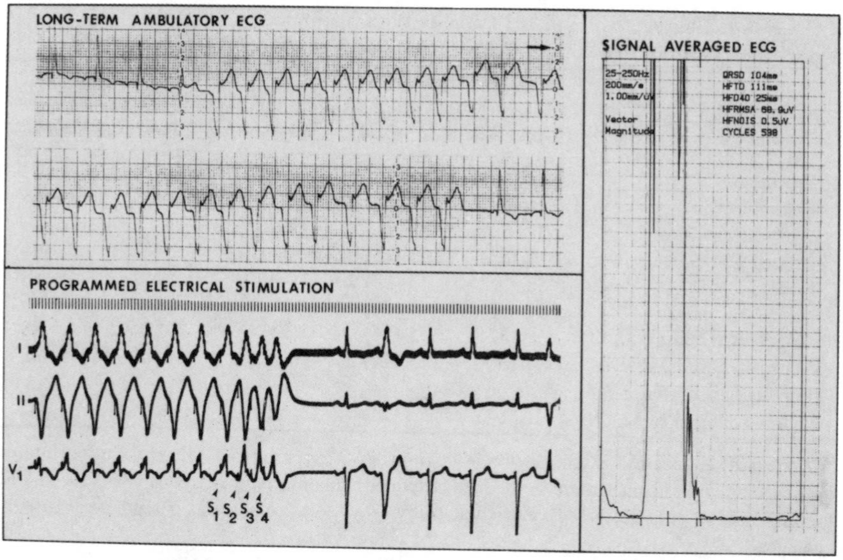

Fig. 6–2. Recordings of ambulatory ECG, programmed electrical stimulation and signal-averaged ECG from a 41-year-old man with idiopathic dilated cardiomyopathy. The patient had no history of syncope/presyncope. The ejection fraction by radionuclide ventriculography was 16%. A 24 hour ambulatory ECG showed frequent ventricular premature complexes (average 240/hour) and six runs of nonsustained monomorphic ventricular tachycardia. The longest one is shown. It comprised 26 beats and had an averaged cycle length of 452 msec. The signal-averaged ECG was normal. There was no inducible arrhythmia on programmed electrical stimulation. (Reproduced from Turitto et al. [33] with permission of the publisher.)

polymorphic nonsustained VT, or no VT were induced. Late potentials were recorded in 23 patients (23%): 14 in group 1, 3 in group 2, and 6 in group 3. The sensitivity, specificity, positive, negative, and total predictive accuracy of late potentials for the induction of sustained monomorphic VT were, respectively, 64%, 89%, 61%, 90%, and 84%. In other words, the probability of inducing sustained monomorphic VT was 61% in patients with late potentials and declined to 10% in those without late potentials. The frequency of late potentials was similar in patients with coronary artery disease (25%) and in those with idiopathic dilated cardiomyopathy (23%). Their predictive accuracy was also comparable in the two groups: 85% in coronary artery disease and 81% in cardiomyopathy patients. Among the 43 patients with prior myocardial infarction, late potentials showed high predictive accuracy both in anterior infarction (73%) and in inferior infarction (88%). Using stepwise discriminant function analysis late potentials proved to be the variable most strongly correlated ($P < 0.00001$) with the induction of sustained monomorphic VT, with an overall predictive accuracy of 84%. No combination of late potentials and other significant variables (ejection fraction and symptoms) provided an improvement in predicting sustained VT

TABLE 6–4. Characteristics of 105 Patients With Spontaneous Nonsustained Ventricular Tachycardia With or Without Induced Ventricular Tachyarrhythmias[a]

	Group 1 (n = 22)	Group 2 (n = 14)	Group 3 (n = 69)	Probability	
				1 vs. 3	2 vs. 3
Heart disease					
Ischemic	16 (73)	7 (50)	37 (54)	NS	NS
With prior MI	12	5	26		
Dilated CMP	5 (23)	3 (21)	18 (26)	NS	NS
None	1 (5)	4 (29)	14 (20)	NS	NS
Syncope/presyncope	11 (50)	7 (50)	15 (22)	<0.05	NS
LV ejection fraction <0.40	19 (86)	5 (36)	25 (36)	<0.0001	NS
LV segmental a/dyskinesia	11 (50)	3 (21)	16 (23)	NS	NS
Late potentials on the signal averaged ECG	14 (64)	3 (21)	6 (9)	<0.00001	NS

[a]CMP, cardiomyopathy; ECG, electrocardiogram; LV, left ventricle; MI, myocardial infarction; NS, not significant. Group 1, induced sustained monomorphic VT; group 2, induced VF; group 3, no induced sustained ventricular tachyarrhythmias. Values in parentheses are percentages.

inducibility compared to late potentials alone. When late potentials were removed from the analysis, the combination of other variables provided a predictive accuracy of 71%. Late potentials could still enter the model, with a probability of improving it of <0.05. Thus the signal-averaged ECG offered predictive information above that found in clinical variables and other noninvasive tests. On the other hand, no single variable or combination of variables predicted the induction of VF.

In our series of 105 patients, concordance between the results of PES and those of the signal-averaged ECG was observed in 84% of cases. The largest subgroup consisted of patients who had no late potentials and no induced sustained monomorphic VT (70%). In these patients, it is reasonable to speculate that the spontaneous arrhythmia may be due to mechanisms other than reentry, e.g., abnormal automaticity [90] or triggered activity [91]. Patients with both late potentials and induced sustained monomorphic VT accounted for 14% of cases. The results of the two tests were discordant in the remaining 16% of cases. Nine patients had late potentials but failed to develop sustained monomorphic VT at PES. This may be explained by electrophysiologic limitations of both PES [55] and signal-averaging techniques [86]. The relationship between myocardial zones with delayed conduction during sinus rhythm and the occurrence of reentrant arrhythmias is complex. Zones showing conduction delay (i.e., late potentials) during basic rhythm may completely block during premature stimulation and not participate in a reentrant pathway [86]. In eight patients a sustained VT was induced in the absence of late potentials. Again, limitations of the signal-averaged ECG, e.g., inability to detect delayed activation potentials with a dynamic Wenckebach sequence, as well as the possibility that some induced VT may have represented a nonspecific response to PES can be invoked. In this regard, four of the eight patients in this group had a cycle length of induced sustained monomorphic VT of 190–195 msec.

Our observation that patients with induced VF could not be distinguished from patients with no induced VT/VF by the signal-averaged ECG or by any other variables suggests that the induction of VF may represent a nonclinical response to PES in this group of patients. Further, the fact that the induction of sustained monomorphic VT rather than that of VF or nonsustained VT was correlated to the presence or absence of late potentials on the signal-averaged ECG provides evidence to the hypothesis that late potentials represent abnormal myocardial zones with delayed activation potentials capable of providing the electrophysiologic substrate for reentrant rhythms [86]. It also emphasizes the specificity of induced sustained monomorphic VT rather than induced nonsustained VT or VF as the endpoint of PES in patients with spontaneous nonsustained VT.

The Use of PES for Risk Stratification

In patients with no documented sustained ventricular tachyarrhythmias, the induction of sustained monomorphic VT by PES may either represent a mere laboratory finding or indicate patients at high risk for future serious arrhythmic events. The latter hypothesis was tested by a number of investigators. However, published reports on the prognostic significance of ventricular tachyarrhythmias induced by PES in patients with complex ventricular arrhythmias and nonsustained VT could be criticized for 1) small sample size [12,14,15,16,18,21,26–30,35], 2) retrospective data collection [18,29,30], 3) study population not representative of the overall population with nonsustained VT (selection was based on the absence of symptoms in two studies) [18,21], and 4) lack of uniform therapeutic approach. The indication for antiarrhythmic therapy varied in different studies. Authors subjected to treatment those patients with induced sustained VT [33,35], with induced nonsustained VT [13,15,18,21] and with induced VF [15]. In some studies, therapy was defined by means of repeat PES [15,21,33,35] while in other studies this was not always the case [18,29]. On the other hand, guidelines for the management of patients without induced VT were disparate; in some instances, these subjects did not receive any antiarrhythmic treatment [21,32,33,35], while in other studies there were subgroups followed on or off antiarrhythmic drugs [14,15,18,29]. In none of the published reports was treatment randomized.

Most studies reported a low risk of sudden cardiac death in patients with nonsustained VT who had no induced VT (Table 6–5) [14–16,21,28,30,32,35–37]. The risk of sudden death was equally low in patients with induced nonsustained VT in studies by Turitto et al. [32,33], Reddy et al. [16], Miles et al. [26], Buxton et al. [29], and Kharsa et al. [35].

TABLE 6–5. Outcome of Patients With Spontaneous Nonsustained Ventricular Tachycardia and/or Complex Ventricular Ectopy Studied With Programmed Stimulation[a]

Authors	No. of patients induced/not induced	Follow-up (months)	Percent sudden death or major arrhythmic events induced/not induced	Relation of induced arrhythmias to sudden death	Role of therapy	Significant risk factors for sudden death
Swerdlow et al., 1982 [12][b]	25/16	?	12/12	NS	Guided by PS; not predictive of outcome	None identified
Gomes et al., 1984 [15]	20/53	30 ± 15	32/2	<0.001	Guided by PS; not effective in preventing SD	Induced VT/VF and ejection fraction <0.40
Reddy and Jivrajka 1984 [16][b]	14/38	23 ± 16	27/5	<0.001	Guided by PS; not effective in preventing SD	Induced sustained VT/VF
Buxton et al., 1984 [14]	15/68	33	27/9	<0.00001	Similar mortality in patients treated empirically or by PS	Induced sustained VT and ejection fraction <0.40
Veltri et al., 1985 [18]	14/19	23 ± 16	21/21	NS	Uncertain	Low ejection fraction
Zheutlin et al., 1986 [21]	33/55	22	12/0	<0.02	Only to induced patients, guided by PS; not effective in preventing SD	Induced VT
Klein and Machell 1986 [27][b]	11/11	2–32	45/9	<0.05	Uncertain	Induced sustained VT
Miles et al., 1986 [26][b]	13/40	8.6 ± 5.3	23/5	=0.08	Only to induced patients when PS-guided, effective in preventing SD	Induced sustained VT and VF by ≤2 extrastimuli

Batsford et al., 1986 [28][b]	53/28	17	17/0	<0.02	Uncertain	Induced VT sustained or nonsustained
Buxton et al., 1987 [29]	28/34	28	25/12	Among induced patients, higher mortality in those treated empirically vs. those receiving PS-guided therapy (<0.001)	PS-guided therapy effective in preventing SD	Induced sustained VT not treated with PS-guided therapy
Sulpizi et al., 1987 [30]	9/52	26	11/6	NS	Uncertain	Low ejection fraction
Kharsa et al., 1988 [35]	8/32	16.2	0/0	Low risk of SD in both untreated patients without induced sustained VT and induced patients on PS-guided therapy	Guided by PS, only to induced patients	
Turitto et al., 1988 [36]	23/87	14 ± 7	4/3	Low risk of SD in both untreated patients without induced sustained VT and induced patients on PS-guided therapy	Guided by PS, only to induced patients	

[a]NS, not significant; PS, programmed stimulation; SD, sudden death; VT, ventricular tachycardia; VF, ventricular fibrillation.
[b]Abstract reports.

Zhetlin et al. [21] followed 52 patients with asymptomatic spontaneous nonsustained VT who had no inducible VT on PES for 22 months off antiarrhythmic therapy and found no instance of sudden cardiac death. Similarly, Kharsa et al. [35] reported no cases of sudden death among 32 patients without induced sustained VT followed for 17 months off antiarrhythmic drugs. In our recent series [37], three sudden deaths occurred in 58 patients who had no induced sustained VT/VF during a follow-up period of 30 ± 10 months off antiarrhythmic drugs. The 3-year sudden death rate was the same (7%) in patients with no induced sustained VT/VF, both in those with ejection fraction ≥ 40% or < 40%. On the other hand, the 3-year total cardiac mortality was significantly higher (27%) in those patients with ejection fraction < 40%, compared to those with ejection fraction ≥ 40%. It is interesting to note that the risk of serious arrhythmic events in the noninducible group of patients was low in both the presence [14,15] and the absence [15,32,35] of antiarrhythmic therapy. In an earlier study from our laboratory, Gomes et al. [15] followed 53 patients without induced VT/VF for 30 ± 15 months: Among them, 27 did not receive any antiarrhythmic drugs, while 26 were randomly assigned to long-term oral antiarrhythmic therapy. No significant differences in the occurrence of sudden death were found between treated and untreated patients. Thus it may be concluded that subjects with spontaneous nonsustained VT and no induced sustained VT can be managed safely without the use of an antiarrhythmic drug [15,21,32,33,35].

There are few follow-up studies on patients with induced VF. In our series [36,37], all patients with spontaneous nonsustained VT who had induced VF remained alive off antiarrhythmic therapy during a follow-up period of 19 ± 8 months. These findings are consistent with the findings of DiCarlo et al. [92] and Mahmud et al. [93], who reported no major arrhythmic events in a total of 27 patients without documented spontaneous sustained VT/VF and with induced VF who were followed for over 2 years. The arrhythmia was considered a nonclinical response to PES in patients without clinical sustained ventricular tachyarrhythmias.

On the other hand, VT inducibility seems to carry an increased risk of sudden death in patients with spontaneous nonsustained VT. The induced arrhythmia that portended a poor prognosis was identified as sustained VT by Buxton et al. [14], Klein et al. [27], Reddy et al. [16], Miles et al. [26], and Turitto et al. [36,37] and as both sustained or nonsustained VT by Gomes et al. [15], Zheutlin et al. [21], and Batsford et al. [28]. In the study by Buxton et al. [14], sudden death occurred in 4 of 15 patients (27%) with induced sustained VT, 2 of 37 (5%) with induced nonsustained VT, and 4 of 31 (13%) without induced VT during a follow-up period of 33 months. Sudden death occurred only in patients with ejection fractions ≤0.40. Using multivariate analysis, patients with one poor prognostic marker (induced sustained VT or low ejection fraction) were characterized by a threefold increased risk of sudden death, while patients with both markers had a sevenfold increased risk. Gomes et al. [15] reported major arrhythmic events in two of eight patients (25%) with induced sustained VT, two of five (40%) with induced VF, two of seven (29%) with induced nonsustained VT, and one of 53 (2%) without induced arrhythmias during a follow-up period of 30 ± 15 months. Actuarial survival curves revealed that, at 1 year, 75% of patients with induced VT/VF and 100% of those without induced VT/VF were alive, while at 2 years the probability of survival declined, respectively, to 65% and 97% ($P < 0.0001$). In a study by Batsford et al. [28], the incidence of serious arrhythmic events was 57% (4/7) in patients with induced sustained VT, 14% (5/36) in those with induced nonsustained VT, and 0 (0/28) in those without induced VT. Differences in survival between patients with and without induced VT were statistically significant ($P < 0.02$). The relationship between outcome and different types of induced arrhythmias was not specified by Zheutlin et al. [21].

Few studies failed to find a correlation between the inducibility of VT and high risk for sudden cardiac death in patients with spontaneous nonsustained VT. Two of these studies were retrospective [18,30], and one was a preliminary report [12]. In the study by Sulpizi et al. [30], the overall probability of sudden death was low (7% during a follow-up period of 26 months) and was not influenced by VT inducibility. On the other hand, poor left ventricular function was an important predictor of mortality. Similar findings were reported by Veltri et al. [18]. In their study, a 21% incidence of serious arrhythmic events was documented over a follow-up period of approximately 2 years. Ejection fraction was significantly lower in the group with than in the group without arrhythmic events (0.49 ± 0.18 vs. 0.31 ± 0.17, $P < 0.04$), while the ability to induce VT was not correlated to outcome.

The available literature on the effects of empirical antiarrhythmic therapy or therapy guided by PES on survival of patients with spontaneous nonsustained VT and induced VT are controversial. Most of the reported studies failed to demonstrate that PES-guided therapy improved survival of patients with induced VT or was superior to empirical therapy [11,12, 14,17,18,27]. Patients with induced VT treated with drug regimens selected by PES maintained an excess mortality, with respect to those without induced VT, in studies by Gomes et al. [15] and Zheutlin et al. [21]. On the other hand, the significance of the finding that PES-guided therapy in patients with induced sustained VT was associated with low risk of sudden death in the study by Kharsa et al. [35] and in our own series [36,37] is limited by the lack of a controlled group followed off antiarrhythmic therapy. It is of interest that a recent report, which only utilized historical controls, suggested that therapy guided by PES in this group was associated with a lower rate of sudden cardiac death compared with empiric therapy [29].

The hypothesis that the induction of sustained VT in patients with complex ventricular arrhythmias and nonsustained VT identifies a subset of patients with increased risk of sudden cardiac death will remain unsubstantiated in the absence of a randomized study that compares the incidence of sudden death on and off antiarrhythmic therapy. The antiarrhythmic protocol probably should be based on the prevention of induction of sustained VT.

RECOMMENDED PROTOCOL FOR RISK STRATIFICATION AND MANAGEMENT OF PATIENTS WITH NONSUSTAINED VT

Our recent studies [36,37] strongly suggest that an optimal protocol for risk stratification and management of patients with organic heart disease and spontaneous nonsustained VT should be based on the results of the signal-averaged ECG, left ventricular ejection fraction, and PES as follows: 1) Patients with no late potentials in the signal-averaged ECG and with an injection fraction >40% do not require testing by PES or long-term antiarrhythmic therapy, since the incidence of inducible sustained monomorphic VT and the risk of sudden death are very low in this group of patients (there was no instance of induced sustained VT in 33 consecutive patients in this group); and 2) patients with no late potentials but with ejection fractions <40% and patients with late potentials should be recommended for electrophysiologic evaluation. The incidence of inducible sustained monomorphic VT was 21% in the former group and 65% in the latter group. In patients with late potentials, the high incidence of inducible VT was independent of the etiology of heart disease and the degree of ejection fraction (50% with ejection fractions >40% vs. 68% with ejection fractions <40%). Based on the results of PES, patients with no inducible nonsustained VT or VF could be followed off antiarrhythmic therapy with a low risk of sudden death. However, if sustained monomorphic VT is induced, these patients should receive antiarrhythmic therapy guided by PES with the understanding that the value of antiarrhythmic therapy in this group has not been definitely established. This could only be achieved through randomization of therapy in a large multicenter study. Considering the magnitude of the problem, such a study is long overdue.

ACKNOWLEDGMENTS

This work was supported by National Institutes of Health grant HL31341 and by Veterans Administration Medical Research Funds.

REFERENCES

1. Lown B: Sudden cardiac death—1978. Circulation 60:1593–1599, 1979.
2. Mason J, Winkle R: Electrode-catheter arrhythmia induction in the selection and assessment of antiarrhythmic drug therapy for recurrent ventricular tachycardia. Circulation 58:971–985, 1978.

3. Horowitz L, Josephson M, Farshidi A, Spielman SR, Michelson EL, Greenspan AM: Recurrent sustained ventricular tachycardia. 3. Role of the electrophysiologic study in selection of antiarrhythmic regimens. Circulation 58:986–997, 1978.
4. Swerdlow CD, Winkle RA, Mason JW: Determinants of survival in patients with ventricular tachyarrhythmias. N Engl J Med 308:1436–1442, 1983.
5. Myerburg RJ, Kessler KM, Estes D, Conde CA, Luceri RM, Zaman L, Kozlovskis PL, Castellanos A: Long-term survival after prehospital cardiac arrest: Analysis of outcome during an 8 year study. Circulation 70:538–546, 1984.
6. Goldstein S, Landis JR, Leighton R, Ritter G, Vasu CM, Wolfe RA, Acheson A, Medendorp SV: Predictive survival models for resuscitated victims of out-of-hospital cardiac arrest with coronary heart disease. Circulation 5:873–880, 1985.
7. Bigger JT Jr, Fleiss JL, Kleiger R, Miller JP, Rolnitzky LM, and the Multicenter Post-Infarction Research Group: The relationships among ventricular arrhythmias, left ventricular dysfunction, and mortality in the 2 years after myocardial infarction. Circulation 69:250–258, 1984.
8. Mukharji J, Rude RE, Poole WK, Gustafson N, Thomas LJ Jr, Strauss HW, Jaffe AS, Muller JE, Roberts R, Raabe DS Jr, Croft CH, Passamani E, Braunwald E, Willerson JT, and the MILIS Group: Risk factors for sudden death after acute myocardial infarction: Two-year follow-up. Am J Cardiol 54:31–36, 1984.
9. Maisel AS, Scott N, Gilpin E, Ahnve S, Winter ML, Henning H, Collins D, Ross J Jr: Complex ventricular arrhythmias in patients with Q wave versus non-Q wave myocardial infarction. Circulation 72:963–970, 1985.
10. Josephson ME: Treatment of ventricular arrhythmias after myocardial infarction. Circulation 74:653–658, 1986.
11. Naccarelli GV, Prystowsky EN, Jackman WM, Heger JJ, Rahilly GT, Zipes DP: Role of electrophysiologic testing in managing patients who have ventricular tachycardia unrelated to coronary artery disease. Am J Cardiol 50:165–171, 1982.
12. Swerdlow CD, Echt DS, Soderholm-Difatte V, Winkle RA, Mason JW: Limited value of programmed stimulation in patients with unsustained VT [abstract]. Circulation 66[Suppl II]:II-145, 1982.
13. Buxton AE, Waxman HL, Marchlinski FE, Josephson ME: Electrophysiologic studies in nonsustained ventricular tachycardia: Relation to underlying heart disease. Am J Cardiol 52:985–991, 1983.
14. Buxton AE, Marchlinski FE, Waxman HL, Flores BT, Cassidy DM, Josephson ME: Prognostic factors in nonsustained ventricular tachycardia. Am J Cardiol 53:1275–1279, 1984.
15. Gomes JAC, Hariman RI, Kang PS, El-Sherif N, Chowdhry I, Lyons J: Programmed electrical stimulation in patients with high-grade ventricular ectopy: Electrophysiologic findings and prognosis for survival. Circulation 70:43–51, 1984.
16. Reddy CP, Jivrajka VB: Is programmed cardiac stimulation useful in risk stratification of patients with high-grade ventricular ectopy [abstract]? Circulation 70[Suppl II]:II-400, 1984.
17. Miles WM, Skale BT, Windle JR, Heger JJ, Prystowsky EN: Electrophysiologic characteristics and follow-up of 139 patients with nonsustained ventricular tachycardia [abstract]. Circulation 70[Suppl II]:II-400, 1984.
18. Veltri EP, Platia EV, Griffith LSC, Reid PR: Programmed electrical stimulation and long-term follow-up in asymptomatic nonsustained ventricular tachycardia. Am J Cardiol 56:309–314, 1985.
19. Spielman SR, Greenspan AM, Kay HR, Discigil KF, Webb CR, Sokolff NM, Rae AP, Morganroth J, Horowitz LN: Electrophysiologic testing in patients at high risk for sudden cardiac death. 1. Nonsustained ventricular tachycardia and abnormal ventricular function. J Am Coll Cardiol 6:31–39, 1985.

20. Meinertz T, Treese N, Kasper W, Geibel A, Hofmann T, Zehender M, Bohn D, Pop T, Just H: Determinants of prognosis in idiopathic dilated cardiomyopathy as determined by programmed electrical stimulation. Am J Cardiol 56:337–341, 1985.
21. Zheutlin TA, Roth H, Chua W, Steinman R, Summers C, Lesch M, Kehoe RF: Programmed electrical stimulation to determine the need for antiarrhythmic therapy in patients with complex ventricular ectopic activity. Am Heart J 111:860–867, 1986.
22. Breithardt G, Borggrefe M, Podczeck A: Electrophysiology and pharmacology of asymptomatic nonsustained ventricular tachycardia. Clin Progr Electrophysiol Pacing 4:81–99, 1986.
23. Das SK, Morady F, DiCarlo L, Jr, Baerman J, Krol R, De Buitleir M, Crevey B: Prognostic usefulness of programmed ventricular stimulation in idiopathic dilated cardiomyopathy without symptomatic ventricular arrhythmias. Am J Cardiol 58: 998–1000, 1986.
24. Poll DS, Marchlinski FE, Buxton AE, Josephson ME: Usefulness of programmed stimulation in idiopathic cardiomyopathy. Am J Cardiol 58:992–997, 1986.
25. Friedman L, Yusuf S: Does therapy directed by programmed electrical stimulation provide a satisfactory clinical response? Circulation 73[Suppl II]:II-59–II-66, 1986.
26. Miles WM, Heger JJ, Zipes DP, Prystowsky EN: Management of patients with asymptomatic nonsustained ventricular tachycardia directed by electrophysiologic study [abstract]. Clin Res 34:326A, 1986.
27. Klein RC, Machell C: Electrophysiologic studies in patients with nonsustained ventricular tachycardia and coronary disease: Relation of ventricular aneurysm to inducible tachycardia and prognosis [abstract]. J Am Coll Cardiol 7:71A, 1986.
28. Batsford WP, Sudbrink L, Stark SI, McPherson CA, Kennedy EE, Rosenfeld LE: Outcome in non-sustained ventricular tachycardia: Relation to clinical factors, spontaneous and induced ventricular arrhythmias [abstract]. J Am Coll Cardiol 7:71A, 1986.
29. Buxton AE, Marchlinski FE, Waxman HL, Flores BT, Miller JM, Doherty JU, Josephson ME: Nonsustained ventricular tachycardia in patients with coronary artery disease: Role of electrophysiologic study. Circulation 75:1178–1185, 1987.
30. Sulpizi AM, Friehling TD, Kowey PR: Value of electrophysiologic testing in patients with nonsustained ventricular tachycardia. Am J Cardiol 59:841–845, 1987.
31. Fontaine JM, Turitto G, El-Sherif N: Prognostic significance of ambulatory electrocardiographic recording, programmed electrical stimulation and signal-averaged electrocardiogram in patients with complex ventricular arrhythmias. J Electrophysiol 1:204–216, 1987.
32. Turitto G, Fontaine J, Caref E, Benhuri M, Howard M, Ibrahim B, El-Sherif N: Low-risk of sudden cardiac death in patients with non-sustained ventricular tachycardia and normal signal averaged electrocardiogram [abstract]. Circulation 76[Suppl IV]:IV-32, 1987.
33. Turitto G, Fontaine JM, Ursell SN, Caref EB, Henkin R, El-Sherif N: Value of the signal-averaged electrocardiogram as a predictor of the results of programmed stimulation in nonsustained ventricular tachycardia. Am J Cardiol 61:1272–1278, 1988.
34. El-Sherif N, Turitto G, Fontaine JM: Risk stratification of patients with complex ventricular arrhythmias. Herz 13:204–214, 1988.
35. Kharsa MH, Gold RL, Moore H, Yazaki Y, Haffajee C, Alpert JS: Long-term outcome following programmed electrical stimulation in patients with high-grade ventricular ectopy. PACE 11:603–609, 1988.
36. Turitto G, El-Sherif N: Role of the signal averaged electrocardiogram and electrophysiologic study in the management of patients with non-sustained ventricular tachycardia. New Trends Arrhythmias 5:431–435, 1988.
37. Turitto G, Fontaine JM, Ursell S, Caref EB, Bekheit S, El-Sherif N: Risk stratification and management of patients with organic heart disease and non-sustained ventricular tachy-

cardia: Role of programmed stimulation, left ventricular ejection fraction and the signal averaged electrocardiogram. Am J Med (In press).
38. Anderson KP, DeCamilla J, Moss AJ: Clinical significance of ventricular tachycardia (3 beats or longer) detected during ambulatory monitoring after myocardial infarction. Circulation 57:890–897, 1978.
39. Bigger JT, Weld FM, Rolinzky LM: Prevalence, characteristics and significance of ventricular tachycardia (three or more complexes) detected with ambulatory electrocardiographic recording in the late hospital phase of acute myocardial infarction. Am J Cardiol 48:815–823, 1981.
40. Kleiger RE, Miller JP, Thanavaro S, Province MA, Martin TF, Oliver GC: Relationship between clinical features of acute myocardial infarction and ventricular runs 2 weeks to 1 year after infarction. Circulation 63:64–70, 1981.
41. Surawicz B: Prognosis of ventricular arrhythmias in relation to sudden cardiac death: Therapeutic implications. J Am Coll Cardiol 10:435–447, 1987.
42. Kennedy HL, Whitlock JA, Sprague MK, Kennedy LJ, Buckingham TA, Goldberg RJ: Long-term follow-up of asymptomatic healthy subjects with frequent and complex ventricular ectopy. N Engl J Med 312:193–197, 1985.
43. Rubin DA, Nieminski KE, Monteferrante JC, Mages T, Reed GE, Herman MV: Ventricular arrhythmias after coronary artery bypass graft surgery: Incidence, risk factors and long-term prognosis. J Am Coll Cardiol 6:307–310, 1985.
44. DeSoyza N, Murphy ML, Bissett JK, Kane JJ, Doherty JE: Ventricular arrhythmia in chronic stable angina pectoris with surgical or medical treatment. Ann Intern Med 89:10–14, 1978.
45. Schultze RA Jr, Strauss HW, Pitt B: Sudden death in the year following myocardial infarction. Relationship to ventricular premature contractions in the late hospital phase and left ventricular ejection fraction. Am J Med 62:192–199, 1977.
46. Packer M: Sudden unexpected death in patients with congestive heart failure: A second frontier. Circulation 72:681–685, 1985.
47. Maskin CS, Siskind SJ, LeJemtel TH: High prevalence of nonsustained ventricular tachycardia in severe congestive heart failure. Am Heart J 107:896–901, 1984.
48. Meinertz T, Hoffman T, Kasper W, Treese N, Bechtold H, Stienen U, Tiberius P, Leitner E, Andersen D, Jurgen M: Significance of ventricular arrhythmias in idiopathic dilated cardiomyopathy. Am J Cardiol 53:902–907, 1984.
49. Holmes J, Kubo SH, Cody RJ, Kligfield R: Arrhythmias in ischemic and non-ischemic dilated cardiomyopathy: Prediction of mortality by ambulatory electrocardiography. Am J Cardiol 55:146–151, 1985.
50. Unverferth DV, Magorien RD, Moeschberger ML, Baker PB, Fetters JK, Leier CV: Factors influencing the one-year mortality of dilated cardiomyopathy. Am J Cardiol 54:147–152, 1984.
51. Furberg CD, May GS: Effect of long-term prophylactic treatment on survival after myocardial infarction. Am J Med 76:76–83, 1984.
52. Woosley RL: Indications for antiarrhythmic therapy: A wealth of controversy, a dearth of data. Ann Intern Med 108:450–452, 1988.
52a. The Cardiac Arrythmia Suppression Trial (CAST) Investigators: Preliminary report: Effect of encainide and flecainide on mortality in a randomized trial of arrhythmia suppression after myocardial infarction. New Engl J Med 321:406–412, 1989.
53. Estes NAM III, Garan H, McGovern B, Ruskin JN: Influence of drive cycle length during programmed stimulation on induction of ventricular arrhythmias: Analysis of 403 patients. Am J Cardiol 57:108–112, 1986.
54. Prystowsky EN, Miles WM, Evans JJ, Hubbard JE, Skale BT, Windle JR, Heger JJ, Zipes DP: Induction of ventricular tachycardia during programmed electrical stimulation: Analysis of pacing methods. Circulation 73[Suppl II]:II-32–II-38, 1986.

55. Mason JW, Anderson KP, Freedman RA: Techniques and criteria in electrophysiologic study of ventricular tachycardia. Circulation 75[Suppl III]:III-125–III-130, 1987.
56. Buxton AE, Waxman HL, Marchlinski FE, Unterker WJ, Waspe LE, Josephson ME: Role of triple extrastimuli during electrophysiologic study of patients with documented sustained ventricular tachyarrhythmias. Circulation 69:532–540, 1984.
57. Brugada P, Wellens HJJ: Comparison in the same patient of two programmed stimulation protocols to induce ventricular tachycardia. Am J Cardiol 55:380–383, 1985.
58. Breithardt G, Borggrefe M, Podczeck A, Budde T: Influence of the cycle length of basic drive on induction of sustained ventricular tachycardia associated with coronary artery disease. Am J Cardiol 60:1306–1310, 1987.
59. Morady F, DiCarlo LA Jr, Baerman JM, de Buitleir M: Comparison of coupling intervals that induce clinical and nonclinical forms of ventricular tachycardia during programmed stimulation. Am J Cardiol 57:1269–1273, 1986.
60. Vandepol CJ, Farshidi A, Spielman SR, Greenspan AM, Horowitz LN, Josephson ME: Incidence and clinical significance of induced ventricular tachycardia. Am J Cardiol 45:725–731, 1980.
61. Morady F, DiCarlo L, Winston S, Davis JC, Scheinman MM: A prospective comparison of the role of triple extrastimuli and left ventricular stimulation in studies of ventricular tachycardia induction. Circulation 70:52–57, 1984.
62. Gottlieb C, Josephson ME: The preference of programmed stimulation guided therapy for sustained ventricular arrhythmias. In Brugada P, Wellens HJJ (eds): "Cardiac Arrhythmias: Where To Go From Here?" Mount Kisco, NY: Futura Publishing Co, pp 421–434, 1987.
63. Zehender M, Brugada P, Geibel A, Waldecker B, Stevenson W, Wellens HJJ: Programmed electrical stimulation in healed myocardial infarction using a standardized ventricular stimulation protocol. Am J Cardiol 59:578–585, 1987.
64. Platia EV, Greene HL, Vlay SC, Werner JA, Gross B, Reid PR: Sensitivity of various extrastimulus techniques in patients with serious ventricular arrhythmias. Am Heart J 106:698–703, 1983.
65. Schoenfeld MH, McGovern B, Garan H, Kelly E, Grant G, Ruskin JN: Determinants of the outcome of electrophysiologic study in patients with ventricular tachyarrhythmias. J Am Coll Cardiol 6:298–306, 1985.
66. El-Sherif N, Mehra R, Gough WB, Zeiler RH: Reentrant ventricular arrhythmias in the late myocardial infarction period. 11. Burst pacing versus multiple premature stimulation in the induction of reentry. J Am Coll Cardiol 4:295–304, 1984.
67. Denker S. Lehmann M, Mahmud R, Gilbert C, Akhtar M: Facilitation of ventricular tachycardia induction with abrupt changes in ventricular cycle length. Am J Cardiol 53:508–515, 1984.
68. Rosenfeld LE, McPherson CA, Kennedy EE, Stark SI, Batsford WP: Ventricular tachycardia induction: Comparison of triple extrastimuli with an abrupt change in ventricular drive cycle length. Am Heart J 111:868–874, 1986.
69. Livelli FD Jr, Bigger JT Jr, Reiffel JA, Gang ES, Patton JN, Noethling PM, Rolnitzky LM, Gliklich JI: Response to programmed ventricular stimulation: Sensitivity, specificity and relationship to heart disease. Am J Cardiol 50:452–458, 1982.
70. Brugada P, Green M, Abdollah H, Wellens HJJ: Significance of ventricular arrhythmias initiated by programmed ventricular stimulation: The importance of the type of ventricular arrhythmia induced and the number of premature extrastimuli required. Circulation 69:87–92, 1984.
71. Morady F, Shapiro W, Shen E, Sung RJ, Scheinman MM: Programmed ventricular stimulation in patients without spontaneous ventricular tachycardia. Am Heart J 107: 875–882, 1984.
72. Stevenson WG, Brugada P, Waldecker B, Zehender M, Wellens HJJ: Can potentially

significant polymorphic ventricular arrhythmias initiated by programmed stimulation be distinguished from those that are nonspecific: Am Heart J 111:1073–1080, 1986.
73. Mann DE, Luck JC, Griffin JC, Herre JM, Limacher MC, Magro SA, Robertson NW, Wyndham CRC: Induction of clinical ventricular tachycardia using programmed stimulation: Value of third and fourth extrastimuli. Am J Cardiol 52:501–506, 1983.
74. Kim SG, Mercando AD, Fisher JD: Comparison of characteristics of nonsustained ventricular tachycardia on Holter monitoring and sustained ventricular tachycardia observed spontaneously or induced by programmed stimulation. Am J Cardiol 60:288–292, 1987.
75. Kammerling JM, Miles WM, Zipes DP, Heger JJ, Klein LS, Chang M-S, Prystowsky EN: Characteristics of spontaneous nonsustained ventricular tachycardia poorly predict rate of sustained ventricular tachycardia [abstract]. Clin Res 34:312A, 1986.
76. Doherty JU, Kienzle MG, Waxman HL, Buxton AE, Marchlinski FE, Josephson ME: Programmed ventricular stimulation at a second right ventricular site: An analysis of 100 patients, with special reference to sensitivity, specificity and characteristics of patients with induced ventricular tachycardia. Am J Cardiol 52:1184–1189, 1983.
77. Lin H-T, Mann DE, Luck JC, Krafchek J, Magro SA, Sakun V, Wyndham CRC: Prospective comparison of right and left ventricular stimulation for induction of sustained ventricular tachycardia. Am J Cardiol 59:559–563, 1987.
78. Denniss RA, Richards DA, Cody DV, Russell PA, Young AA, Cooper MJ, Ross DL, Uther JB: Prognostic significance of ventricular tachycardia and fibrillation induced at programmed stimulation and delayed potentials detected on the signal-averaged electrocardiograms of survivors of acute myocardial infarction. Circulation 74:731–745, 1986.
79. Roy D, Arenal A, Godin D, Marchand E, Cassidy D, Theroux P, Waters DD: The Canadian experience on the identification of candidates for sudden cardiac death after myocardial infarction. In Brugada P, Wellens HJJ (eds): "Cardiac Arrhythmias: Where To Go From Here?" Mount Kisco, NY: Futura Publishing Co, pp 343–351, 1987.
80. Wellens HJJ, Brugada P, Stevenson WG: Programmed stimulation of the heart in life-threatening ventricular arrhythmias: What is the significance of induced arrhythmias and what is the correct stimulation protocol? Circulation 72:1–7, 1985.
81. Buxton AE, Simson MS, Falcone RA, Marchlinski FE, Doherty JU, Josephson ME: Results of signal-averaged electrocardiography and electrophysiology study in patients with nonsustained ventricular tachycardia after healing of acute myocardial infarction. Am J Cardiol 60:80–85, 1987.
82. Marchlinski FE, Buxton AE, Waxman HL, Josephson ME: Identifying patients at risk of sudden death after myocardial infarction: Value of the response to programmed stimulation, degree of ventricular ectopic activity and severity of left ventricular dysfunction. Am J Cardiol 52:1190–1196, 1983.
83. Nalos PC, Gang ES, Mandel WJ, Ladenheim ML, Lass Y, Peter T: The signal-averaged electrocardiogram as a screening test for inducibility of sustained ventricular tachycardia in high risk patients: A prospective study. J Am Coll Cardiol 9:539–548, 1987.
84. Gradman AH, Batsford WP, Rieur EC, Leon L, Van Zetta AM: Ambulatory electrocardiographic correlates of ventricular inducibility during programmed electrical stimulation. J Am Coll Cardiol 5:1087–1093, 1985.
85. Simson MB: Use of signals in the terminal QRS complex to identify patients with ventricular tachycardia after myocardial infarction. Circulation 64:235–242, 1981.
86. El-Sherif N, Gomes JAC, Restivo M, Mehra R: Late potentials and arrhythmogenesis. PACE 8:440–462, 1985.
87. Denes P, Uretz E, Santarelli P: Determinants of arrhythmogenic ventricular activity detected on the body surface QRS in patients with coronary artery disease. Am J Cardiol 53:1519–1523, 1984.

88. Freedman RA, Gillis AM, Keren A, Soderholm-Difatte V, Mason JW: Signal-averaged electrocardiographic late potentials in patients with ventricular fibrillation or ventricular tachycardia: Correlation with clinical arrhythmia and electrophysiologic study. Am J Cardiol 55:1350–1353, 1985.
89. Lindsay BD, Ambos HD, Schechtman KB, Cain ME: Improved selection of patients for programmed ventricular stimulation by frequency analysis of signal-averaged electrocardiograms. Circulation 73:675–683, 1986.
90. Hoffman BF, Rosen MR: Cellular mechanisms for cardiac arrhythmias. Circ Res 49: 1–15, 1981.
91. El-Sherif N, Gough WB, Zeiler RH, Mehra R: Triggered ventricular rhythms in 1-day-old myocardial infarction in the dog. Circ Res 52:566–579, 1983.
92. DiCarlo LA Jr, Morady F, Schwartz AB, Shen EN, Baerman JM, Krol RB, Scheinman MM, Sung RJ: Clinical significance of ventricular fibrillation-flutter induced by ventricular programmed stimulation. Am Heart J 109:959–963, 1985.
93. Mahmud R, Denker S, Lehmann MH, Tchou P, Dongas J, Akhtar M: Incidence and clinical significance of ventricular fibrillation induced with single and double ventricular extrastimuli. Am J Cardiol 58:75–79, 1986.

Chapter 7

β-Adrenergic Blockade in the Prevention of Sudden Cardiac Death

William H. Frishman, M.D.

Departments of Medicine, Epidemiology, and Social Medicine, Albert Einstein College of Medicine, and Department of Medicine, Hospital of the Albert Einstein College of Medicine, Bronx, New York 10461

INTRODUCTION

The introduction of β-adrenoceptor-blocking drugs to clinical medicine 35 years ago ushered in a new era of pharmacologic intervention that revolutionized the management of cardiovascular disease. In addition to becoming a therapeutic mainstay for the treatment of hypertension, angina, and various arrhythmias, beta-blockers have now been shown to reduce the risk of mortality after myocardial infarction, and these drugs have numerous applications well beyond the cardiovascular sphere [1]. The use of beta-blockers in prevention of sudden death is discussed below. It is important first to review some basic pharmacologic actions of β-adrenergic blocking drugs.

ELECTROPHYSIOLOGIC EFFECTS

β-Adrenoreceptor-blocking drugs have two main effects on the electrophysiologic properties of specialized cardiac tissue (Table 7–1). The first effect of beta-blockers results from the specific blockade of adrenergic stimulation of cardiac pacemaker potentials. This is undoubtedly important in the

The Prevention of Sudden Cardiac Death, pages 139–153

TABLE 7–1. Antiarrhythmic Mechanisms for Beta-Blockers[a]

Beta-blockade
Electrophysiology: depress excitability; depress conduction
Prevention of ischemia: decrease automaticity; inhibit reentrant mechanisms
Membrane-stabilizing effects
Local anesthetic ''quinidine-like'' properties: depress excitability; prolong refractory period; delay conduction

[a]Special pharmacologic properties (β_1-selectivity, intrinsic sympathomimetic activity) do not appear to contribute to antiarrhythmic effectiveness.

control of arrhythmias caused by enhanced automaticity. In concentrations causing significant inhibition of adrenergic receptors, the beta-blockers produce little change in the transmembrane potentials of cardiac muscle. However, by competitively inhibiting adrenergic stimulation, beta-blockers decrease the slope of phase 4 depolarization and the spontaneous firing rate of sinus or ectopic pacemakers and thus decrease automaticity. Arrhythmias occurring in the setting of enhanced automaticity, as encountered in myocardial infarction, digitalis toxicity, hyperthyroidism, and pheochromocytoma, would therefore be expected to respond well to beta-blockade [2].

The second electrophysiologic effect of beta-blockers is membrane-stabilizing action, also known as the ''quinidine-like'' or ''local anesthetic'' action. This property of source beta-blockers is unrelated to inhibition of catecholamine action and is possessed equally by both the d- and l-isomers of the drugs (d-isomers have almost no beta-blocking activity) [3]. Characteristic of this effect is a reduction in the rate of rise of the action potential without an effection duration [4]. Associated features include an elevated electrical threshold of excitability, a delay in conduction velocity, and a significant increase in the effective refractory period. This effect and its attendant changes have been explained by an inhibition of the depolarizing inward sodium current.

Sotalol is unique among the beta-blockers in that it alone possesses class III antiarrhythmic properties, causing prolongation of the action potential period and thereby delaying repolarization [5]. Clinical studies have verified the efficacy of sotalol in control of arrhythmias [6–9], but additional investigation will be required to determine whether its class III antiarrhythmic properties contribute significantly to its efficacy as an antiarrhythmic agent.

The most important mechanism underlying the antiarrhythmic effect of beta-blockers (with the possible exclusion of sotalol) is believed to be beta-blockade, with resultant inhibition of pacemaker potentials. The contribution of membrane-stabilizing action does not appear to be clinically significant. This is borne out by at least two separate lines of evidence. The plasma concentration of propranolol necessary for arrhythmia control is far less than the level required for membrane stabilization. In vitro experiments with human ventricular muscle have shown that the concentration of propranolol required for membrane stabilization is 50–100 times the concentration usually associated with inhibition of exercise-induced tachycardia and at which only beta-blocking effects occur [10]. Moreover, d-propranolol, which possesses membrane-stabilizing properties but no beta-blocking action, is a weak antiarrhythmic agent in high doses, whereas beta-blockers devoid of membrane-stabilizing action (atenolol, metoprolol, nadolol, pindolol) have been shown to be effective antiarrhythmic drugs.

If, indeed, beta-blockade is the major mechanism for antiarrhythmic effect, with the contribution of membrane-stabilizing properties being negligible, then one would expect all beta-blockers to be similarly effective at a comparable level of beta-blockade. In fact, this appears to be the case. No superiority of one beta-blocking agent over another in the therapy of arrhythmias has yet been convincingly demonstrated. Differences in overall clinical usefulness are related to their other associated pharmacologic properties [11].

Beta-blockers slow the rate of discharge of sinus and ectopic pacemakers and increase the effective refractory period of the atrioventricular (AV) node by their β-adrenergic blocking actions. They also slow both antegrade and retrograde conduction in anomalous pathways [12]. Inasmuch as all beta-blockers studied thus far cause an increase in AV conduction time, advancing AV block is a potential complication when beta-blockers are used. Agents with partial agonist activity [intrinsic sympathomimetic activity (ISA)], such as acebutolol and pindolol, may provide some protection from the AV conduction impairment induced by beta-blockade [13].

In high doses, beta-blockers can induce sinus node dysfunction and lead to sinoatrial block or sinus arrest. These drugs are, therefore, best avoided in patients with "sick sinus syndrome," a condition that can be exacerbated by β-adrenergic blockade [12].

THERAPEUTIC USES

β-Adrenergic-blocking drugs have become an important treatment modality for various cardiac arrhythmias [1]. Although it has long been acknowledged that beta-blockers are more effective in treating supraventricular than ventricular arrhythmias, it has been appreciated only recently that these agents can be quite useful in the treatment of ventricular tachyarrhythmias (Table 7–2), especially in the setting of myocardial ischemia.

Ventricular Arrhythmias

β-Adrenoreceptor-blocking drugs can decrease the frequency of or abolish ventricular ectopic beats in various conditions (Table 7–3) [14–23]. They are particularly useful if these arrhythmias are related to excessive

TABLE 7–2. Effects of Beta-Blockers on Ventricular Arrhythmias

Premature ventricular contractions	Variable response to beta-blockers, except digitalis-induced, exercise (ischemia)-induced, mitral valve prolapse, or hypertrophic cardiomyopathy
Ventricular tachycardia	Usually not effective, except in digitalis toxicity or exercise (ischemia)-induced
Ventricular fibrillation	Electrical defibrillation is treatment of choice; beta-blockers can be used to prevent recurrence in cases of excess digitalis or sympathomimetic amines; appear to be effective in reducing the incidence of ventricular fibrillation and sudden death after myocardial infarction

TABLE 7–3. Beta-Blocking Agents in Chronic Ventricular Ectopy: Efficacy Determined by Holter Monitoring [14]

			Efficacy	
Study	Dx.	Drug/dose	No. (%) of patients responding	Percent decrease in PVCs
Winkle et al. [15]	Mixed	Propranolol/240[a]	2/16 (50)	>70[b]
Winkle et al. [16]	MVP	Propranolol/40–320	5/9 (56)	>75
Pratt et al. [17]	CAD	Metoprolol/100–200	7/13 (54)	>75
Woosley et al. [18]	Mixed[c]	Propranolol/up to 960	24/32 (75)	>70
deSoyza et al. [19]	Mixed	Acebutolol/300	11/20 (55)	>70
Koppes et al. [20]	Acute MI	Propranolol/80–480	18/32 (56)	>70
Schlemann et al. [21]	Mixed	Nadolol/80–640	7/13 (54)	>75
Morganroth [22]	Mixed	Atenolol/50–200	7/12 (58)	>70
Podrid and Lown [23]	Mixed	Pindolol/20–80	21/42 (50)[d] 15/45 (33)[e]	50–90

[a]Dose range studied (in milligrams daily).
[b]Percentage reduction required to define drug efficacy.
[c]Several cardiac diseases studied.
[d]Acute drug testing.
[e]Chronic drug testing.

catecholamines (e.g., exercise, halothane anesthesia, pheochromocytoma, exogenous catecholamines), myocardial ischemia, or digitalis excess.

Premature ventricular contractions. The response of these arrhythmias to beta-blockade is variable. The best response can be expected in coronary heart disease, particularly when the arrhythmia is secondary to an ischemic event. Because beta-blockers are effective in preventing ischemic episodes, arrhythmias generated by these episodes may be prevented.

Beta-blockers are also quite effective in controlling the frequency of premature ventricular contractions in hypertrophic cardiomyopathy and in mitral valve prolapse [16]. In these conditions, a beta-blocker is generally the antiarrhythmic drug of choice.

Ventricular tachycardia. Beta-blocking drugs should not be considered agents of choice in the treatment of acute ventricular tachycardia, although their efficacy in the setting of myocardial ischemia may warrant early use. Cardioversion or other antiarrhythmic drugs (lidocaine, quinidine, procainamide) should be the initial mode of therapy. Beta-blockers, however, have been shown to be of benefit for prophylaxis against recurrent ventricular tachycardia, particularly if sympathetic stimulation appears to be a precipitating cause. Several studies have been reported showing the prevention of exercise-induced ventricular tachycardia by beta-blockers; in many cases, there had been a poor response to digitalis or quinidine [24–26].

Prevention of ventricular fibrillation. Beta-blocking agents can attenuate cardiac stimulation by the sympathetic nervous system and perhaps reduce the potential for reentrant ventricular arrhythmias and sudden death [2,27]. Experimental studies have shown that beta-blockers raise the ventricular fibrillation threshold in the ischemic myocardium [2,27]. Placebo-controlled clinical trials have shown that beta-blockers reduce the number of episodes of ventricular fibrillation and cardiac arrest during the acute phase of myocardial infarction [28,29]. The long-term beta-blocker postmyocardial infarction trials and other clinical studies with beta-blockers have demonstrated that there is a significant reduction of simple and complex ventricular arrhythmias [20–34].

POSSIBLE MECHANISMS OF BENEFIT FROM β-ADRENERGIC BLOCKADE IN THE PREVENTION OF SUDDEN DEATH

Although no one has demonstrated that suppression of ventricular ectopy reduces sudden cardiac death in humans, several clinical trials have evaluated the efficacy of β-adrenergic-blocking drugs in reducing the incidence of sudden cardiac death after myocardial infarction [30,35–40]. β-Adrenergic blocking drugs have several pharmacologic actions that might make them protective against sudden death after myocardial infarction (Table 7–4). First, beta-blockers interfere with the adverse electrophysiologic effects of the autonomic nervous system during myocardial ischemia and by this mechanism can raise the ventricular fibrillation threshold [2,27,41]. Second, some beta-blockers have direct, intrinsic antiarrhythmic activity [2,41,42]. However, the antiarrhythmic effects of the different beta-blockers are similar and appear to be related to their common β_1-adrenergic blocking actions, not to their ancillary properties: membrane-stabilizing or partial agonist activities [1]. Third, beta-blockers can reduce the myocardial workload by their hemodynamic actions, reducing myocardial ischemia and the potential for arrhythmogenesis [1]. Fourth, in the postinfarction trials, a higher serum potassium was noted and a shorter corrected electrocardiographic QT interval was observed in patients receiving beta-blockers compared to those receiving placebo [43–45]. Beta-blockers, specifically those with β_2-adrenoceptor-blocking activity, have been observed to attenuate in-

TABLE 7–4. Possible Mechanisms by Which Beta-Blockers May Prevent Sudden Cardiac Death in Patients With Myocardial Infarction

Antiarrhythmic (anticatecholamine action)
Raising threshold for ventricular fibrillation
Ventricular premature contraction suppression
Reducing myocardial wall tension
Prevention of free-wall rupture
Antiischemic effects
Reduction of platelet aggregability
Improved collateral blood flow
Reduction of coronary wall tension
Reducing risk of plaque fissure and rupture
Reduction in myocardial infarct size
Metabolic actions
Reducing intracellular transmembrane potassium flux
Reducing lipolysis and free fatty acid production

tracellular transmembrane potassium fluxes in response to high catecholamine levels [46]. Perhaps part of the antiarrhythmic effect of beta-blockers comes from their ability to preserve normokalemia, especially in those patients receiving diuretics [45]. Fifth, during myocardial infarction, adrenergic activity stimulates lipolysis, resulting in increased circulating free fatty acids [47,48]. This, in turn, may augment free fatty acid uptake by the heart, an effect which can increase the risk of arrhythmogenesis [47]. β-Adrenergic blockade can decrease catecholamine-induced lipolysis and myocardial free fatty acid uptake, with a shift in myocardial substrate utilization toward glucose [47].

Although propranolol can markedly reduce the late two- to threefold increase in ventricular arrhythmias observed in patients with myocardial infarction [32], death among myocardial infarction patients is not significantly reduced [49]. Therefore, arrhythmias are not the only important cause of sudden death. Some of these deaths might be caused by free myocardial wall rupture, a risk that could be diminished by beta-blocker-induced attenuation of ventricular wall tension [50].

Other possible mechanisms include a decrease in the size of scar, an increase in vascularity of the myocardium, and an antiplatelet effect [50,51]. The fact that nonsudden cardiac death and reinfarction are decreased by beta-blockade suggests that antiischemic actions of these drugs may be important [52].

There is autopsy evidence that sudden death in patients with ischemic heart disease is sometimes accompanied by fissuring of coronary atheromatous plaques, giving rise to intraluminal thrombosis. It has been proposed that beta-blockers, by diminishing vascular wall tension, could decrease the risk of plaque fissuring and the resultant thrombosis, which might lead to reinfarction or sudden death. Davies et al. [54] demonstrated that the hearts of patients who died suddenly had scattered areas of focal nerosis, predominantly subendocardial: Such lesions might have arisen from either platelet emboli or catecholamine-induced necrosis. Experimentally, it has been shown that similar lesions arising in high catecholamine states might be prevented by beta-blockade [56,57].

CLINICAL TRIALS OF β-ADRENERGIC-BLOCKING DRUGS IN THE PREVENTION OF SUDDEN DEATH

Clinical trials designed to study the effects of beta-blockers on survival have focused on two population groups. The first group of studies examined the effects of beta-blockers in patients during the hyperacute and early phases of myocardial infarction. These acute-phase studies were directed toward influencing the immediate in-hospital mortality and reducing myocardial infarct size [58,59]. It was postulated that the reduction of myocardial infarct size by beta-blockers could favorably affect long-term mortality [58]. Three large, early-intervention clinical trials with beta-blockers showed benefit on survival [60–62]; however, a reduction in the number of episodes of in-hospital ventricular fibrillation [28] compared to placebo was observed in only one of these trials [28,60].

The second group of studies enrolled patients who had survived the early phase of myocardial infarction, and these studies compared survival in those subjects given chronic beta-blocker therapy vs. placebo [63–66]. Although prevention of sudden cardiac death was considered a potential beneficial action of beta-blockade in these trials, most studies focused on all-cause mortality as the primary endpoint. This may have resulted from the difficulty in defining and establishing sudden cardiac death and, in part, the importance of all-cause death.

Included in this review are the findings from randomized, long-term, controlled clinical trials that report on the effects of beta-blocker therapy on the risk of all-cause mortality and sudden cardiac death in patients who had survived an acute myocardial infarction [30,35–40]. Excluded from this review are those trials in which sudden cardiac death was not reported [67,68] and studies that were too small in size to achieve any statistical power.

Study results are presented using the intent-to-treat approach; that is, all randomized patients are accounted for in the group to which they had been assigned. Some of the studies have used other primary statistical analyses, and this explains why the results reported here may differ from those published elsewhere. In the seven trials meeting our review criteria, the beta-blocker intervention was started after patients had been stabilized, usually 7–3 weeks after infarction, with therapy continued for at least 1 year [30,35–40]. Study design features, including the beta-blocker and the dose used, the

TABLE 7–5. Selected Design Features of Long-Term Beta-Blocker Trials

Trial	Patients randomized	Beta-blocker	Daily dose (mg)	Entry time[a] (days)	Mean follow-up (months)
Wilhelmsson et al. [35]	230	Alprenolol	400	7–21[b]	24
Ahlmark et al. [36]	393	Alprenolol	400	14	24
Multicenter International Study [39]	3,053	Practolol	400	13.2	14
Norwegian Multicenter Study [37]	1,884	Timolol	20	11.5	17
BHAT [38]	3,837	Propranolol	180–240	13.8	25
Hansteen et al. [40]	560	Propranolol	160	4–6	12
Julian et al. [30]	1,456	Sotalol	320	8.3	12

[a]Entry into study from time of hospitalization for myocardial infarction.
[b]From discharge following hospitalization for myocardial infarction.

time when treatment was initiated, and the length of treatment, are shown in Table 7–5.

Definition of Sudden Cardiac Death

The primary endpoint in all the trials was death, that is, all-cause mortality. Sudden cardiac death according to various definitions was also an endpoint. In essence, each trial utilized the onset of premonitory symptoms or new symptoms as the starting point for measurement of time. Death occurring within 24 hours of symptom onset constituted the definition in three trials [35–37]. Death occurring within 1 hour of symptoms and excluding only violent deaths was used in the fourth study [38]. A fifth trial reported all nonviolent deaths for both the 24 hour and the 1 hour definitions [30]. Another study divided the cardiac deaths known to have taken place within 24 hours into four time segments: first hour, second hour, 1–12 hours, and 12–24 hours [39]. The seventh report applied the following three definitions: witnessed instantaneous death, death witnessed but preceded by chest pain of less than 1 hour's duration, and patients found dead but seen alive and free of chest pain less than 12 hours earlier [40]. Three trials reported data on the frequency of instantaneous death [37,38,40].

Antiarrhythmic Effects of Beta-Blockers

Three of the seven trials obtained 24 hour ambulatory electrocardiographic (ECG) recordings on a subset of their participants both at trial entry and at a subsequent follow-up visit [30,37,38]. The findings of these three trials are similar. In the subgroup of survivors who entered the trial with frequent ventricular premature beats, fewer patients demonstrated this arrhythmia at a later follow-up visit than in the placebo group [30,32,34].

Among patients with frequent ventricular premature beats at entry, many continued to have this arrhythmia at follow-up, although fewer patients on beta-blockers than on placebo [14,30,32,34]. Although the recorded episodes of ventricular tachycardia were few in all trials at follow-up, this arrhythmia was less common in patients on beta-blockers than on placebo.

Effects on All-Cause Mortality and Sudden Cardiac Death

All-cause mortality was lower in the beta-blocker group compared with the control group for all seven long-term trials [37–39]. The relative differences in mortality rates are expressed as risk ratios (intervention group mortality divided by control group mortality), which ranged from 0.51 to 0.82. When all data are combined, the weighted mean is 0.72, which indicates an overall reduction of 28% in all-cause mortality in the trials.

The rate of sudden cardiac deaths is also lower in the beta-blocker groups for all seven trials. There seems to be a trend toward a greater overall reduction in sudden cardiac death than in all-cause mortality resulting from beta-blocker treatment (Table 7–6). The weighted risk ratios of sudden cardiac death vary between 0.15 and 0.84, with a weighted mean of 0.67, indicating an overall reduction of 33% in sudden cardiac deaths. Indeed, if the sudden cardiac deaths are subtracted from all-cause mortality, the remaining death rate is 3.5% in the intervention group and 4.4% in control, which represents an intervention/control risk ratio for nonsudden death of 0.80. Thus, whereas nonsudden deaths are reduced by 20% in these trials, the sudden cardiac death rate is reduced to a greater extent.

In the five largest trials, the intervention/control risk ratio for nonsudden death ranged from 0.75 to 1.02 [37–39]. The two smallest trials had the most favorable risk ratios of intervention-to-control, that is, 0.51 and 0.61 for all-cause mortality and 0.25 and 0.15 for sudden cardiac death [35,36]. However, these same studies had intervention-to-control risk ratios of 1.4 and 2.8 for nonsudden death. Although it may be argued that this unfavorable difference in nonsudden cardiac death may relate to the specific beta-blocker used, a more probable explanation is the potential for chance associated with small patient numbers.

For witnessed instantaneous deaths, an even larger relative benefit from beta-blocker therapy was recorded. The reduction was 59% in one study [37], 46% in the second [40], and 37% in the third [38], corresponding to an average reduction in instantaneous death of 46%. For these three trials, the pooled reduction in all-cause mortality was 31%, indicating that the relative reduction in instantaneous death is about 50% higher than that of all-cause mortality. When, as above, the instantaneous deaths are removed from the all-cause mortality, the pooled reduction in death in the remaining patients is 23% and the relative reduction in instantaneous deaths twice as great.

TABLE 7–6. Selected Results of Long-Term Beta-Blocker Trials [35]

	Patients randomized		All-cause mortality			Sudden cardiac death			
Trial	Intervention	Control	Intervention (%)	Control (%)	Risk ratio (I/C) (%)	Definition (hr)	Intervention (%)	Control (%)	Risk ratio (I/C) (%)
Wilhelmsson et al. [35]	114	116	6.1	12.1	0.51	≤24	2.6	9.5	0.28
Ahlmark et al. [36]	69[a]	93[a]	7.2	11.8	0.61	≤24	1.4	9.7	0.15
Multicentre Inter-National Study [39]	1,533	1,520	6.7	8.4	0.80	≤1	2.9[b]	4.2[b]	0.70
Norwegian Multicenter Study [37]	945	939	10.4	16.2	0.64	≤24	7.0	11.7	0.60
BHAT [38]	1,916	1,921	7.2	9.8	0.74	≤1	3.3	4.6	0.72
Hansteen et al. [40]	278	282	9.0	13.1	0.69	≤1	4.0	8.2	0.49
Julian et al. [30]	873	583	7.3	8.9	0.82	≤24	5.5	6.5	0.84

[a]Incomplete reporting.
[b]Sudden cardiac death rates underestimated because of missing information.

CONCLUSIONS AND CLINICAL IMPACT

The varied definitions and the difficulty in ascertaining sudden cardiac death have been recognized. When the results of these seven trials involving 11,182 patients are combined, 344 (59%) of the 584 deaths in the placebo-treated group are considered sudden. The results of these long-term beta-blocker trials in survivors of acute myocardial infarction who qualified for treatment demonstrate a clinically and statistically significant reduction in both all-cause mortality and sudden cardiac death of 28% and 33%, respectively. Whether certain beta-blockers are more effective than others has not been well defined. The three beta-blockers approved by the FDA for reducing mortality in infarct survivors (metoprolol, propranolol, and timolol) are without partial agonism; two of these drugs (both nonselective) have also been shown to affect favorably the risk of sudden cardiac death (propranolol and timolol) [37,38].

Continued efforts are needed to subdivide the population of myocardial infarction survivors into those who will have relatively greater and lesser benefits from chronic β-adrenergic blockade. The prognosis of some patient subgroups may be sufficiently favorable without this prophylactic therapy, so any improvement on survival with beta-blockers may not outweigh the potential side effects, costs, and inconvenience [69–71]. Others believe that all postinfarction patients should be treated, even the low-risk subgroup [52,72]. When treating patients with beta-blockers, the length of time following myocardial infarction for which such therapy continues to yield clinical benefit remains undefined. Consensus seems to be that therapy for at least 2–3 years is warranted.

Although some details of patient selection may undergo refinement, the role of β-adrenergic blockers in the management of most survivors of myocardial infarction is now established as a means for decreasing the risk of both sudden and nonsudden cardiac death. Whether similar protective benefits on mortality and sudden cardiac death can be achieved in high-risk coronary patients who have not yet had a myocardial infarction remains to be determined.

REFERENCES

1. Frishman WH, Sonnenblick EH: The beta-adrenergic blocking drugs. In Hurst JW (ed): "The Heart, 7th ed." New York: McGraw-Hill, pp 1712–1731, 1990.
2. Pratt C, Lichstein E: Ventricular antiarrhythmic effects of beta-adrenergic blocking drugs: A review of mechanism and clinical studies. J Clin Pharmacol 22:335–347, 1982.
3. Levy JV, Richards V: Inotropic and chronotropic effects of a series of β-adrenergic blocking drugs: Some structure activity relationships. Proc Soc Exp Biol Med 122:373, 1966.
4. Vaughan Williams EM, Papp J: The effect of oxprenolol on cardiac intracellular potentials in relation to its antiarrhythmic local anesthetic and other properties. Postgrad Med J 46:22–32, 1970.

5. Frishman WH: β-Adrenergic blockade in the treatment of coronary artery disease. In "Clinical Essay on the Heart, Vol. II." New York: McGraw-Hill, 1983, pp 25–63.
6. Latour Y, Dumont G, Brosseau A, et al.: Effects of sotalol in twenty patients with cardiac arrhythmias. Int J Clin Pharmacol 15:275, 1977.
7. Prakash R, Allen HN, Condo F, et al.: Clinical evaluation of the antiarrhythmic effects of sotalol (abstract). Am J Cardiol 26:654, 1970.
8. Simon A, Berman E: Long-term sotalol therapy in patients with arrhythmias. J Clin Pharmacol 19:547–556, 1979.
9. Burckhardt D, Pfisterer M, Hoffman A, et al.: Effects of the beta-adrenoceptor blocking agent sotalol on ventricular arrhythmias in patients with chronic ischemic heart disease: A placebo-controlled, double-blind crossover study. Cardiology 70[Suppl I]:114, 1983.
10. Coltart DJ, Gibson DG, Shand DG: Plasma propranolol levels associated with suppression of ventricular ectopic beats. Br Med J 3:731–734, 1970.
11. Gibson DG: Pharmacodynamic properties of β-adrenergic receptor blocking drugs in man. Drugs 7:8–38, 1974.
12. Frishman W, Silverman R: Clinical pharmacology of the new β-adrenergic blocking drugs: Part 3. Comparative clinical experience and new therapeutic applications. Am Heart J 98:119–131, 1979.
13. Giudicelli JF, Lhoste F, Bossier JR: β-Adrenergic blockade and atrioventricular conduction impairment. Eur J Pharmacol 31:216–225, 1975.
14. Morganroth J: Clinical antiarrhythmic effects of adrenergic blocking agents (class II). In Reiser HJ, Horowitz LN (eds): "Mechanisms and Treatment of Cardiac Arrhythmias." Baltimore: Urban and Schwrzenberg, 1985, pp 249–257.
15. Winkle RA, Gradman AH, Fitzgerald JW, Bell PA: Antiarrhythmic drug effect assessed from ventricular antiarrhythmic reduction in the ambulatory ECG and treadmill test. Comparison of propranolol, procainamide and quinidine. Am J Cardiol 42:473–480, 1978.
16. Winkle RA, Lopes MG, Goodman DJ, Fitzgerald JW, Schroeder JS, Harrison DC: Propranolol for patients with mitral valve prolapse. Am Heart J 93:422–430, 1977.
17. Pratt CB, Matlack J, Carney S, et al.: Effect of metoprolol in suppression of ventricular ectopic beats (abstract). Circulation 62:III–180, 1980.
18. Woosley RL, Kornhause D, Smith R, et al.: Suppression of chronic ventricular arrhythmias with propranolol. Circulation 60:819–827, 1979.
19. deSoyza N, Kane JJ, Murphy ML, Laddu AR, Doherty JE, Bissett JK: The long-term suppression of ventricular arrhythmias by oral acebutolol in patients with coronary artery disease. Am Heart J 100:631–638, 1980.
20. Koppes GM, Beckmann CH, Jones FG: Propranolol therapy for ventricular arrhythmias two months post acute myocardial infarction. Am J Cardiol 46:322–328, 1980.
21. Schlemann M, Morganroth J, Reid P: Beta-blockade for suppression of high grade ventricular arrhythmias (abstract). J Am Coll Cardiol 1:613, 1983.
22. Morganroth J: Short-term evaluation of atenolol in hospitalized patients with chronic ventricular arrhythmias. Drugs 5:181–185, 1983.
23. Podrid PJ, Lown B: Pindolol for ventricular arrhythmias. Am Heart J 104:491–496, 1982.
24. Taylor RR, Halliday EJ: β-Adrenergic blockade in the treatment of exercise-induced paroxysmal ventricular tachycardia. Circulation 32:778–782, 1965.
25. Sloman G, Stannard M: β-Adrenergic blockade and cardiac arrhythmias. Br Med J 4: 508–512, 1967.
26. Gettes LS, Surawicz B: Long-term prevention of paroxysmal arrhythmias with propranolol therapy. Am J Med Sci 254:256–265, 1967.
27. Anderson JL, Rodier HE, Green LS: Comparative effects of beta-adrenergic blocking drugs on experimental ventricular fibrillation threshold. Am J Cardiol 51:1196–1202, 1983.

28. Ryden L, Ariniego R, Arnman K, et al.: A double-blind trial of metoprolol in acute myocardial infarction: Effects on ventricular tachyarrhythmias. N Engl J Med 308: 614–618, 1983.
29. Yusuf S, Sleight P, Rossi P: Reduction in infarct size, arrhythmias, and chest pain by early intravenous beta-blockade in suspected acute myocardial infarction. Circulation 67[Suppl 1]:32–41, 1983.
30. Julian DG, Prescott RJ, Jackson FS, et al.: Controlled trial of sotalol for one year after myocardial infarction. Lancet 1:1142–1147, 1982.
31. Hjalmarson A, Herlitz J, Holmberg S, et al.: The Goteberg metoprolol study: Effects on mortality and morbidity in acute myocardial infarction. Circulation 67[Suppl 1]:I26–32, 1983.
32. Lichstein E, Morganroth J, Harrist R, et al.: Effects or propranolol on ventricular arrhythmias: The Beta-Blocker Heart Attack Trial. Circulation 67[Suppl 1]:I5–10, 1983.
33. Koppes GM, Beckmann CH, Jones FG: Propranolol therapy for ventricular arrhythmias two months after acute myocardial infarction. Am J Cardiol 46:322–328, 1980.
34. von der Lippe G, Lund-Johansen P: Effect of timolol on late ventricular arrhythmias after myocardial infarction. Acta Med Scand 65[Suppl]:253–258, 1981.
35. Wilhelmsson C, Vedin JA, Wilhelmsen L, et al.: Reduction of sudden deaths after myocardial infarction by treatment with alprenolol: Preliminary results. Lancet 2:1157–1160, 1974.
36. Ahlmark G, Saetre H: Long-term treatment with beta-blockers after myocardial infarction. Eur J Clin Pharmacol 10:77–83, 1976.
37. Norwegian Multicenter Study Group: Timolol-induced reduction in mortality and reinfarction in patients surviving acute myocardial infarction. N Engl J Med 304:801–807, 1981.
38. Beta-Blocker Heart Attack Trial Research Group: A randomized trial of propranolol in patients with acute myocardial infarction. I. Mortality results. JAMA 247:1707–1714, 1981.
39. Multicentre International Study: Reduction in mortality after myocardial infarction with long-term beta-adrenoreceptor blockade: Supplementary report. Br Med J 2:419–421, 1977.
40. Hansteen V, Moinichen E, Lorentsen E, et al.: One year's treatment with propranolol after myocardial infarction: Preliminary report of Norwegian Multicentre Trial. Br Med J 284:155–160, 1982.
41. Singh BN, Jewitt DE: β-Adrenergic receptor drugs in cardiac arrhythmias. Drugs 7: 426–446, 1974.
42. Frishman W: β-Adrenoceptor antagonists: New drugs and new indications. N Engl J Med 305:500–506, 1981.
43. Furberg CD, Byington RP, Prineas RJ: Potassium, $beta_2$-receptor blockade and mortality, the BHAT experience (abstract). Circulation 70[Suppl II]:II–7, 1984.
44. Jardine RM, Obel IW, Smith AM: Intravenous acebutolol raises serum potassium in acute myocardial infarction. Eur Heart J 7:140–145, 1986.
45. Nordehaug JE, Johannessen KA, von der Lippe G, et al.: Effect of timolol on changes in serum potassium concentration during acute myocardial infarction. Br Heart J 53:388–393, 1985.
46. Brown MJ, Brown DC, Murphy MB: Hypokalemia from $beta_2$ receptor stimulation by circulating epinephrine. N Engl J Med 309:1414–1419, 1983.
47. The International Collaborative Study Group: Reduction of infarct size with the early use of timolol in acute myocardial infarction. N Engl J Med 310:9–15, 1984.
48. Opie LH: Myocardial infarct size: Part 1. Basic considerations. Am Heart J 100:355–372, 1980.
49. Friedman LM, Byington RP, Capone RJ, Furberg CD, Goldstein S, Lichstein E: Effect of

propranolol in patients with myocardial infarction and ventricular arrhythmia. J Am Coll Cardiol 7:1–8, 1986.
50. Cruickshank JM, Prichard BNC: "Beta Blockers in Clinical Practice." Edinburg: Churchill Livingstone, 1987, pp 435–504.
51. Frishman WH: Multifactorial actions of β-adrenergic blocking drugs in ischemic heart disease: Current concepts. Circulation 67[Part 2]:I–11–18, 1983.
52. Frishman WH, Furberg CD, Friedewald WT: The use of β-adrenergic blocking drugs in patients with myocardial infarction. Curr Prob Cardiol 9:1–50, 1984.
53. Davies MJ, Thomas AC: Plaque fissuring—The cause of acute myocardial infarction, sudden ischemic death and crescendo angina. Br Heart J 53:363–373, 1985.
54. Davies MJ, Thomas AC, Knapman PA, Hangartner JR: Intramyocardial platelet aggregation in patients with unstable angina suffering sudden ischemic cardiac death. Circulation 73:418–427, 1986.
55. Falk E: Unstable angina with fatal outcome: Dynamic coronary thrombosis leading to infarction and/or sudden death. Atuopsy evidence of recurrent mural thrombosis with peripheral embolization culminating in total vascular occlusion. Circulation 71:699–708, 1985.
56. Neil-Dwyer G, Walter P, Cruickshank JM, Doshi B, O'Gorman P: Effect of propranolol and phentolamine on myocardial necrosis after subarachnoid hemorrhage. Br Med J 2:990–992, 1978.
57. Cruickshank JM, Degaute JP, Kuurne T, et al.: Reduction of stress/catecholamine-induced cardiac necrosis by $beta_1$-selective blockade. Lancet 2:585–589, 1987.
58. May GS: A review of acute-phase beta-blocker trials in patients with myocardial infarction. Circulation 67[Suppl 1]:I21–25, 1983.
59. Muller J, Roberts R, Stone P, et al.: Failure of propranolol administration to limit infarct size in patients with acute myocardial infarction (abstract). Circulation 68[Suppl III]: 294, 1983.
60. Hjalmarson A, Elmfeldt D, Herlitz J, et al.: Effect on mortality of metoprolol in acute myocardial infarction: A double-blind randomized trial. Lancet 2:823–827, 1981.
61. MIAMI Trial Research Group: Metoprolol in acute myocardial infarction (MIAMI). A randomized, placebo-controlled international trial. Eur Heart J 6:199–226, 1985.
62. ISIS-I (First International Study of Infarct Survival) Collaborative Group: Randomized trial of intravenous atenolol among 16,027 cases of suspected acute myocardial infarction: ISIS-I. Lancet 2:57–66, 1986.
63. May GS: A review of long-term beta-blocker trials in survivors of myocardial infarction. Circulation 67[Suppl 1]:I46–49, 1983.
64. Taylor SH, Silke B, Ebbutt A, et al.: A long-term prevention study with oxprenolol in coronary heart disease. N Engl J Med 307:1293–1301, 1982.
65. Australian and Swedish Pindolol Study Group: The effect of pindolol on the two year mortality after complicated myocardial infarction. Eur Heart J 4:367–375, 1983.
66. European Infarction Study Group: European Infarct Study (EIS): A secondary beta-blocker prevention trial after myocardial infarction (abstract). Circulation 68[Suppl III]:294, 1983.
67. Baber NS, Wainwright-Evans D, Howitt G, et al.: Multicentre post-infarction trial of propranolol in 49 hospitals in the United Kingdom, Italy and Yugoslavia. Br Heart J 44:96–100, 1980.
68. Coronary Prevention Research Group: An early intervention secondary prevention study with oxprenolol following myocardial infarction. Eur Heart J 2:389, 1981.
69. Chamberlain DA: Beta-adrenoceptor antagonists after myocardial infarction—Where are we now? Br Heart J 49:105–110, 1983.
70. Griggs TR, Wagner GS, Gettes LS: Beta-adrenergic blocking agents after myocardial

infarction: An undocumented need in patients at lowest risk. J Am Coll Cardiol 1: 1530–1533, 1983.
71. Goldman L, Sia STB, Cook EF, et al.: Costs and effectiveness of routine therapy with long-term beta-adrenergic antagonists after myocardial infarction. N Engl J Med 319: 152–157, 1988.
72. Frishman WH, Furberg CD, Friedewald WT: Beta-adrenergic blockade for survivors of acute myocardial infarction. N Engl J Med 310:830–836, 1984.

Chapter 8

Pharmacologic Prevention of Sudden Cardiac Death: Role of Antiarrhythmic Drugs

J. Thomas Bigger, Jr., M.D.

Arrhythmia Control Unit, Columbia–Presbyterian Medical Center, New York, New York 10032

INTRODUCTION

In this chapter, we discuss the prevention of sudden cardiac death by using drugs to treat ventricular arrhythmias. We do not discuss the potential of β-adrenergic blocking drugs to prevent sudden cardiac death because Dr. Frishman has discussed this topic in the previous chapter. To plan an attack on sudden cardiac death, the prognostic significance of ventricular arrhythmias should be assessed prior to initiating drug treatment. Prognostic classification requires determination of the presence and etiology of heart disease, quantitative measurement of left ventricular dysfunction, as well as categorization of the ventricular arrhythmias [1,2]. Table 8–1 shows the methodology for classifying ventricular arrhythmias by prognosis. The scientific basis for the classification is the independent predictive value of left ventricular dysfunction and spontaneous ventricular arrhythmias for cardiac death [3–5]. In descending order of risk for sudden cardiac death are: 1) malignant ventricular arrhythmias, with severe left ventricular dysfunction; 2) malignant ventricular arrhythmias, with mild left ventricular dysfunction; 3) potentially malignant ventricular arrhythmias, with severe left ventricular dysfunction; and 4) potentially malignant ventricular arrhythmias, with mild left ventricular dysfunction. As discussed in previous chapters, the presence

The Prevention of Sudden Cardiac Death, pages 155–195

TABLE 8–1. Prognostic Classification of Ventricular Arrhythmias[a]

	Benign	Potentially malignant	Malignant
Risk for sudden death	Very low	Low to moderate	High
Clinical presentation	Palpitations; detected by routine exam	Palpitations; detected by routine exam or screening	Palpitations; syncope; cardiac arrest
Heart disease	Usually absent	Present	Present
Cardiac scarring and/or hypertrophy	Absent	Present	Present
Left ventricular ejection fraction	Normal	Low to very low	Low to very low
VPD frequency	Low to moderate	Moderate to high	Moderate to high
Sustained VT	Absent	Absent	Present
Hemodynamic effects of arrhythmia	Absent	Absent to mild	Moderate to severe

[a]The characteristics listed in this table are typical but do not represent the full range of observations. For example, benign ventricular arrhythmias can be frequent, and occasionally, repetitive. VPD, ventricular premature depolarization(s); VT, ventricular tachycardia.

or absence of late potentials in the signal-averaged electrocardiogram (ECG) increases the likelihood of future sustained ventricular arrhythmias or sudden cardiac death in patients with potentially malignant ventricular arrhythmias [6–12]. The prognostic classification of ventricular arrhythmias is a powerful tool for managing these diverse rhythm disturbances. It provides a reasonably accurate measure of the risk/benefit ratio, efficacy rate, and rates of several adverse effects, e.g., proarrhythmia and aggravation of congestive heart failure. Also, the prognostic classification provides information useful for selecting from the ever-widening array of antiarrhythmic drugs. For example, for potentially malignant ventricular arrhythmias but with good left ventricular function, drugs with class IC action have the best risk/benefit ratio, whereas for malignant ventricular arrhythmias but with poor left ventricular function, drugs with class IA action or combinations of drugs with class IA and IB actions have the best risk/benefit ratio.

The prognostic classification is used together with symptoms and knowledge about the potential risks and benefits of treatment to make management decisions. For example, patients with malignant ventricular arrhythmias and poor left ventricular function have a high risk of dying and usually have severe symptoms during episodes of sustained ventricular arrhythmias. Also, it has been shown beyond reasonable doubt that adequate treatment with antiarrhythmic drugs can reduce the frequency of symptomatic sustained ventricular arrhythmias and can prolong life. Therefore, patients with malignant ventricular arrhythmias and poor left ventricular function should all be treated. The principal issue with these patients is how to evaluate treatment (see below). On the other hand, patients with potentially malignant ventricular arrhythmias, regardless of left ventricular function, have no known benefit from treatment in terms of prolonging life. Therefore, they have no indication for treatment unless arrhythmic symptoms are present. It is almost impossible to make an asymptomatic patient feel better with antiarrhythmic drug treatment. A special cautionary note is in order for patients who have potentially malignant ventricular arrhythmias and poor left ventricular function, especially those with a clinical heart failure syndrome. The use of antiarrhythmic drugs in this group is inadequately studied, but it is apparent that special problems attend the use of antiarrhythmic drugs in this group of patients [13]. First, antiarrhythmic drugs are less likely to be effective in patients with left ventricular dysfunction. Second, the pharmacokinetic properties of antiarrhythmic drugs are altered substantially in patients with significant left ventricular dysfunction. Absorption of drugs may be slowed due to reduced splanchnic blood flow. The volume of distribution of antiarrhythmic drugs usually is reduced substantially in patients with congestive heart failure. Elimination of drugs is slowed in heart failure due to reduced splanchnic or renal blood flow or to slowed hepatic metabolism. Adverse effect rates tend to be higher in patients with heart failure, at least for some drugs. Aggravation of congestive heart failure by drugs is strongly dependent on the degree of left ventricular dysfunction, and proarrhythmia may be. A detailed review of the pharmacology of antiarrhythmic drugs is beyond the scope of this discussion and recent reviews should be consulted for information on this topic.

In this chapter, we discuss the evidence that drug treatment improves outcome (i.e., prevents symptomatic ventricular arrhythmias and sudden cardiac death) as well as how to evaluate drug therapy for patients with malignant ventricular arrhythmias. Then, we discuss previously completed and ongoing trials of antiarrhythmic drug treatment in patients with potentially malignant ventricular arrhythmias.

PREDICTION OF ANTIARRHYTHMIC DRUG EFFICACY IN PATIENTS WITH MALIGNANT VENTRICULAR ARRHYTHMIAS

A number of studies have shown that drugs that prevent initiation of ventricular tachycardia (VT) or ventricular fibrillation during programmed ventricular stimulation have a high degree of efficacy during long-term follow-up, whereas those that do not prevent sustained ventricular arrhythmias are associated with a much higher rate of arrhythmia recurrence and sudden death during long-term follow-up [14–25]. One group has reported that a programmatic evaluation using ECG monitoring, 24 hour ECG recording, and exercise testing also has predictive accuracy for long-term efficacy of drug therapy for malignant ventricular arrhythmias [26–30].

Selection of Long-Term Drug Treatment for Malignant Ventricular Arrhythmias

The efficacy of antiarrhythmic drug treatment has been demonstrated for patients with malignant ventricular arrhythmias, i.e., sustained VT or cardiac arrest due to ventricular fibrillation. More and more patients with malignant ventricular arrhythmias have been salvaged from their initial event as community programs have been developed to deal with out-of-hospital cardiac arrest. Patients who are resuscitated after an episode of sustained VT have a recurrence rate for sustained ventricular arrhythmias of 25–50% per year, and many recurrences are fatal. Thus, these patients must be treated aggressively with the best means at hand. The first line of treatment is antiarrhythmic drugs. Arbitrary drug therapy, i.e., giving a patient an antiarrhythmic drug and discharging him, is associated with high recurrence and fatality rates. Although arbitrary drug treatment is still used for malignant ventricular arrhythmias, it is giving way to methods that utilize programmatic evaluation of drug efficacy before selecting an agent for long-term treatment. Drug/dose finding in patients with malignant ventricular arrhythmias must be evaluated with rigorous methods shown to have an excellent predictive accuracy for a good long-term clinical response. Patients with malignant ventricular arrhythmias are admitted to hospital and monitored in a telemetry facility or intensive care unit while the sequelae of the most recent episode of sustained ventricular arrhythmia are treated and a search is made for a reversible and temporary cause for the arrhythmia, e.g., myocardial infarction, electrolyte derangement, or drug toxicity. If no reversible cause is found, further work-up should proceed under the assumption that the condition that caused the sustained arrhythmia is chronic and that the arrhythmia will recur. Antiarrhythmic drugs should be discontinued, and the arrhythmia substrate should be characterized with a baseline evaluation that includes 48 hours of continuous ECG recording, exercise testing, and electrophysiologic studies. In addition, left ventricular function and coronary anatomy should be evaluated. This initial evaluation not only will clarify the biology of the arrhythmia but also will indicate how drug/dose finding should proceed. If sustained ventricular tachycardia is recurring several times a day, then evaluation with ECG recordings and exercise testing is preferred. This situation is rare. If ventricular ectopic activity is infrequent, e.g., fewer than 10 ventricular premature depolarizations (VPD) per hour on the average over the 48 hour recording period, treatment guided by electrophysiologic studies is preferred. This situation is common. The standard method for drug/dose finding is endocardial electrical stimulation (programmed ventricular stimulation) [14–25]. Recent studies suggest that a programmatic noninvasive approach using 24 hour continuous ECG recordings and exercise tests can be used to evaluate treatment of malignant ventricular arrhythmias [26–30].

Twenty-Four Hour Continuous ECG Recordings and Exercise Tests in Patients With Malignant Ventricular Arrhythmias

Continuous 24 hour ECG recording has the following advantages for evaluating drug efficacy. Computerized arrhythmia detectors can provide accurate quantification of drug effects on ventricular ectopic activity [31–34]. During dose ranging, i.e., doses can be adjusted until efficacy is achieved. Dose response information is the best way to establish the causal role of a drug in suppressing ventricular ectopy [35,36]. The 24 hour continuous ECG recording is useful for predicting long-term efficacy, detecting cardiac electrical adverse effects, and monitoring treatment effects during follow-up.

The disadvantages of 24 hour ECG recording for judging drug efficacy are: 1) many patients with malignant ventricular arrhythmias have too few ventricular arrhythmias to use this method; 2) spontaneous variability of ventricular arrhythmias can mimic either efficacy or toxicity, making judgments difficult in individual patients [37–39]; 3) the response of spontaneous ventricular ectopy to drugs provides no insight into the effect of drugs on the substrate for sustained ventricular arrhythmias or on the ventricular fibrillation threshold; and 4) it is technically difficult and expensive to perform a series of accurate quantitative analyses of 24 hour ECG recordings for antiarrhythmic drug evaluation. As many as 30–50% of patients with malignant ventricular arrhythmias have fewer than 10–30 VPDs per hour in a 24–48 hour ECG recording [40,41]. Swerdlow and Peterson [40] compared baseline 24 hour ECG recordings and electrophysiologic studies in 43 consecutive patients with coronary heart disease who had sustained ventricular tachyarrhythmias to compare the suitability of each method for guiding drug therapy. A 24 hour ECG recording with ≥30 VPDs per hour was found in only 50% of patients. Electrophysiologic studies induced sustained, uniform VT suitable for electropharmacologic testing in 82%. Thus, in these 43 consecutive patients with coronary heart disease and sustained ventricular tachyarrhythmias, electrophysiologic studies were suitable for guiding therapy more frequently than 24 hour ECG recordings. Kim et al. [41] found that only 52 of 112 patients (46%) with sustained ventricular arrhythmias were suitable for testing with both electrophysiologic studies and 24 hour ECG recordings. About 40% had fewer than 30 VPDs per hour in their 24 hour ECG recording. The arrhythmia response to exercise is even less reproducible than 24 hour continuous ECG recordings, but exercise testing can be useful by provoking arrhythmias on drugs that have been judged efficacious on the basis of Holter criteria [42]. Also, exercise can reveal drug-associated aggravation of ventricular arrhythmias. The Holter/exercise method can be very expensive because of the extended hospitalization needed for drug/dose finding.

The Holter/exercise method is very likely to identify an effective drug. It is not yet clear whether this is an advantage, because the relative predictive accuracy of the tests is not established.

Electrophysiologic Studies in Malignant Ventricular Arrhythmias

Programmed ventricular stimulation is the most commonly used quantitative method to evaluate antiarrhythmic drug efficacy in patients with malignant ventricular arrhythmias. Programmed ventricular stimulation will provoke a sustained VT suitable for drug evaluation in about 80% of patients with coronary heart disease and malignant ventricular arrhythmias [43]. The sensitivity of programmed ventricular stimulation is less, about 60%, in patients with cardiomyopathy [43]. This technique can be used when spontaneous ventricular arrhythmias are infrequent or absent. Programmed ventricular stimulation is sensitive [44], reproducible [43,45], and accurate for predicting the outcome of treatment [16–25]. Also, programmed ventricular stimulation is quite useful for detecting adverse drug effects on the sinus node, atrioventricular node, and His-Purkinje system [46] and for detecting the proarrhythmic effects of antiarrhythmic drugs [47]. The electrophysiologic technique is safe, having about the same morbidity as insertion of a Swan-Ganz catheter under direct fluoroscopic guidance. Programmed ventricular stimulation requires only a venapuncture and can be repeated when, in the course of therapy, the physician wants to evaluate new symptoms or to determine the arrhythmic status after new events, e.g., myocardial infarction or coronary bypass graft surgery. Also, electrophysiologic studies should be used during follow-up for evaluating changes in antiarrhythmic drugs or doses or a change in concomitant therapy in patients with malignant ventricular arrhythmias.

Electrophysiologic studies also have disadvantages. Patients who are not inducible during baseline drug-free cannot have drug efficacy evaluated by this technique. About 10–15% of the patients whose spontaneous clinical event was sustained VT, and 30–40% of the patients who survive an episode of ventricular fibrillation cannot be induced by programmed ventricular stimulation. The likelihood of inducing sustained VT with programmed ventricular stimulation in patients with malignant ventricular arrhythmias is substantially less if the etiologic heart disease is cardiomyopathy rather than coronary heart disease. It is impractical to evaluate a full range of oral doses of an antiarrhythmic drug using programmed ventricular stimulation. Even though programmed ventricular stimulation is simpler and can be less expensive than 24 hour ECG recordings [48,49], the expense of serial drug evaluation with electrophysiologic studies is substantial because of extended hospitalization required to complete drug testing in drug resistant patients. The results of programmed ventricular stimulation provide no further information about drug effect on ambient ventricular ectopy. It is current practice to hospitalize patients for a day for programmed ventricular stimulation when the test needs to be repeated during follow-up, making this test less convenient than Holter recordings for evaluation during long-term follow-up.

Programmed ventricular stimulation is less likely to identify a successful treatment than Holter/exercise [41,50–52]. It remains to be seen which technique more accurately predicts future events.

Sequencing Tests and Drugs for Malignant Ventricular Arrhythmias

The rationale and process of evaluating drug efficacy in malignant ventricular arrhythmias is similar for the noninvasive method and the invasive electrophysiologic method [17,18,26,51]. With either method, the patient is stabilized, and baseline drug-free studies are carried out to determine the biologic nature of the arrhythmia and the techniques that can be used to evaluate the patient. Patients who are not evaluable by one method are evaluated by the alternate method or are treated empirically. Patients who are evaluable are then tested with a series of drugs until the efficacy criteria are satisfied. For the noninvasive method, efficacy usually is defined as a 50–80% reduction in VPD frequency, 80–90% reduction in paired VPD, and 90–100% reduction in runs of unsustained ventricular tachycardia (three or more consecutive VPDs) [26,51]. When a drug or drug combination is predicted to be successful by these criteria, the patient is discharged on this regimen and followed.

The criterion for efficacy using programmed ventricular stimulation is conversion of inducible, sustained ventricular tachycardia to unsustained or no ventricular tachycardia. There is some variability in the definition of ventricular tachycardia among clinical electrophysiology laboratories: >10 complexes, >100 complexes, >15 seconds, and >30 seconds have all been used. At present, there is no theoretical or experimental basis for choosing among these definitions. Some other electrophysiologic endpoints have been used to define drug efficacy, e.g., increased difficulty in inducing sustained ventricular tachycardia [53] or induction of a slower, better tolerated ventricular tachyarrhythmia [24,25].

The most convincing evidence that changing the characteristics of the induced VT can be used as a predictor of favorable long-term outcome was reported by Waller et a. [25]. These workers studied 258 patients who were referred for electrophysiologic studies and had inducible sustained VT or ventricular fibrillation. The two most common etiologic forms of heart disease were coronary heart disease (210 patients, 81%) and cardiomyopathy (19 patients, 11%). These authors used slowing of the ventricular arrhythmia and lack of severe symptoms during the induced arrhythmia as indicators of a good long-term outcome. For patients with sustained VT, the cycle length of the tachycardia had to increase by at least 100 msec. For patients with ventricular fibrillation, the absolute cycle length of the VT had to be 300 msec or greater. Severe symptoms were defined as syncope, near syncope, dizziness, angina, or dyspnea. At the baseline study, the induced arrhythmia

TABLE 8–2. Response to Electrophysiologic Drug Testing and Outcome[a]

Drug response	N	Recurrence of sustained ventricular arrhythmia (%)	Total mortality (%)	Sudden cardiac death[b] (%)
Uninducible	103	7	13	3
Beneficial	51	39	12	4
No benefit	104	50	39	34

[a]Reproduced from Waller et al. [25] with permission of the publisher.
[b]Unexpected, witnessed death occurring within 1 hour of the onset of symptoms not otherwise explained. Patients who were resuscitated from cardiac arrest during follow-up also were considered as suffering sudden cardiac death. These events occurred during an average follow-up of 21 months.

was sustained VT in 221 patients (86%) and ventricular fibrillation in 37 patients (14%). Severe symptoms were present in 241 patients (93%) during tachycardia in the baseline study. Using these responses, the patients were divided into three groups: 1) those who were rendered uninducible (n = 103), 2) those who remained inducible but had a response considered beneficial (n = 51), and 3) those who had no benefit predicted (n = 104). Patients were followed up to three years (mean of 21 months).

Table 8–2 shows the follow-up findings in the three groups. The patients who became noninducible had a low rate of recurrence of VT and a low mortality rate. Patients who were inducible but showed a beneficial response had a high rate of recurrence of VT but a low mortality rate. Patients who showed no beneficial response had a high rate of recurrence of VT and a high mortality rate. Half of the patients were treated with amiodarone alone, 37% with a drug with class I action alone, and the remainder with drug combinations or other classes of drugs. The response to programmed ventricular stimulation was equally predictive for amiodarone vs. other drugs. It is interesting that neither the increase in VT cycle length nor the change in severity of symptoms during tachycardia alone was predictive of clinical outcome. Thus the combined endpoint seemed necessary for accurate prediction. The recommendation made on the basis of these findings is that patients who do not become uninducible on drugs or have a beneficial response should not be treated with drugs if any other form of treatment is an option. Patients who are inducible but have a beneficial response to one of a series of drugs can be treated with the drug that slows their tachycardia and renders them asymptomatic. However, half of these patients will experience a nonfatal recurrence of their tachycardia within 1 year. This probability should be discussed candidly with the patient and his family. The endpoints reported by Waller et al. [25] are promising but require additional study and independent validation.

The usual sequence for drugs that are tested in patients with malignant ventricular arrhythmias is substantially different from the sequence used in benign or potentially malignant ventricular arrhythmias [54]. First in the sequence is a drug with class IA action (e.g., quinidine or procainamide), followed by a combination of class IA and IB drugs (e.g., quinidine and mexiletine), drugs with class IC action (e.g., encainide, flecainide, or propafenone), and finally drugs with class III action (amiodarone). Drugs with class IC action are used later in the treatment sequence in patients with malignant ventricular arrhythmias, because, although IC drugs are more efficacious than IA drugs, they also are more likely to aggravate the arrhythmia and left ventricular dysfunction [55,56]. These latter adverse effects are disease-related. For patients with benign arrhythmias or patients with potentially malignant ventricular arrhythmias without severe left ventricular dysfunction, drugs with class IC action are least likely to aggravate ventricular arrhythmias. For patients with benign ventricular arrhythmias and for most patients with potentially malignant ventricular arrhythmias, aggravation of left ventricular dysfunction is not an issue. Amiodarone is used last because of its frequent and severe toxicity [57]. dl-Sotalol is an interesting drug that will be marketed in the United States in the near future. This drug has class II (beta-blockade) and class III antiarrhythmic action [58]. It is more likely than either class I drugs or amiodarone to render patients with malignant ventricular arrhythmias uninducible; it will convert about 40%. Its tolerance and long-term adverse effects need to be better defined in this group of patients.

Patients in Whom Drugs Cannot Be Evaluated

About 10% of patients with malignant ventricular arrhythmias are not evaluable with either noninvasive or electrophysiologic methods, i.e., have low frequency of spontaneous ventricular ectopic activity and are not inducible by programmed ventricular stimulation [40,41]. This situation is much more common in survivors of cardiac arrest due to ventricular fibrillation than in patients who have had recurrent, sustained ventricular tachycardia. Patients who are not evaluable by either the Holter/exercise method or the electrophysiologic method present difficult judgements. Patients who have ischemia demonstrated on exercise/perfusion studies should be revascularized aggressively with percutaneous transluminal coronary angioplasty (PTCA) or coronary artery bypass graft surgery on the likelihood that an ischemic episode may have been responsible for the cardiac arrest. This approach is encouraged further if ischemic symptoms preceded the cardiac arrest and left ventricular function is good. Patients with previous myocardial infarction and poor left ventricular function and particularly those with left ventricular aneurysms are more likely to have had a scar-related sustained ventricular arrhythmia. Additional attempts should be made to induce them, including stimulation of left ventricular sites and use of maneuvers that increase cardiac sympathetic activity, e.g., isoproterenol infusion [59]. If none of these maneuvers elicits a sustained arrhythmia, the most effective empirical treatment should be selected. For patients with coronary heart and previous myocardial infarction, this usually is the automatic implantable cardioverter defibrillator. Currently, this is not an approved indication for the device, but it should be.

Are All Drugs Evaluable by Acute Drug Testing?

The concern has been raised that some drugs may not be evaluable by the tests that are used currently to predict efficacy, i.e., that the predictive value of either 24 hour continuous ECG recordings or electrophysiologic studies is lower for some drugs. Thus the drug may fail during long-term treatment even though success is predicted by acute drug testing. Conversely, the drug may succeed during long-term treatment even though failure is predicted by acute drug testing. Amiodarine is a prominent example of this latter concern. Early reports suggested that a negative electrophysiologic test in patients with malignant ventricular arrhythmias had low predictive accuracy; i.e., patients who were still inducible on amiodarone did well during follow-up. There are a number of possible explanations for this finding. First, the test may have been done improperly. Amiodarone has bizarre pharmacokinetic properties, accumulating in the body over many weeks. It is possible therefore that a test done too early could be uninformative. Second, without a control group, it is difficult to conclude whether a drug is altering the natural history of an arrhythmia. In many patients, recurrences of sustained ventricular arrhythmias are infrequent so that an ineffective drug could give a false impression of efficacy. There were never any controlled studies done for amiodarone treatment of malignant ventricular arrhythmias.

Contrary to early opinion, recent studies show that electrophysiologic studies have excellent predictive accuracy for amiodarone [22,24,60–65]. The largest study is that of Horowitz et al. [24], who studied 100 patients with coronary heart disease, 97 of whom had experienced a previous myocardial infarction. All the patients were inducible, i.e., had sustained ventricular arrhythmias in response to programmed ventricular stimulation during their baseline electrophysiologic study. Patients were studied about 2 weeks after a 10–13 g loading dose of amiodarone had been administered. In 20 patients, the ventricular tachyarrhythmia was no longer inducible after amiodarone; no recurrent arrhythmia occurred in this group during an average follow-up period of 18 ± 10 months. In 80 patients, the arrhythmia remained inducible after amiodarone; 38 of these patients (48%) had arrhythmia recurrence during a follow-up of 12 ± 9 months. The dose of amiodarone at the time of recurrence was 600 mg/day in 21 patients, 400 mg/day in 14 patients, and <400 mg/day in three patients. The dose and plasma concentration of amiodarone was higher in the group of patients with recurrences during follow-up than in those without recurrences. Additional prognostic information was obtained from analysis of the rate of the sustained ventricular arrhythmia induced by programmed ventricular stimulation and the symptoms experienced during the tachyarrhythmia. Of 24 patients who had cardiovascular collapse or other severe symptoms during electrophysiologic study after amiodarone treatment, 12 had sudden death during follow-up. Of 56 patients who had moderate symptoms during the induced ventricular arrhythmia, 26 (46%) had a spontaneous sustained arrhythmia during follow-up, but there were no fatal arrhythmias or sudden cardiac deaths in this group. This study showed that electrophysiologic testing provides clinical guidance and predicts prognosis in patients treated with amiodarone as it does for the evaluation of other antiarrhythmic agents. These findings suggest that patients who develop rapid symptomatic ventricular arrhythmias during an electrophysiologic evaluation of amiodarone should be taken off amiodarone and managed with another treatment, e.g., surgical ablation or implantation of an automatic cardioverter defibrillator.

Because of its peculiar pharmacokinetic properties, the electrophysiologic and antiarrhythmic effects of amiodarone continue to accumulate over the first weeks of treatment [66]. Because of logistical constraints, it is common practice to give large loading doses of amiodarone and to evaluate the efficacy of treatment with an electrophysiologic study after about 2 weeks of treatment. If the study indicates efficacy, the patient is often placed on a lower maintenance dose and then followed. Also, adverse effects often prompt lowering of the maintenance dose. Unfortunately, the antiarrhythmic effect of amiodarone against sustained ventricular arrhythmias can be lost when the dose is reduced during maintenance therapy [67]. When doses are reduced during the course of follow-up, serious consideration should be given to reevaluation with an electrophysiologic study.

Direct Comparison of Noninvasive Methods and Invasive Electrophysiologic Studies

Until head-to-head comparisons of electrophysiologic studies and noninvasive methods are done, we will not know which method is preferable for drug evaluation in patients with malignant ventricular arrhythmias. These two methods need to be compared for predictive accuracy, efficiency, and cost. To make a valid comparison, patients who are evaluable by both noninvasive and electrophysiologic methods must be studied. Patients must have a sufficient level of ambient ectopy in their baseline 24 or 48 hour continuous ECG recordings and should have sustained, uniform ventricular tachycardia as a response to programmed ventricular stimulation. To avoid bias in the allocation of patients and to ensure the validity of statistically significant tests, patients who are comparable at enrollment must be randomized to the two approaches for evaluating treatment [68]. Only two such comparisons have been done: a recently completed small study by investigators in Calgary, Canada [50], and an ongoing multicenter study called ESVEM [51].

TABLE 8–3. Comparison of the Calgary Study and ESVEM

	Calgary study	ESVEM[a]
Presented with clinical arrhythmia	124	1,114
Not excluded	105	779
Randomized	57	232
No drug found effective	13	63
Discharged on drug predicted effective	44	136

[a]As of April 30, 1988.

Some of the major features of these two important trials are given in Table 8–3.

The Calgary Trial

Between February, 1983, and April, 1986, Mitchell et al. [50] in Calgary, Canada, randomized patients with symptomatic potentially malignant or malignant ventricular arrhythmias to therapy selected either with noninvasive (Holter recordings and exercise tests) or with electrophysiologic studies. During the study period, 124 patients presented, of whom 105 survived, were not excluded, and consented to participate. After written consent was obtained, baseline studies were done without antiarrhythmic drugs. The baseline studies included a 24 hour continuous ECG recording, exercise test, electrophysiologic study, and radionuclide ventriculogram. To qualify for the noninvasive evaluation, patients had to have an average of ≥30 VPDs/hour or reproducible exercise induced VT (i.e., five or more consecutive VPDs at a rate >120/min). To qualify for the invasive evaluation, patients had to have VT (five or more consecutive VPDs at a rate >120/min) representative of their clinical arrhythmia induced by programmed ventricular stimulation. Of the 105 patients who enrolled, 57 qualified for both noninvasive evaluation and invasive evaluation, 30 qualified for only the invasive evaluation, 14 for only the noninvasive evaluation, and four qualified for neither method of evaluation (see Fig. 8–1). Of the 57 patients who qualified for both methods of evaluation, 29 were randomized to the noninvasive approach and 28 to the invasive approach. Randomization was stratified on left ventricular ejection fraction (<40% vs. ≥40%) and on the type of VT induced by programmed ventricular stimulation (five consecutive complexes to 30 sec vs. >30 sec). The two groups of patients were well matched on age, sex, etiologic heart disease, ventricular arrhythmia frequency, and left ventricular ejection fraction. The group assigned to noninvasive assessment had 326±363 VPDs/hour and 34%±13% left ventricular ejection fraction compared with

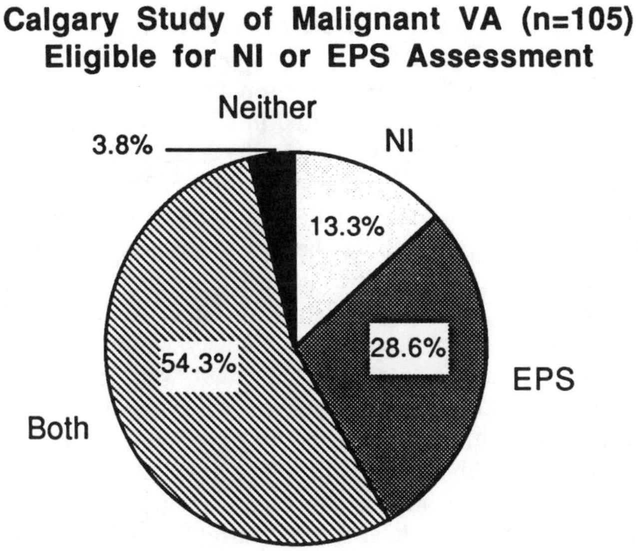

Fig. 8–1. Proportion of patients eligible for noninvasive or electrophysiologic studies in the Calgary study.

203±220 VPDs/hour and 39%±16% left ventricular ejection fraction for the group assigned to electrophysiologic assessment.

The drug sequence by drug action usually was: class IA or IB (mexiletine), IA + IB, II, and III (sotalol). When no drug predicted to be effective was found, patients were given amiodarone and followed. Efficacy in the noninvasive approach was defined as an 80% decrease in VPD frequency, 90% decrease in paired VPD, and 100% decrease in repetitive VPD of three or more complexes plus absence of two or more repetitive VPDs during the exercise test. A drug treatment predicted to be efficacious was found for all 29 patients (100%) assigned to the noninvasive approach; none were given amiodarone. However, seven patients in the noninvasive limb were switched to amiodarone during follow- up. Efficacy in the invasive approach was defined as fewer than six consecutive VPDs induced by programmed ventricular stimulation. A drug treatment predicted to be efficacious was found for 15 patients (54%) assigned to the invasive approach; 13 patients (46%) were given amiodarone. Electrophysiologic testing done on amiodarone showed that all patients treated with this drug had inducible, sustained VT. When patients developed intolerable adverse effects of their drug treatment, they were rehospitalized for the selection of an alternate therapy using the approach to which they were originally randomized.

The average follow-up in the Calgary study was 27±13 months. The primary endpoints for the study were the occurrence of symptomatic, sustained ventricular tachycardia or sudden cardiac death. Deaths that were not sudden were censored. During follow-up, 11 patients in the noninvasive limb and six in the invasive limb were rehospitalized for the selection of an alternate therapy. Sustained VT occurred in 45% of the noninvasive group and 18% of the invasive group. Sudden death occurred in two patients in the noninvasive group and in one of the invasive group. The total mortality was 19% in both groups. Thus, this small study showed fewer nonfatal recurrences of VT in the group whose therapy was selected by programmed ventricular stimulation, but there was no difference in sudden death or total mortality between the groups. It remains for larger studies to confirm the lower VT recurrence rates seen in the Calgary study and to determine whether a lower mortality rate accompanies the lower recurrence rate.

The trend toward less frequent recurrence of symptomatic sustained VT in the group treated with drugs selected by programmed ventricular stimulation was not due to treatment with amiodarone. As predicted by their electrophysiologic assessment, the amiodarone-treated patients in the invasive group actually tended to have more recurrences than those in the same group treated with antiarrhythmic drugs predicted to be effective by programmed ventricular stimulation.

Electrophysiologic Study vs. Electrocardiographic Monitoring (ESVEM)

ESVEM is a 13 center trial supported by the National Heart, Lung, and Blood Institute to determine if electrophysiologic studies or noninvasive methods (24 hour continuous ECG recordings and exercise tests) give more accurate predictions of efficacy for antiarrhythmic drug treatment in patients who have survived one or more episodes of cardiac arrest or sustained VT [51]. ESVEM began enrolling patients on October 1, 1985, and follow-up is scheduled to be completed in 1991. The number of patients to be enrolled in the ESVEM trial is predicated on the assertion that a 60% difference in the median time to arrhythmia occurrence between the two methods of selecting antiarrhythmic drugs will be found. About 70 patients with arrhythmia recurrence will provide a power of 0.80 to detect a 60% difference at a significance level of 0.05. Estimating the annual recurrence rate to be 25%, it was calculated that 285 patients will have to be enrolled, randomized, discharged on a drug predicted to be successful, and followed an average of 2.5 years. A summary of the protocol is depicted in Figure 8–2. After qualifying with a spontaneous episode of sustained ventricular arrhythmia, eligible patients are evaluated further with a continuous 48 hour ECG recording, an exercise test, and an electrophysiologic study (Table 8–4 outlines the ESVEM stimulation protocol). Patients who have sustained, uniform ventricular tachycardia in response to programmed ventricular stimulation and average at least 10 VPDs/hour during a 48 hour baseline recording period are randomized to be evaluated either by noninvasive methods or by programmed ventricular stimulation. The six stratifying variables used for ran-

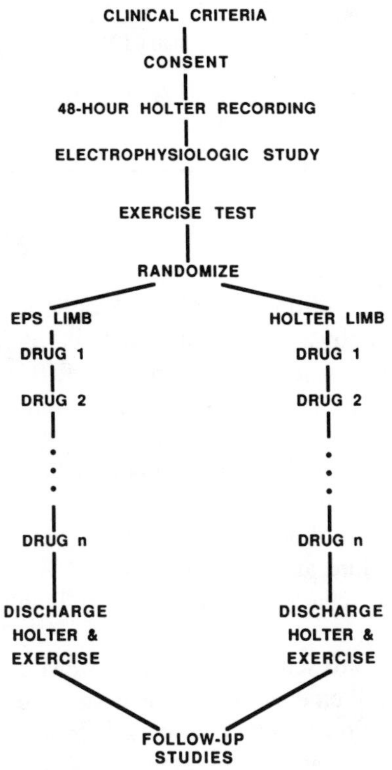

Fig. 8–2. Design of the ESVEM trial.

TABLE 8–4. ESVEM Stimulation Protocol

Pacing mode	Pacing site	Cycle length (msec)
V2	RVA	Sinus
V2V3	RVA	Sinus
V1V2	RVA	600, 500, 400
V1V2V3	RVA	600, 500, 400
V1V2	RVOT	600, 500, 400
V1V2V3	RVOT	600, 500, 400
V1V2V3V4	RVOT	600, 500, 400
V1V2V3V4	RVA	600, 500, 400

domizing patients for ESVEM are given in Table 8–5. Drugs from a set of six are randomly assigned one at the time; the investigator does not know which drug will be assigned next until the evaluation of the current drug is

TABLE 8–5. ESVEM Stratifying Variables

Institution (13)
Coronary heart disease vs. other etiologies
Cardiac arrest or ventricular fibrillation vs. sustained VT or syncope with sustained inducible VT
VPD (10–29/hour vs. ≥30/hour)
SAS class of CHF (class 1 vs. classes 2–4)
Amiodarone level (≤0.3 mg/ml vs. >0.3 mg/ml)

completed. The drugs and doses used in ESVEM are given in Table 8–6. Efficacy in the electrophysiologic limb is defined as failure to induce a run of VT longer than 15 consecutive complexes. Efficacy in the noninvasive limb is a ≥70% reduction in VPD frequency, ≥80% reduction in paired VPD, ≥90% reduction in unsustained VT, and 100% reduction in runs of VT >15 complexes. When analysis of 24 hour ECG recordings indicates the efficacy of an antiarrhythmic drug, a treadmill exercise test is done using the Bruce protocol. If a run of VT >15 complexes occurs during exercise, the drug is declared a failure and titration resumes. When an effective drug is found, the patient is discharged and followed until an endpoint occurs or the end of the study.

Follow-up visits are scheduled at an ESVEM enrolling center at 1, 3, 6, and 12 months and then every 6 months until the end of study is reached. The following evaluation is obtained at each follow-up visit: 1) symptom assessment, 2) physical examination, 3) plasma level of the study drug, 4) 12 lead ECG, and 5) 24 hour ECG recording. Study drugs can be changed for intolerable adverse effects occurring within 1 month of discharge. Study drug doses can be adjusted during follow-up to control adverse effects or to bring the plasma concentration into the target range. The endpoint criteria for evaluation of patients in this comparison study is the occurrence of sudden death or the recurrence of symptomatic sustained ventricular arrhythmias during follow-up. The primary analysis will be an actuarial analysis of the accuracy of drug efficacy predictions based on the "intention to treat" principle. Secondary analyses will include comparisons of the two methods for frequency of declaring efficacy, time to find a drug predicted to be effective, safety, and cost. Also, the relative efficacy of the study drugs and the accuracy of the methods for predicting the outcome with each drug will be evaluated.

In addition to revealing whether one of the two methods recommended for the evaluation of antiarrhythmic drug treatment for malignant ventricular arrhythmias is substantially better than the other, the Calgary study and ESVEM will produce important information about the sequencing of tests and treatments. For example, if drugs predicted to fail by noninvasive meth-

TABLE 8–6. Antiarrhythmic Drugs Used in ESVEM

Drug	Initial dose (mg/kg/day)	Target plasma concentration range (μg/ml)	Target dose range (mg/kg/day)
Imipramine	1.5	100–300	—
Mexiletine	8.5	1–2	—
Procainamide	25–60	4–12	—
Quinidine	20	2–6	—
Pirmenol	2.8	—	2.8–5.6
Propafenone	8.6	—	6.4–12.9
dl-Sotalol	3.5	—	3.5–7.0

ods were always predicted to fail by electrophysiologic studies, then electrophysiologic studies can be reserved for patients who have noninvasive criteria predicting drug success.

OBSERVATIONAL STUDIES TO DETERMINE THE ASSOCIATION BETWEEN VENTRICULAR ARRHYTHMIAS AND MORTALITY INDEPENDENT OF LEFT VENTRICULAR DYSFUNCTION

By 1981, several studies had established a statistically significant and reasonably strong association between ventricular arrhythmias detected between 7 and 90 days after myocardial infarction and subsequent mortality [69–72]. These studies also indicated that the prediction of mortality by ventricular arrhythmias was independent of clinical manifestations of heart failure. However, these studies did not clarify definitively the relationships among ventricular arrhythmias, left ventricular dysfunction, and mortality after myocardial infarction. These relationships were clarified by two large multicenter studies that performed 24 hour continuous ECG recordings and radionuclide ventriculograms prior to discharge from hospital after myocardial infarction.

The Multicenter Postinfarction Program (MPIP)

MPIP was conducted by four university cardiology groups in nine affiliated hospitals, located in New York City, Rochester, St. Louis, and Tucson [73]. Between January 1, 1979, and December 31, 1980, 4,093 patients were screened; 1,422 patients were eligible, i.e., had myocardial infarction, survived the coronary care unit, were under 70 years of age, and resided within the catchment area of a participating hospital [73]. Of the 1,422 eligible patients, 867 lacked exclusion criteria and enrolled. The MPIP hospitals included both primary community hospitals and tertiary hospitals. MPIP was an observational study that attempted to enroll all patients less than age 70 years with myocardial infarction. Thus, the sample is not systematically biased by the drug-related exclusion criteria that characterize intervention studies. A large fraction of the eligible patients, i.e., 61%, were enrolled. Thus the sample seems not to be biased by patient selection; the mortality experience of the enrolled patients was very similar to that of the patients who were eligible but not enrolled [73]. For all of these reasons, the findings in the MPIP study are likely to be nonbiased estimates of the prevalence and significance of ventricular arrhythmias and left ventricular dysfunction in the postinfarction population in the United States.

Three special tests, i.e., radionuclide ejection fraction, 24 hour continuous ECG recording, and exercise test, were performed prior to hospital discharge. The objective of these tests was to assess the relationships among three functional risk factors (left ventricular systolic function, ventricular arrhythmias, and myocardial ischemia) and total or cause-specific mortality.

Of the 867 patients enrolled, 820 had a 24 hour ECG recording and 767 patients had both a 24 hour ECG recording and a radionuclide ventriculogram. The group who underwent both tests permitted analyses to determine the relationships among ventricular arrhythmias, left ventricular dysfunction, and mortality during follow-up [3].

During the 31 month average follow-up, 144 patients died on or before December 31, 1982. To assign a mechanism to each death, the classification by Hinkle and Thaler [74] was used. The major categories in this classification are arrhythmic death, death due to circulatory failure, and deaths that are not classifiable as being either arrhythmic or the result of circulatory failure.

The findings of MPIP that provide a rationale for a full-scale clinical trial to test the ability of antiarrhythmic drug treatment to reduce sudden cardiac death are as follows. Frequent and/or repetitive ventricular arrhythmias were associated with total, sudden, and arrhythmic mortality. Ventricular arrhythmias had a stronger association with arrhythmic death than with nonarrhythmic death [3]. Low values of left ventricular ejection fraction also were associated with total, sudden, and arrhythmic mortality [75,76]; the association of left ventricular ejection fraction with arrhythmic death was substantially stronger than with nonarrhythmic death [75,76]. There was only a weak association between left ventricular ejection fraction and ventricular arrhythmias after myocardial infarction. For example, 70% of the patients with ventricular tachycardia had left ventricular ejection fraction ≥30% [3,75]. There was no interaction between ventricular arrhythmias and left ventricular dysfunction with respect to their mortality effects [3,77]. Table 8–7 shows that the fractional step up in mortality rate in patients with ventricular arrhythmias is identical for those with low and high left ventricular ejection fraction indicating a lack of a statistical interaction between ventricular arrhythmias and left ventricular dysfunction with respect to subsequent mortality.

TABLE 8–7. Relationships Among Left Ventricular Dysfunction, Ventricular Arrhythmias, and Mortality Rate in the MPIP Observational Study and for the MILIS Trial

		MPIP[b]		MILIS[c]	
Left ventricular ejection fraction	Ventricular arrhythmias[a]	No.	Mortality rate (%)	No.	Mortality rate (%)
<40%	Present	72	41	40	18
	Absent	184	20	141	10
≥40%	Present	78	16	30	8
	Absent	433	8	314	2

[a]VPD frequency ≥10/hour.
[b]Kaplan-Meier estimate of 30 month mortality rate.
[c]Average follow-up 18 months.

The Multicenter Investigation of the Limitation of Infarct Size (MILIS)

MILIS was a randomized, placebo-controlled trial to determine whether hyaluronidase or propranolol treatment given within 18 hours of the onset of myocardial infarction could limit the extent of myocardial necrosis [4]. MILIS was conducted in five hospitals: Barnes Hospital, Brigham and Women's Hospital, Massachusetts General Hospital, Medical Center of Vermont, and Parkland Memorial Hospital. Patients under age 75 years with myocardial infarction within 18 hours were enrolled. A positive creatine kinase MB evaluation, measured in a core laboratory, was required for documentation of myocardial infarction. About 55% of the eligible patients were enrolled and randomized. Obviously, MILIS is biased by the treatment-related exclusion criteria and by the effects of treatment. However, since the overall treatment effect was weak, it is not likely to have obscured the effects of such strong predictor variables as left ventricular ejection fraction and ventricular arrhythmias. Radionuclide ventriculograms and 24 hour continuous ECG recordings were obtained prior to hospital discharge about 10 days after myocardial infarction, and the results were used to evaluate the relationships among ventricular arrhythmias, left ventricular ejection fraction, and sudden cardiac death [4]. The average follow-up in the MILIS report was 18 months. Of the 66 deaths in MILIS, 29 were judged to be sudden, defined as death occurring within 1 hour of terminal symptoms (n = 16), patients found dead in bed (n = 9), or patients who collapsed at home (n = 4).

The patients were divided into four groups based on ventricular arrhythmias and left ventricular ejection fraction. The cut points for dichotomizing the two predictor variables were: left ventricular ejection fraction ≤40% vs. >40% and VPD <10 vs. ≥10 per hour [4]. The results obtained in the MILIS sample are shown in Table 8–7. The step up in mortality rate attributable to ventricular arrhythmias is slightly higher in patients with left ventricular ejection fraction >40% than in those with left ventricular ejection fraction ≤40%, but the difference is not significant. Again, these results suggest that ventricular arrhythmias are related to mortality independent of any relationship with left ventricular ejection fraction.

Since MPIP and MILIS both showed that the prediction of mortality by left ventricular ejection fraction and ventricular arrhythmias are independent of one another, the risks attributable to these two indicators should be multiplied to obtain the overall risk of dying. For example, if the increase in risk is increased threefold by left ventricular ejection fraction and 2.5-fold by ventricular arrhythmias, then the risk of dying during a period of follow-up would be the product of the two individual risks, i.e., 7.5-fold [77].

The MPIP study clarified the prevalence and significance of ventricular arrhythmias after myocardial infarction and showed that they were associated with death independent of their weak association with left ventricular dysfunction [3,75,77]. The MILIS study confirmed the significance and independence of ventricular arrhythmias in predicting sudden death after myocardial infarction [4]. These two studies considerably strengthened the scientific rationale for a large-scale clinical trial to determine if treatment of ventricular arrhythmias after myocardial infarction would reduce sudden cardiac death.

PREVIOUS POSTINFARCTION CLINICAL TRIALS WITH ANTIARRHYTHMIC DRUGS

May et al. [78] and Furberg [79] reviewed clinical trials of antiarrhythmic drug therapy after myocardial infarction when they met the following criteria: 1) 100 or more patients were enrolled in the trial, 2) subjects were randomly assigned to treatment or control groups, and 3) all-cause mortality was reported. These scientists recognized that a sample size of 100 is far too small to show an effect on mortality, but they thought that a trend might be observed in studies this small. However, no trend suggesting benefit was found in the long-term postinfarction antiarrhythmic drug trials.

Table 8–8 summarizes several important features of eight long-term clinical trials with antiarrhythmic drugs after myocardial infarction [80–88]. Six of the eight studies used an antiarrhythmic drug with class IB action, i.e., phenytoin, tocainide, or mexiletine, and the other two used aprindine, a drug that is not marketed in the United States. All studies were much too small to have the power to detect treatment effects of reasonable magnitude, e.g., 25%. Only the aprindine studies required that patients have ventricular arrhythmias to be eligible for enrollment in the clinical trial [87,88]. Since only 20% or less of patients have significant ventricular arrhythmias after myocardial infarction, the other six studies are, for practical purposes, one-fifth as large as their total number of patients, i.e., none of these six studies has more than 200 relevant patients. Also, the drugs with class IB action are not likely to suppress ventricular arrhythmias in patients with a recent myocardial

TABLE 8–8. Long-Term Randomized Trials of Antiarrhythmic Treatment After Myocardial Infarction[a]

Drug	Dose (mg/day)	No. of patients	Placebo control	Double blind	Arrhythmia required to enroll	Dose titrated to suppress arrhythmia	Months of follow-up	Mortality (%)	
								Controls	Treated
Phenytoin [80]	300–400	568	No (low-dose phenytoin)	Yes	No	No	12	9.1	8.1
Phenytoin [81]	—[b]	150	No (usual therapy)	No (open)	No	No	24	18.4	24.3
Tocainide [82]	1,200	112	Yes	Yes	No	No	6	8.9	8.9
Tocainide [83]	600	146	Yes	Yes	No	No	6	4.1	5.6
Mexiletine [84]	600–750	344	Yes	Yes	No	No	4	11.7	13.3
Mexiletine [85,86]	720	630	Yes	Yes	No	No	12	4.8	7.6
Aprindine [87]	100–200[c]	300	Yes	Yes	Yes	Yes	12	12.1	7.3
Aprindine [88]	100–200[c]	143	Yes	Yes	Yes	Yes	12	22.2	17.1

[a]All studies enrolled patients within 3 weeks of the index myocardial infarction.
[b]Dose adjusted to achieve plasma concentration of 40–80 μmol/liter.
[c]Dose adjusted to achieve suppression of ventricular arrhythmias.

infarction. Only the aprindine studies modified the dose of the active study drug in the attempt to suppress ventricular arrhythmias [87,88], and none of the eight studies permitted a change of active drug to achieve efficacy or avoid adverse effects. The drop-out rates were high in these trials, ranging from 20% to 30%, even though the follow-up period was relatively short, 1 year or less in seven of the eight trials. The number of deaths was small in all the studies; therefore, the precision of the estimates of mortality rates is very low. For what they are worth, three of the studies had almost identical mortality rates in the control and active treatment groups, three studies showed a mortality rate that was 32–58% higher in the group treated with antiarrhythmic drug, and the aprindine studies showed 40% and 23% lower mortality rates in the groups treated with antiarrhythmic drug. It is interesting that the two studies that showed encouraging results only enrolled patients who had ventricular arrhythmias and attempted to suppress ventricular arrhythmias by dose ranging with the active treatment [87,88].

The results of the eight small studies summarized in Table 8–8 fail to suggest any benefit of treatment with antiarrhythmic drugs in unselected patients after myocardial infarction. Table 8–9 gives the reasons discussed by Furberg [79] for a lack of positive treatment effect in the preliminary

TABLE 8–9. Reasons Randomized Controlled Trials With Antiarrhythmic Drugs after Myocardial Infarction Have Not Shown Improved Survival

Treatment with antiarrhythmic drugs does not improve survival
Suppression of ventricular arrhythmias may be required
Suppression of ventricular arrhythmias may not reduce mortality rates
Suppression of ventricular arrhythmias does improve survival, but the effect was not detected in previous clinical trials
Patients without arrhythmias were enrolled
The studies were too small to detect benefit
Suppression of ventricular arrhythmias was not documented
Study designs permitted too many drop-outs
Drug-induced proarrhythmia was not carefully monitored/controlled

studies. It may be that treatment with antiarrhythmic drugs does not improve survival. However, since the studies carried out so far do not have nearly enough power to detect a treatment effect, a negative conclusion is not warranted. All the previous studies were far too small to make statements about lack of benefit, and they must be regarded as preliminary. No long-term postinfarction study of over 1,000 patients has been performed to date. A future study of appropriate size and design that showed no improvement in survival after effective suppression of postinfarction ventricular arrhythmias would have a strong impact on the diagnosis and approach to treatment of ventricular arrhythmias after myocardial infarction. The second possibility given by Furberg is that suppression of ventricular arrhythmias improves survival, but the effect was not detected in previous clinical trials. Some of the reasons for this explanation are listed in Table 8–9. In all but one previous study, patients without drug-related exclusions were enrolled, including those without ventricular arrhythmias. Since only 15–20% of patients have significant ventricular arrhythmias at the time of discharge after myocardial infarction [3–5], a policy of enrolling all postinfarction patients yields a study sample in which most individuals may have more risk than benefit from antiarrhythmic drug treatment. Also, single-dose studies are likely to result in lower efficacy and higher levels of adverse effects and drop-out rates than studies that permit dose changes. Only one previous study attempted to document suppression of ventricular arrhythmias. Unfortunately, therefore, previous studies do not tell us whether it is feasible to suppress ventricular arrhythmias after myocardial infarction under clinial trial conditions. Both efficacy and drop-outs due to adverse effects should improve if changes in drugs and doses are permitted in the study protocol. Because of large interpatient variability in response to treatment, flexibility in dosing with antiarrhythmic drugs is important to achieve a high level of arrhythmia suppression and to avoid drop-out due to adverse effects in a study that plans to treat a group of patients. Finally, previous studies were done before the problem of drug-induced proarrhythmia and aggravation of

TABLE 8–10. Objectives of the Cardiac Arrhythmia Pilot Study

Develop effective screening and enrollment methods
Determine natural history and variability of VPD after infarction
Determine feasibility of 24 hour ECG to determine drug efficacy
Evaluate therapeutic strategies to suppress ventricular arrhythmias
Dose ranging (three doses)
Drug changes
Evaluate adverse effects rates of antiarrhythmic drugs
Proarrhythmia
Congestive heart failure
Other adverse effects
Drop-out rates
Evaluate stress and behavioral effects
On ventricular arrhythmia rates
On response to treatment

heart failure was widely appreciated, so these potentially negative effects of treatment were not carefully detected and controlled.

THE CARDIAC ARRHYTHMIA PILOT STUDY (CAPS)

Therefore, for a variety of reasons, previous studies of antiarrhythmic treatment after myocardial infarction do not shed much light on the efficacy or adverse effect rates. The National Heart, Lung, and Blood Institute recognized that these trials did not establish the feasibility of a full-scale trial to determine whether treatment or suppression of ventricular arrhythmias after myocardial infarction with antiarrhythmic drugs will improve survival. Moreover, there was not enough information available to permit the design of such a trial. Therefore, CAPS was initiated to provide information on feasibility and on how to design a full-scale trial [89].

CAPS Objectives

Some of the CAPS objectives are listed in Table 8–10 [89]. One goal of CAPS was to develop effective screening and enrolling methods in order to find and enroll patients with significant ventricular arrhythmias. Another goal was to determine the natural history of ventricular arrhythmias and the variability over a year after myocardial infarction in order to determine when best to screen patients and how to assess drug effect. The study also determined the feasibility of changing drugs and doses to achieve efficacy and to minimize adverse effects in a placebo-controlled, blinded clinical trial. Also, CAPS evaluated adverse effect rates, especially for proarrhythmia and aggravation of left ventricular dysfunction, and methods for detecting and controlling adverse effects. The need for hospitalization to detect serious adverse drug effects during the first days of antiarrhythmic drug treatment was evaluated. The effect of flexible dosing strategies on drop-out rates was evaluated, and the placebo group was especially important for assessing drug-associated drop-out rates. Finally, CAPS studied behavioral factors and measures of stress to determine how these were related to ventricular arrhythmias and treatment response.

CAPS was divided into three phases: 1) patient screening and recruitment, 2) drug/dose selection, and 3) follow-up [89]. To be eligible, patients had to be younger than 75 years of age, have acute myocardial infarction, have ≥10 VPDs per hour in a 24 hour ECG recording made between 6 and 60 days after myocardial infarction, have a left ventricular ejection fraction (LVEF) >20%, and give written informed consent. The CAPS patients were recruited primarily from coronary care units at participating hospitals, but patients referred from other hospitals, clinics, and private physicians also were included.

The screening process to determine patient eligibility included several steps: 1) review of the chart to determine that the patient was not ineligible, 2) documentation that the myocardial infarction met the CAPS definition, 3) a 24 hour continuous ECG obtained between 6 and 60 days after infarction arrhythmia, and 4) the ejection fraction measured no sooner than 48 hours after infarction. If a patient did not qualify on the first screening 24 hour ECG, a second 24 hour ECG could be done anytime within 60 days of the qualifying myocardial infarction to take advantage of the increase in ventricular arrhythmias during the weeks after myocardial infarction [72,90]. Only two screening Holter recordings were permitted for any patient.

Results of Screening

In the 27 hospitals comprising the 10 clinical sites, 3,957 patients were screened for CAPS; 687 patients (17.4%) were eligible, and 502 patients were randomized. For the 502 patients who were randomized, the average time from myocardial infarction to the qualifying 24 hour ECG was 26 days, and the average time from qualifying 24 hour ECG to randomization was 4.7 days.

Baseline Characteristics of the CAPS Population

Between July 25, 1983, and August 21, 1985, 502 patients, 418 men and 84 women with mean age of 59±9 years were enrolled [91]. Descriptive statistics of selected factors for patients participating in CAPS are shown in Table 8–11. In general, there was excellent balance among the five treatment groups. Not all factors are uniformly distributed across initial treatment groups. For example, the prevalence of cardiac enlargement was substantially lower in patients assigned to the encainide-imipramine-moricizine arm (23%) than in patients assigned to the placebo arm (39%). The only maldistribution of nonstudy drugs across the treatment arms at baseline was for calcium antagonists; overall 40% of the patients were on calcium antagonists,

TABLE 8–11. Comparison of Baseline Characteristics of CAPS Patients by Treatment Track

Variable	First drug in treatment arm				
	Encainide (N = 99)	Flecainide (N = 103)	Imipramine (N = 102)	Moricizine (N = 98)	Placebo (N = 100)
Mean age (years)	59	59	59	59	60
Men (%)	85	82	84	85	81
Previous infarction (%)	27	35	26	31	31
VPD/hour ≥30 (%)	54	64	71	68	70
Runs of 3 to 9 VPDs (%)[a]	38	35	38	28	32
LVEF <40 (%)	35	37	34	35	33
Drugs at baseline					
Beta-blockers (%)	46	36	43	37	41
Calcium-channel blockers (%)	34	51	42	38	34
Diuretics (%)	33	35	27	36	30
Digitalis (%)	18	25	26	26	20

[a]Baseline Holter for drug dosing.

ranging from 51% in the flecainide-imipramine-moricizine arm to 34% in the encainide-imipramine-moricizine and placebo arms.

Twenty-Four Hour Ambulatory ECG and LVEF

The analyzable recording time in the qualifying 24 hour ECG averaged 23±1.6 hours. The VPD average hourly rate was 10–29.9 in 35%; 30–99.9 in 29%; and ≥100 in 36%; 34% of recordings had at least one run of unsustained VT (three to nine consecutive VPD at a rate ≥100); there was an average of 13 runs; 51% had only one run. The baseline LVEF was measured by radionuclide ventriculography in 86% of the randomized patients and by dye angiography in 14% [91]. The overall LVEF was 0.45±0.13, and 35% of the patients had an LVEF <0.40. Very few correlations were found between VPD frequency, expressed as ln(VPD+1), and more than 150 baseline variables. The correlation between VPD frequency (ln[VPD/hour + 1]) and LVEF was very low ($r = -0.07$).

Drug/Dose Selection Phase

CAPS participants were randomized to one of the five treatment "tracks" shown in Figure 8–3, 100 patients to each track [89]. The placebo track provided a comparison with the active treatment strategies and a control for spontaneous VPD variability. The four active drug treatments were selected on the basis of potential efficacy, safety, and the prospect of developing new information for planning a full-scale trial [89]. "Standard" antiarrhythmic drugs were not chosen because the information about them was considered adequate to determine their relative worth for a full-scale trial. Unapproved drugs were evaluated for their efficacy, convenience of use, lack

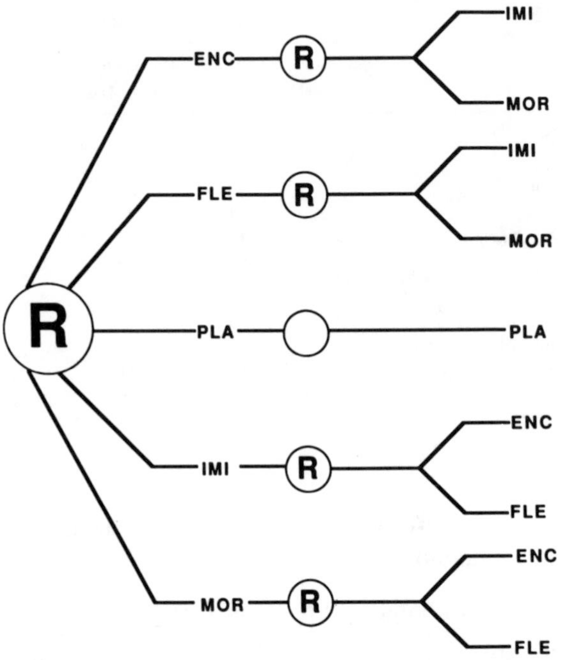

Fig. 8–3. Design of the Cardiac Arrhythmia Pilot Study. R, randomization. The drug abbreviations are as follows: ENC, encainide; FLE, flecainide; PLA, placebo; IMI, imipramine; MOR, moricizine. Note that drugs with class IA action (imipramine or moricizine) always cross over to drugs with class IC action (encainide or flecainide) and vice versa.

of known adverse effects, and likelihood of ultimately being marketed in the United States. Based on these considerations, encainide, moricizine, flecainide, and imipramine were selected for CAPS. All these drugs were judged to be at least as effective as quinidine or procainamide but more convenient to use or less likely to cause serious adverse effects. Note that CAPS was designed as a two-tiered strategy. Patients assigned to either of the drugs with class IC action, encainide and flecainide, always crossed over to drugs with class IA action, imipramine and moricizine, and vice versa. Thus encainide and flecainide were never compared in the same patient; likewise, imipramine and moricizine were never compared.

Each of the four active treatment tracks permitted up to three doses of the first drug to be evaluated. The rationale for three doses was to minimize adverse effects and to maximize ventricular arrhythmia suppression [89]. The doses used in CAPS are listed in Table 8–12. The criteria for efficacy were: a 70% reduction in VPD frequency, and a 90% reduction in runs of VT. If the first drug failed to achieve efficacy or caused intolerable adverse

TABLE 8–12. Doses of Drugs Used in CAPS

	Dose (mg) three times per day		
Drug	Low	Medium	High
Encainide	35	50	60
Flecainide	67	100	133
Imipramine	50	75	125
Moricizine	200	250	300

effects, the patient was crossed over to the second drug in the track by random assignment to one of two possible drugs. Then, dose ranging resumed at the lowest dose of drug 2 in the treatment track. If efficacy was reached, the patient was treated for the rest of the year on that drug and dose.

Patient flow during the drug dose selection phase. Two patients withdrew early, so 500 patients began the drug dose selection phase. The number of days required to complete drug/dose selection was shorter for active treatment (16 days) than for placebo (32 days) [92]. During treatment with the first drug, 64% (320) of patients achieved efficacy and lacked intolerable adverse effects, 4.2% (21 of 500) of patients withdrew, and 1.2% (6 of 500) of patients died. There were 153 patients (31%) who lacked efficacy or had intolerable adverse effects on CAPS drug 1 and were randomized to CAPS drug 2. By the completion of the drug/dose selection phase, 89% (448 of 502) of the patients were assigned to a CAPS drug for follow-up.

Efficacy during the drug dose selection phase. Figure 8–4 shows the efficacy of CAPS drugs during the drug/dose selection phase. As the first drug in the treatment arms, encainide (79%) and flecainide (83%), together had higher overall efficacy rates compared to imipramine (52%), moricizine (66%), and placebo (37%) as a group. The relatively high efficacy rate for placebo is explained by the greater number of ''drug'' trials in that group (3.0 compared to 1.7 for active treatment) and the correspondingly greater number of 24 hour ECG recordings to assess efficacy. The larger the number of recordings analyzed, the larger the chance of achieving apparent efficacy due to spontaneous variability in VPD frequency. LVEF before treatment was a significant determinant of drug efficacy (see Fig. 8–5).

Adverse effects during the drug dose selection phase. Patients were hospitalized and carefully monitored for at least the first 48 hours of treatment [92]. There were no differences between active treatments and placebo with respect to adverse events. Serious adverse effects were rare, and no early deaths could be ascribed to CAPS treatment. Orthostatic hypotension in patients taking imipramine (five instances) was the most frequent early adverse effect. During dose titration on drug 1, there was no difference among the five treatments for the frequency of serious adverse cardiac effects con-

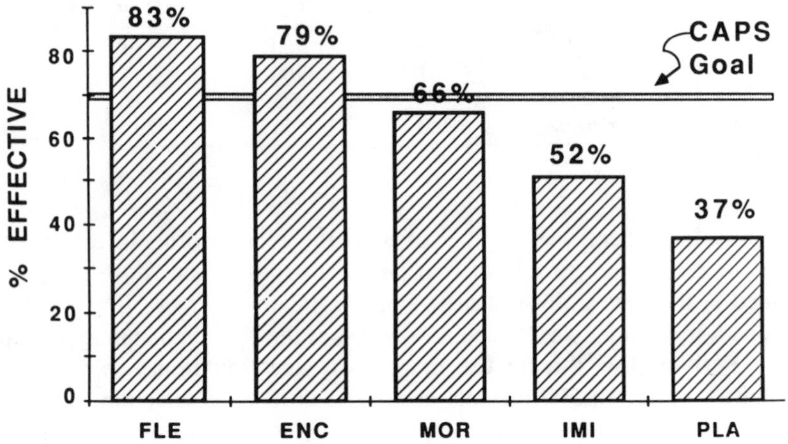

Fig. 8–4. Efficacy of the drugs in CAPS at the end of the drug/dose selection phase. Flecainide and encainide exceeded the goal for suppression of ventricular premature complexes, and moricizine was close.

firmed by drug washout, such as proarrhythmic effect (2%), disqualifying VT (≥10 consecutive VPD at a rate >100/minute) (3%), conduction abnormalities (3%), or heart failure (2%). Imipramine had a 26% incidence of intolerable adverse effects documented by drug washout, contrasted with a 5% incidence for the other active drugs and placebo taken together.

The Follow-Up Phase of CAPS

After the drug and dose selection phase, the patients were followed for 1 year to assess efficacy and adverse effects of treatment. At the beginning of follow-up, the assignments to drug treatment were encainide, 108; flecainide, 119; imipramine, 57; moricizine, 77; and placebo, 87 [92]. About 75% of the patients remained on their assigned drug for 1 year. Encainide and flecainide achieved the CAPS goal for long-term efficacy (≥70% reduction in VPD frequency), and moricizine was close (61%). The adverse effect rates for active drugs were similar to those for placebo. The incidence of any adverse effect was lower for encainide (49%) and flecainide (55%) than for imipramine (67%), moricizine (64%), or placebo (60%). Imipramine was the only treatment discontinued because of adverse symptoms more frequently (18%) than with placebo (7%). The discontinuation rates for the other drugs were encainide, 2%; flecainide, 3%; and moricizine, 6%. Disqualifying VT, proarrhythmic effect, or syncope that occurred during the follow-up phase, prompted withdrawal from CAPS drug 1, and disappeared during drug wash-

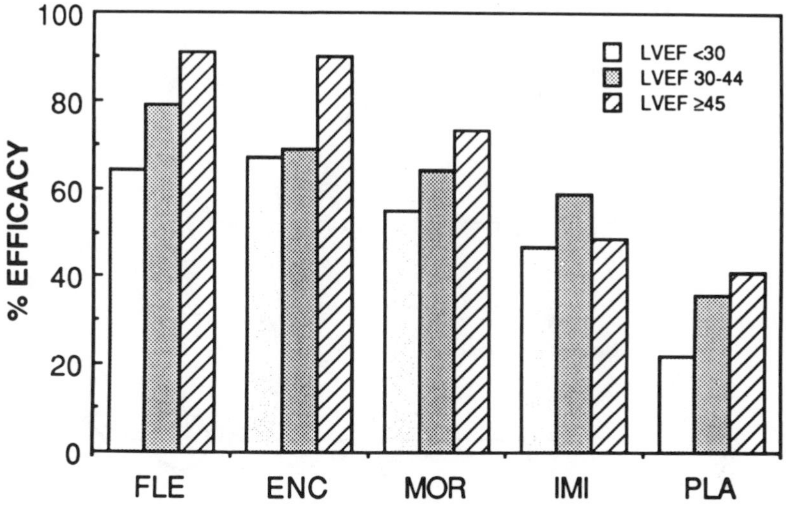

Fig. 8–5. Relationship between LVEF and efficacy rates in CAPS. Except for imipramine, efficacy rates are a direct positive function of LVEF. The dependence of "efficacy" on LVEF in the placebo group indicates that there is less spontaneous variability in patients with left ventricular dysfunction.

out was seen in 7% of the patients on encainide, 7% on flecainide, 2% on imipramine, 6% on moricizine, and 9% on placebo.

The actuarial 1 year incidence of heart failure was 25%. There was no statistically significant difference in the incidence of heart failure between the active treatments taken together and placebo. Similarly, there was no differences between encainide and placebo or between flecainide and placebo in the incidence of heart failure.

Dry mouth and constipation were seen most often after imipramine (44%) [92]. Neurologic adverse effects (poor coordination, clumsiness or stumbling, dizziness or lightheadedness, numbness or tingling) were common for all treatments but were most common for placebo (38%).

Summary of CAPS Findings

CAPS showed that 1) it is possible to identify and recruit suitable subjects for a definitive trial to test the hypothesis that suppression of ventricular arrhythmias after myocardial infarction will significantly improve survival; 2) several antiarrhythmic agents were found to be well tolerated and highly efficacious for suppressing ventricular arrhythmias after acute myocardial infarction; 3) dose titration with multiple drugs is feasible under clinical trial conditions and improves the chance of finding effective, well-tolerated treatment; 4) two doses perform as well as three doses of encainide, flecainide, or moricizine during titration; and 5) patient compliance and

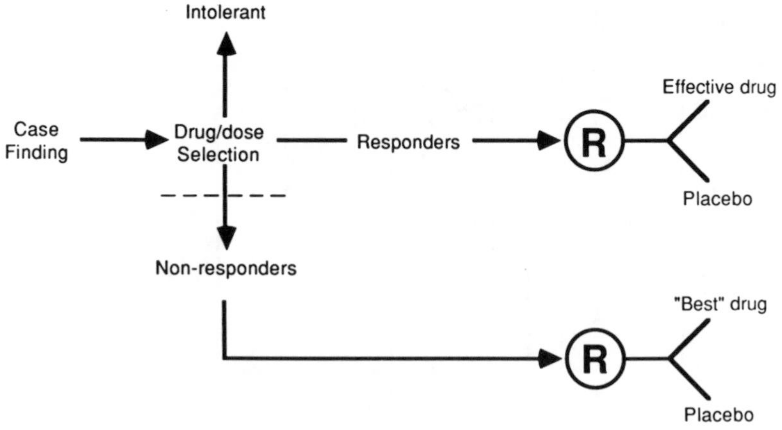

Fig. 8–6. Design of the Cardiac Arrhythmia Suppression Trial (CAST). Patients with ventricular arrhythmias and reduced LVEF have an antiarrhythmic drug and dose selected during open-label titration. Patients who are adequately suppressed are randomized to the effective drug or a placebo (above the dotted line). Patients who do not achieve enough arrhythmia suppression to enter the main trial are randomized to best treatment or placebo in a substudy (below the dotted line).

follow-up can be maintained for at least 1 year in a postinfarction cohort [92]. It is important to recognize that, because of the exclusion criteria used in CAPS, one cannot extrapolate the results to the entire postinfarction population. CAPS excluded patients with VT ≥10 complexes and LVEF ≤20%. Aggravation of heart failure or proarrhythmia might occur more frequently if patients with LVEF ≤20% or sustained VT were exposed to the these drugs [55,56].

THE CARDIAC ARRHYTHMIA SUPPRESSION TRIAL (CAST)

The findings of CAPS were valuable for planning of the Cardiac Arrhythmia Suppression Trial (CAST), a large-scale clinical trial initiated in 1987 to determine whether suppression of ventricular arrhythmias with antiarrhythmic drug treatment after myocardial infarction will significantly reduce arrhythmic death [93]. The design of CAST is uniquely suitable for testing the suppression hypothesis (see Fig. 8–6). During an open-label drug treatment period, an effective treatment is sought using three antiarrhythmic drugs, encainide, flecainide, or moricizine. If suppression is achieved during open label treatment, patients are then randomized to the therapy that suppressed their arrhythmia during open-label drug selection or to a matched placebo. If suppression is not achieved, patients may be eligible for a sub-

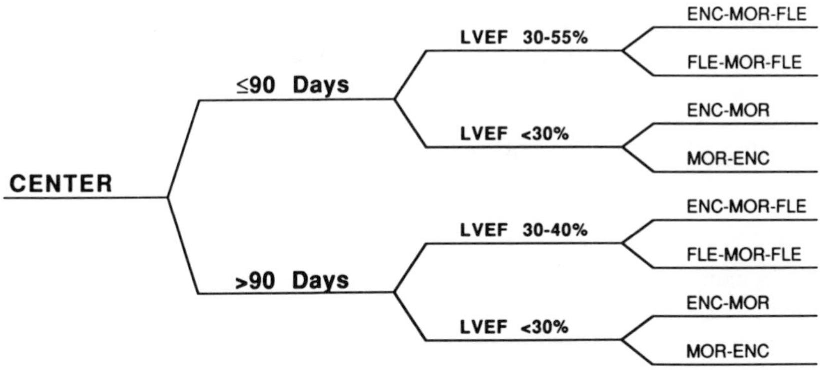

Fig. 8–7. CAST stratification process. Patients are assigned to treatment in accordance with their center, time of randomization with respect to the index myocardial infarction, and their LVEF. The abbreviations of drug names are the same as for Figure 8–3.

study that randomizes them to the best therapy found during open-label titration or to a matching placebo.

Patient Eligibility

Survivors of myocardial infarction who are <80 years of age and have six or more VPDs per hour on a 24 hour continuous ECG recording obtained between 6 days and 2 years after myocardial infarction are eligible for CAST (Fig. 8–7). Patients enrolled between 6 and 90 days after the infarction must have a LVEF ≤55%; if the screening 24 hour ECG recording is obtained more than 90 days after the onset of myocardial infarction, the LVEF must be ≤40%. Patients with runs of VT ≥15 consecutive complexes at a rate of ≥120 per minute or patients with symptomatic hemodynamically important ventricular tachycardia are excluded from CAST.

Open-Label Drug/Dose Selection Phase

During the open-label drug/dose selection phase, three active drugs are used, in a number of sequences that are randomly assigned. For patients with an ejection fraction ≥30%, the sequence will contain all three drugs, encainide, flecainide, or moricizine, in one of two sequences: encainide → moricizine → flecainide and flecainide → moricizine → encainide. For patients with LVEF <30%, two drugs, encainide and moricizine, are used. Patients are randomly assigned to start encainide or moricizine first. Each drug has two dose levels, and dosing always proceeds from the low to the high dose. The two doses used are the same as the two lower doses used in CAPS (see Table 8–12). Suppression is assessed by a 24 hour continuous ECG recording. Suppression is defined as a ≥80% reduction in VPD frequency and

≥90% suppression of runs of unsustained VT (three to 14 consecutive VPDs at a rate of ≥120 per minute). Patients whose arrhythmia is suppressed and who tolerate their treatment are randomized to the drug that suppressed their arrhythmia or to a matching placebo. Randomization is stratified on 1) clinical center, 2) LVEF ≥30% or <30%, 3) time of enrollment <90 days or ≥90 days. Randomization to blinded treatment with drug or placebo begins the trial. Enrollment will continue for 3 years (1987–1990) and follow-up for 2–5 years (until 1992).

Sample Size

A sample of 4,200 patients was calculated for the main study using the following assumptions. The average follow-up will last 3 years. The primary endpoint, arrhythmic death or cardiac arrest, has a 3 year incidence of 11% in the placebo group. Suppression of ventricular arrhythmias with antiarrhythmic drugs will reduce sudden death by 30%. The type I(α) error was set at a one-tail level of 0.025. The power ($1 - \beta$) of the study was set at 0.85. A drop-in rate of 6% and a drop-out rate of 30% were projected. These assumptions led to a calculation that 2,100 patients would need to be enrolled in the placebo group and 2,100 in the treatment group. Assuming an 80% suppression rate during open-label antiarrhythmic titration, about 1,000 patients will be enrolled into the substudy for patients who do not achieve adequate suppression of VPDs during open-label titration. It is recognized that 1,000 patients is not enough to detect a definitive conclusion about the treatment hypothesis, but it was thought that important trends should be demonstrable. Also, the relationship between the reduction in the arrhythmic death and the degree of VPD suppression will improve the interpretation of the findings in the main trial. If the degree of VPD suppression is related monotonically and directly to survival rate, it will strongly suggest that suppression of ventricular arrhythmias is causally related to the improvement in survival.

Encainide and Flecainide Increase Mortality in CAST

The CAST protocol permits drugs to be removed from or added to the trial. On April 17, 1989, the Data and Safety Monitoring Board held its regular semiannual meeting; reviewed mortality data complete as of March 30, 1989; and recommended that encainide and flecainide be removed from CAST because it had become virtually impossible to establish any beneficial effect from these drugs if they were continued to the end of study and because of strong evidence that these drugs increased the death rate compared to placebo. The Data and Safety Monitoring Board also recommended that CAST be continued with moricizine, which still has a significant chance of showing benefit, and that other antiarrhythmic drugs be reviewed as possible additions to CAST.

The National Heart, Lung, and Blood Institute and the CAST Executive Committee reviewed the April 17, 1989, recommendation by the Data and Safety Monitoring Board and decided that same day to remove encainide and flecainide from CAST immediately. On April 18, 1989, a message was sent to each CAST clinical center to discontinue treatment in all patients who had been assigned to encainide, flecainide, or their corresponding placebos. This process was started on April 19, 1989, and was completed by April 24, 1989. Patients whose encainide or flecainide was stopped had a 24 hour ECG recording done 7–30 days after discontinuing their study drug. Those who still had sufficient ventricular arrhythmia frequency to qualify after washout of their original CAST medication, had an LVEF ≤40%, and did not have exclusions were invited to cross over to moricizine or its corresponding placebo. The CAST Drug Selection Committee was reactivated to review drugs that might be added to the CAST. Until such time as other drugs are selected and added to the trial, newly enrolled patients are being randomized to moricizine or placebo.

The data reviewed by the Data and Safety Monitoring Board on March 30, 1989, were on 730 patients randomized to encainide or flecainide and 725 randomized to a corresponding placebo. With an average of about 300 days of exposure to CAST treatment, there were 78 deaths or nonfatal cardiac arrests in the group treated with encainide, flecainide, or the corresponding placebos (event rate 5.4%). Of the 78 events, 54% were primary arrhythmic events. The primary endpoint for the trial, arrhythmic death or nonfatal cardiac arrest, was experienced by 4.5% of the patients randomized to encainide or flecainide compared to 1.2% of the patients randomized to placebo. Patients taking encainide or flecainide were 3.6 times as likely to experience arrhythmic death or nonfatal cardiac arrest as those treated with placebo. The chance of experiencing death of any cause (48 patients) or cardiac arrest (eight patients) was 7.7% in patients treated with encainide or flecainide compared to 3.0% for placebo, an increase in risk of 2.5.

There were no imbalances between the group treated with encainide or flecainide and the group treated with placebo with respect to baseline risk variables that might confound the apparent adverse treatment effect. Age, history of previous infarction, angina pectoris, congestive heart failure, hypertension, diabetes, sustained arrhythmias, baseline LVEF, ventricular arrhythmia frequency, electrocardiographic intervals, therapy in hospital, and discharge medications all were closely matched in patients randomized to encainide or flecainide and those randomized to placebo. The increase in death rate for patients treated with encainide or flecainide was observed consistently in the various subgroups within the study; i.e., there was no interaction with age; time from myocardial infarction to enrollment; ejection fraction; baseline ventricular arrhythmia frequency; baseline QRS duration; or the use of digitalis, diuretics, beta-blockers, or calcium-channel blockers. The relative risk of dying or experiencing a nonfatal cardiac arrest was almost identical for both drugs (2.3 for encainide and 2.7 for flecainide), although the mortality rate was lower for flecainide and its corresponding placebo because patients with LVEF <30% were not randomized to flecainide. Also, 88% of the patients who died or experienced a nonfatal cardiac arrest were taking their assigned study medication at the time of the event.

The finding that treatment of patients who have asymptomatic or minimally symptomatic ventricular arrhythmias during the 2 years after myocardial infarction with encainide and flecainide increases the death rate was totally contrary to the hypothesis being tested in CAST. Since the Data and Safety Monitoring Board found no cause for concern about moricizine, it seems that this adverse effect has been demonstrated only for two drugs with class IC antiarrhythmic action. It is possible that encainide and flecainide, which decrease ventricular arrhythmias substantially, would have reduced mortality if they had not also had toxic effects. However, the CAST finding clearly indicates that marked suppression of ventricular arrhythmias after myocardial infarction by drugs with class IC antiarrhythmic action does not necessarily predict improved survival. A mortality effect of the magnitude found in CAST could not be detected without a controlled clinical trial. Other drugs in common use also may carry a similar increased risk of dying. It is also worth noting that a recent survey showed that more than half of the cardiologists surveyed treated patients like those enrolled in CAST with antiarrhythmic drugs, often with encainide or flecainide. Although this practice had a strong rationale, a controlled clinical trial showed that this common practice was harmful to patients. The knowledge that encainide and flecainide are harmful should save thousands of lives each year. The CAST result should make physicians more conservative about treating postinfarction arrhythmias with unproved drugs even though these arrhythmias are known to pose a substantial risk.

The hypothesis that suppression of ventricular arrhythmias using antiarrhythmic drugs from other classes will improve survival is worthy of continued investigation. In the future, CAST and other trials should tell us whether suppressing asymptomatic ventricular arrhythmias using antiarrhythmic drugs with other mechanisms of action will significantly reduce life-threatening arrhythmic events during long-term follow-up after myocardial infarction. A positive result from CAST using moricizine or other drugs will increase the use of the successful antiarrhythmic drugs almost overnight. A negative result with moricizine or other drugs that may be added to CAST will constrict a dwindling use of drugs with class I antiarrhythmic action even further and turn our diagnostic and therapeutic efforts for controlling sudden cardiac death in coronary heart disease in new directions.

SPANISH TRIAL OF SUDDEN DEATH

The Spanish are conducting a controlled multicenter trial of antiarrhythmic treatment in patients with previous myocardial infarction. The com-

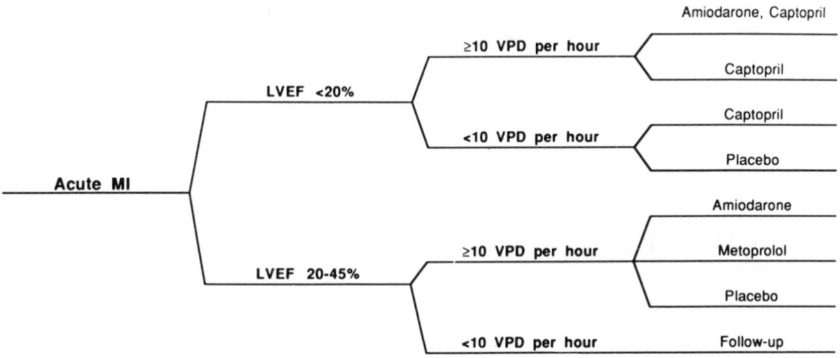

Fig. 8–8. Spanish Trial of Sudden Cardiac Death. The stratification of randomization depends on the level of LVEF and on the presence of ventricular arrhythmias.

plex randomization scheme is shown in Figure 8–8. The value of LVEF and the presence of ventricular arrhythmias are the keys to randomization. Patients with LVEF >45% are followed without treatment; those with LVEF 20–45% and ventricular arrhythmias are randomized to placebo, metoprolol, or amiodarone; and those with LVEF <20% and ventricular arrhythmias are randomized to amiodarone or placebo. All patients with LVEF <20% are treated with captopril. About 3,000 patients will be randomized and followed an average of 2 years. This trial will provide information on the efficacy of amiodarone (reduction of arrhythmias and sudden cardiac death) in patients with coronary heart disease and reduced LVEF. This information will complement the information about suppression of ventricular arrhythmias with antiarrhythmic drugs having class I action that will be developed by CAST. Also, a direct, randomized comparison of drugs with class II (metoprolol) and class III (amiodarone) actions will be obtained in patients with moderately reduced ejection fraction. This trial has been enrolling patients for about 1 year and will be completed about the same time as CAST, i.e., in 1992 or 1993.

CONCLUSIONS

There have been previous trials to test the hypothesis that suppression of ventricular arrhythmias after myocardial infarction will reduce mortality. The preliminary studies have not been encouraging, but they are so flawed that they do not count for much. CAPS showed the feasibility of performing full-scale trials and maintaining a good level of suppression over a long period of time. CAST is testing the suppression hypothesis using antiarrhythmic drugs with class IA and IC actions. A Spanish trial is testing amiodarone (class III antiarrhythmic action) in a similar setting. Until these two definitive studies are completed and reported in the mid 1990s, the best conventional treatment of postinfarction ventricular arrhythmia is with β-adrenergic blocking drugs (class II antiarrhythmic action).

ACKNOWLEDGMENTS

This study was supported in part by contracts HV-28006 and HC-65048 from the National Heart, Lung, and Blood Institute, National Institutes of Health, Bethesda, MD; in part by grants HL-22982, HL-70204, HL-41552 from the National Heart, Lung, and Blood Institute, and RR-00645 from the Research Resources Administration, National Institutes of Health, Bethesda, MD; and in part by grants from the Milstein Family Foundation and the Henry and Shirlee Benach Foundation, New York, New York.

REFERENCES

1. Bigger JT Jr: Antiarrhythmic drug treatment. An overview. Am J Cardiol 53:8B–16B, 1984.
2. Morganroth J: Premature ventricular complexes: diagnosis and indication for therapy. JAMA 252:673–676, 1984.
3. Bigger JT Jr, Fleiss JL, Kleiger R, Miller JP, Rolnitzky LM, The Multicenter Post-Infarction Group: The relationship between ventricular arrhythmias, left ventricular dysfunction and mortality in the 2 years after myocardial infarction. Circulation 69: 250–258, 1984.
4. Mukharji J, Rude RE, Poole WK, Gustafson N, Thomas LJ Jr, Strauss HW, Jaffe AS, Muller JE, Roberts R, Raabe DS Jr, Croft CH, Passamani E, Braunwald E, Willerson JT, The MILIS Study Group: Risk factors for sudden death after acute myocardial infarction: Two year follow-up. Am J Cardiol 54:31–36, 1984.
5. Bigger JT Jr: Management of ventricular arrhythmias in patients with congestive heart failure. Am J Cardiol 57:1b–2b, 1986.
6. Breithardt G, Borggrefe M, Haerten K: Role of programmed ventricular stimulation and noninvasive recording of ventricular late potentials for the identification of patients at risk of ventricular tachyarrhythmias after acute myocardial infarction. In Zipes DP, Jalife J (eds): "Cardiac Electrophysiology and Arrhythmias." New York: Grune & Stratton, Inc. 1985, pp 553–561.
7. Roy D, Marchand E, Theroux P, Waters DD, Pelletier GB, Bourassa MG: Programmed ventricular stimulation in survivors of an acute myocardial infarction. Circulation 72: 487–494, 1985.
8. Denniss AR, Richards DA, Cody DV, Russell PA, Young AA, Cooper MJ, Ross DL, Uther JB: Prognostic significance of ventricular tachycardia and fibrillation induced at programmed stimulation and delayed potentials detected on the signal-averaged electrocardiograms of survivors of acute myocardial infarction. Circulation 74:731–745, 1986.
9. Breithardt G, Borggrefe M: Recent advances in the identification of patients at risk of ventricular tachyarrhythmias: role of ventricular late potentials. Circulation 75:1091–1096, 1987.

10. Breithardt G, Borggrefe M, Podczek A, Schwarzmaier J, Karbenn U: Prognostic significance of late potentials in patients with coronary heart disease (abstract). Circulation 76[Suppl IV]:IV-344, 1987.
11. Gomes JA, Winters SL, Stewart D, Targonski A, Barreca P: A new noninvasive index to predict ventricular tachycardia and sudden death in the first year after myocardial infarction: based on signal averaged electrocardiogram, radionuclide ejection fraction and Holter monitoring. J Am Coll Cardiol 10:349–357, 1987.
12. Kuchar DL, Thorburn CW, Sammel NL: Prediction of serious arrhythmic events after myocardial infarction: signal-averaged electrocardiogram, Holter monitoring and radionuclide ventriculography. J Am Coll Cardiol 9:531–538, 1987.
13. Woosley RL, Echt DS, Roden DM: Effects of congestive heart failure on the pharmacokinetics and pharmacodynamics of antiarrhythmic agents. Am J Cardiol 57:25B–33B, 1986.
14. Fisher JD, Cohen HL, Mehra R, Altschuler H, Escher DJW, Furman S: Cardiac pacing and pacemakers. II. Serial electrophysiologic-pharmacologic testing for control of recurrent tachyarrhythmias. Am Heart J 93:658–668, 1977.
15. Horowitz LN, Josephson ME, Farshidi A, Spielman SR, Michaelson EL, Greenspan AM: Recurrent sustained ventricular tachycardia. 3. Role of the electrophysiologic study in selection of antiarrhythmic regimens. Circulation 58:986–997, 1978.
16. Mason JW, Winkle RA: Electrode-catheter arrhythmia induction in the selection and assessment of antiarrhythmic drug therapy for recurrent ventricular tachycardia. Circulation 58:971–985, 1978.
17. Mason JW, Winkle RA: Accuracy of the ventricular tachycardia induction study for predicting long-term efficacy and inefficacy of antiarrhythmic drugs. N Engl J Med 303:1073–1077, 1980.
18. Horowitz LN, Josephson ME, Kastor JA: Intracardiac electrophysiologic studies as a method for the optimization of drug therapy in chronic ventricular arrhythmia. Prog Cardiovasc Dis 23:81–98, 1980.
19. Ruskin JN, DiMarco JP, Garan H: Out-of-hospital cardiac arrest. Electrophysiologic observations and selection of long-term antiarrhythmic therapy. N Engl J Med 303:607–613, 1980.
20. Swerdlow CD, Winkle RA, Mason JW: Determinants of survival in patients with ventricular tachyarrhythmias. N Engl J Med 308:1436–1442, 1983.
21. Benditt DG, Benson DW, Klein GJ, Prtzker MR, Kriett JM, Anderson RW: Prevention of recurrent sudden cardiac arrest: Role of provocative electropharmacologic testing. J Am Coll Cardiol 2:418–425, 1983.
22. McGovern B, Garan H, Malacoff RF, DeMarco JP, Grant G, Sellers TD, Ruskin JN: Long term clinical out-come of ventricular tachycardia or fibrillation treated with amiodarone. Am J Cardiol 53:1558–1563, 1984.
23. Rae AP, Greenspan AM, Spielman SR, Sokoloff NM, Webb CR, Kay HR, Horowitz LN: Antiarrhythmic drug efficacy for ventricular tachyarrhythmias associated with coronary artery disease as assessed by electrophysiologic studies. Am J Cardiol 55:1494–1499, 1985.
24. Horowitz LN, Greenspan AM, Spielman SR, Webb CR, Morganroth J, Rotmensch H, Sokoloff NM, Rae AP, Segal BL, Kay HR: Usefulness of electrophysiologic testing in evaluation of amiodarone therapy for sustained ventricular tachyarrhythmias associated with coronary heart disease. Am J Cardiol 55:367–372, 1985.
25. Waller TJ, Kay HR, Spielman SR, Kutlaek SP, Greenspan AM, Horowitz LN: Reduction in sudden death and total mortality by antiarrhythmic therapy evaluated by electrophysiologic drug testing: criteria of efficacy in patients with sustained ventricular tachyarrhythmia. J Am Coll Cardiol 10:83–89, 1987.
26. Graboys TB, Lown B, Podrid PJ, DeSilva R: Long-term survival of patients with malig-

nant ventricular arrhythmia treated with antiarrhythmic drugs. Am J Cardiol 50:437–443, 1982.
27. Hoffman A, Schutz E, White R, Follath F, Burckhardt D: Suppression of high-grade ventricular ectopic activity by antiarrhythmic drug treatment as a marker for survival in patients with chronic coronary artery disease. Am Heart J 107:1103–1108, 1984.
28. Vlay SC, Kallman LH, Reid PR: Prognostic assessment of survivors of ventricular tachycardia and ventricular fibrillation with ambulatory monitoring. Am J Cardiol 54:87–90, 1984.
29. Hohnloser SN, Raeder EA, Podrid PJ, Graboys TB, Lown B: Predictors of antiarrhythmic drug efficacy in patients with malignant ventricular tachyarrhythmias. Am Heart J 114:1–7, 1987.
30. Lampert S, Lown B, Graboys TB, Podrid PJ, Blatt CM: Determinants of survival in patients with malignant ventricular arrhythmias associated with coronary artery disease. Am J Cardiol 61:791–797, 1988.
31. Oliver GC, Ripley KL, Miller JP, Thomas LJ Jr: A critical review of computer arrhythmia detection. In Pordy L (ed): "Computer Electrocardiography: Current Status and Criteria." Mount Kisco, NY: Futura Press, 1977, pp 319–325.
32. Hermes RE, GC Oliver: Use of the American Heart Association database. In Wenger NK, Mock MB, Ringqvist I (eds): "Ambulatory Electrocardiography Recording." Chicago: Year Book Medical Publishers, Inc., 1981, pp 165–181.
33. Clark KW, Rolnitzky LM, Miller JP, DeCamilla JJ, Kleiger RE, Thanavaro S, Bigger JT Jr, Other MPIP Participants: Ambulatory ECG analysis shared by two independent computer labs in the multicenter post-infarction program (MPIP). In: "Computers in Cardiology 1980." Long Beach, CA: IEEE 1981, pp 271–275.
34. Bigger JT Jr, Reiffel JA, Coromilas J: Ambulatory electrocardiography. In Platia EV (ed): "Cardiac Arrhythmias—Non Pharmacologic Management." Philadelphia: JB Lippencott Co., 1986, pp 49–80.
35. Bigger JT Jr, Rolnitzky LM, Leahey EB Jr, LaPook J: Ambulatory ECG recording: duration of recording and activity protocol. In Wenger NK, Mock MB, Ringqvist I (eds): "Ambulatory Electrocardiographic Recording." Chicago: Year Book Medical Publishers, 1981, pp 87–102.
36. Bigger JT Jr, Rolnitzky LM: The evaluation of antiarrhythmic drug efficacy. In Reiser HJ, Horowitz LN (eds): "Mechanisms and Treatment of Cardiac Arrhythmias: Relevance of Basic Studies to Clinical Management." Baltimore: Urban & Schwarzenberg, 1985, pp 117–135.
37. Winkle RA: Antiarrhythmic drug effect mimicked by spontaneous variability of ventricular ectopy. Circulation 57:1116–1121, 1978.
38. Morganroth J, Michelson EL, Horowitz LN, Josephson ME, Pearlman AS, Dunkman WB: Limitations of routine long-term monitoring to assess ventricular ectopic frequency. Circulation 58:408–414, 1978.
39. Thomas LJ, Miller JP: Long-Term ambulatory ECG recording in the determination of antidysrhythmic drug efficacy. In Lucchesi BR, Dingell JV, Schwartz RP Jr (eds): "The Clinical Pharmacology of Antiarrhythmic Drugs." New York: Raven Press, 1984, pp 249–265.
40. Swerdlow CD, Pederson J: Prospective comparison of Holter monitoring and electrophysiologic study in patients with coronary artery disease and sustained ventricular tachyarrhythmias. Am J Cardiol 56:577–580, 1985.
41. Kim SG, Seiden SW, Felder SD, Waspe LE, Fisher JD: Is programmed stimulation of value in predicting the long-term success of antiarrhythmic therapy for ventricular tachycardias? N Engl J Med 315:356–362, 1986.
42. Podrid PJ, Graboys TB, Lampert S, Clatt C: Exercise stress testing for exposure of arrhythmias. Circulation 75[Suppl III]:III-60–III-65, 1987.

43. Bigger JT Jr, Reiffel JA, Livelli FD Jr, Wang PJ: Sensitivity, specificity, and reproducibility of programmed ventricular stimulation. Circulation 73[Suppl II]:II-73–II-78, 1986.
44. Livelli FD, Bigger JT Jr, Reiffel JA, Gang ES, Patton JN, Noethling PM, Rolnitzky LM, Gliklich JI: Response to programmed ventricular stimulation: Sensitivity, specificity and relationship to heart disease. Am J Cardiol 50:452–458, 1982.
45. Schoenfeld MH, McGovern B, Garan H, Ruskin JN: Long-term reproducibility of responses to programmed cardiac stimulation in spontaneous ventricular tachyarrhythmias. Am J Cardiol 54:564–568, 1984.
46. Bigger JT Jr, Livelli FD Jr, Gang ES, Reiffel JA: Use of clinical electrophysiologic studies in antiarrhythmic drug development. In Coltar J, Jewitt D (eds): "Recent Developments in Cardiovascular Drugs." Edinburgh: Churchill Livingstone, 1982, pp 78–93.
47. Ruskin JN, McGovern B, Garan H, DiMarco JP, Kelly E: Antiarrhythmic drugs; a possible cause of out-of-hospital cardiac arrest. N Engl J Med 309:1302–1306, 1983.
48. Bigger JT Jr: Identification of patients at high risk for sudden cardiac death. Am J Cardiol 54:3d–8d, 1984.
49. Saksena S, Greenberg E, Ferguson D: Prospective reimbursement for state-of-the-art medical practice: the case for invasive electrophysiologic evaluation. Am J Cardiol 55:963–967, 1985.
50. Mitchell LB, Duff HJ, Manyari DE, Wyse DG: A randomized clinical trial of the noninvasive and invasive approaches to drug therapy of ventricular tachycardia. N Engl J Med 317:1681–1687, 1987.
51. Bigger JT Jr: Holter/exercise and electrophysiologic methods for evaluating drug therapy for malignant ventricular arrhythmias: do we need both models? In Morganroth J, Moore EN (eds): "Cardiac Arrhythmias: New Therapeutic Drugs and Devices." Boston: Martinus Nijhoff, 1985, 211–221.
52. Anderson JL, Mason JW: Testing the efficacy of antiarrhythmic drugs. N Engl J Med 315:391–393, 1986.
53. Breithardt G, Borggrefe M, Seipel L: Selection of optimal drug treatment of ventricular tachycardia by programmed electrical stimulation of the heart. Ann NY Acad Sci 427:49–65, 1984.
54. Bigger JT Jr: Cardiac arrhythmias. In Wyngaarden JB, Smith HK (eds): "Cecil's Textbook of Medicine." Philadelphia: W.B. Saunders Co., 1988, pp 250–274.
55. Morganroth J, Anderson JL, Gentzkow GD: Classification by type of ventricular arrhythmia predicts frequency of adverse cardiac events from flecainide. J Am Coll Cardiol 8:607–615, 1986.
56. de Paola AAV, Horowitz LN, Morganroth J, Senior S, Spielman SR, Greenspan AM, Kay HR: Influence of left ventricular dysfunction on flecainide therapy. J Am Coll Cardiol 9:163–168, 1987.
57. Mason JW: Amiodarone. N Engl J Med 316:455–466, 1987.
58. Kienzle MG, Martins JB, Wendt DJ, Constantin L, Hopson R, McCue ML: Enhanced efficacy of oral sotalol for sustained ventricular tachycardia refractory to type I antiarrhythmic drugs. Am J Cardiol 61:1012–1017, 1988.
59. Freedman RA, Swerdlow CD, Echt DS, Winkle RA, Soderholm Difatte V, Mason JW: Facilitation of ventricular tachyarrhythmia induction by isoproterenol. Am J Cardiol 54:765–770, 1984.
60. McGovern B, Ruskin JN: The efficacy of amiodarone for ventricular arrhythmias can be predicted with clinical electrophysiological studies. Int J Cardiol 3:71–76, 1983.
61. Borggrefe M, Breithardt G: Predictive value of electrophysiologic testing in the treatment of drug-refractory ventricular arrhythmias with amiodarone. Eur Heart J 7:735–742, 1986.
62. Naccarelli GV, Fineberg NS, Zipes DP, Heger JJ, Duncan G, Prystowsky EN: Amio-

darone: Risk factors for recurrence of symptomatic ventricular tachycardia identified at electrophysiologic study. J Am Coll Cardiol 6:814–821, 1985.
63. Fisher JD, Kim SG, Waspe LE, Johnston DR: Amiodarone: Value of programmed electrical stimulation and Holter monitoring (review). PACE 9:422–435, 1986.
64. Kadish AH, Buxton AE, Waxman HL, Flores B, Josephson ME, Marchlinski FE: Usefulness of electrophysiologic study to determine the clinical tolerance of arrhythmia recurrences during amiodarone therapy. J Am Coll Cardiol 10:90–96, 1987.
65. Schmitt C, Brachmann J, Waldecker B, Rizos I, Senges J, Kubler W: Amiodarone in patients with recurrent sustained ventricular tachyarrhythmias: Results of programmed electrical stimulation and long-term clinical outcome in chronic treatment. Am Heart J 114:279–283, 1987.
66. Krafchek, J, Lin HT, Beckman KJ, Nielsen AP, Magro SA, Hargis J, Wyndham CR: Cumulative effects of amiodarone on inducibility of ventricular tachycardia: Implications for electrophysiological testing. PACE 11:434–444, 1988.
67. Sahar DI, Bigger JT Jr, Reiffel JA, Ferrick K, Giardina EGV, Livelli FD Jr, Gliklich JI: Effects of amiodarone dosage changes on ventricular tachycardia inducibility in patients with life-threatening arrhythmias. Circulation 74[Suppl II]:II–213, 1986.
68. Friedman LM, Furberg CD, DeMets DL: "Fundamentals of Clinical Trials." Littleton, MA: PSG Publishers, 1985, pp 83–107.
69. Ruberman W, Weinblatt E, Goldberg JD, Frank CW, Shapiro S: Ventricular premature beats and mortality after myocardial infarction. N Engl J Med 297:750–757, 1977.
70. Moss AJ, Davis HT, DeCamilla J, Bayer LW: Ventricular ectopic beats and their relation to sudden and nonsudden cardiac death after myocardial infarction. Circulation 60: 998–1003, 1978.
71. Bigger JT Jr, Weld FM, Rolnitzky LM: The prevalence and significance of ventricular tachycardia detected by ambulatory ECG recording in the late hospital phase of acute myocardial infarction. Am J Cardiol 48:815–823, 1981.
72. Kleiger RE, Miller JP, Thanavaro S, Marin TF, Province MA, Oliver GC: Relationship between clinical features of acute myocardial infarction and ventricular runs two weeks to one year following infarction. Circulation 63:64–70, 1981.
73. The Multicenter Postinfarction Research Group: Risk stratification and survival after myocardial infarction. N Engl J Med 309:331–336, 1983.
74. Hinkle LE, Thaler JT: Clinical classification of cardiac deaths. Circulation 65:457–464, 1982.
75. Bigger JT Jr, Fleiss JL, Rolnitzky LM, The Multicenter Post Infarction Research Group: Prevalence, characteristics and significance of ventricular tachycardia detected by 24-hour continuous electrocardiographic recordings in the late hospital phase of acute myocardial infarction. Am J Cardiol 58:1151–1160, 1986.
76. Marcus FI, Cobb LA, Edwards JE, Kuller L, Moss AJ, Bigger JT Jr, Fleiss JL, Rolnitzky LM, Serokman R, The Multicenter Postinfarction Research Group: Mechanism of death and prevalence of myocardial ischemic symptoms in the terminal event after acute myocardial infarction. Am J Cardiol 61:8–15, 1988.
77. Bigger JT Jr: Relation between left ventricular dysfunction and ventricular arrhythmias after myocardial infarction. Am J Cardiol 57:8b–14b, 1986.
78. May GS, Eberlein KA, Furberg CD, Passamini ER, DeMets DL: Secondary prevention after myocardial infarction: A review of long-term trials. Prog Cardiovasc Dis 24: 331–352, 1982.
79. Furberg CD: Effect of antiarrhythmic drugs on mortality after myocardial infarction. Am J Cardiol 52:32C–36C, 1983.
80. Collaborative Group: Phenytoin after recovery from myocardial infarction. Controlled trial in 568 patients. Lancet 2:1055–1057, 1971.
81. Peter T, Ross D, Duffield A, Luxton M, Harper R, Hunt D, Sloman G: Effect on survival

after myocardial infarction of long-term treatment with phenytoin. Br Heart J 40:1356–1360, 1978.
82. Ryden L, Arnman K, Conradson TB, Hofvendahl S, Mortensen O, Smedgard P: Prophylaxis of ventricular tachyarrhythmias with intravenous and oral tocainide in patients with and recovering from acute myocardial infarction. Am Heart J 100:1006–1012, 1980.
83. Bastian BC, Macfarlane PW, McLauchlan JH, Ballantyne D, Clark R, Hillis WS, Rae AP, Hutton I: A prospective randomized trial of tocainide in patients following myocardial infarction. Am Heart J 100:1017–1022, 1980.
84. Chamberlain DA, Jewitt DE, Julian DG, Campbell RWF, Boyle DMcC, Shanks RG: Oral mexiletine in high-risk patients after myocardial infarction. Lancet 2:1324–1327, 1980.
85. IMPACT Research Group: International Mexiletine and Placebo Antiarrhythmic Coronary Trial (IMPACT):II. Results from 24-hour electrocardiograms. Eur Heart J 7:749–759, 1986.
86. IMPACT Research Group: International mexiletine and placebo antiarrhythmic coronary trial: I. Report on arrhythmia and other findings. J Am Coll Cardiol 4:1148–1163, 1984.
87. Hagemeijer F, Glaser B, van Durme JP, Bogaert M: Design of a study to evaluate drug therapy of serious ventricular rhythm disturbances after an acute myocardial infarction. Eur J Cardiol 6:299–310, 1977.
88. Gottlieb SH, Achuff SC, Mellits D, Gerstenblith G, Baughman KL, Becker L, Chandra NC, Henley S, Humphries J O'N, Heck C, Kennedy MM, Weisfildt ML, Reid PR: Prophylactic antiarrhythmic therapy of high-risk survivors of myocardial infarction: lower mortality at 1 month but not at 1 year. Circulation 75:792–799, 1987.
89. The CAPS Investigators: The Cardiac Arrhythmia Pilot Study. Am J Cardiol 57:91–95, 1986.
90. Lichstein E, Morganroth J, Harrist R, Hubble E, for the BHAT Study Group: Effect of propranolol on ventricular arrhythmia. The Beta-Blocker Heart Attack Trial experience. Circulation 67:5–10, 1983.
91. The CAPS Investigators: Recruitment and baseline description of patients in the Cardiac Arrhythmia Pilot Study. Am J Cardiol 61:704–713, 1988.
92. The CAPS Investigators: Effects of encainide, flecainide, imipramine, and moricizine on ventricular arrhythmias during the year after acute myocardial infarction: CAPS. Am J Cardiol 61:501–509, 1988.
93. Bigger JT Jr: Methodology for clinical trials with antiarrhythmic drugs to prevent cardiac death: US experience. Cardiology 74[Suppl 2]:40–56, 1987.

Chapter 9

Therapeutic Electrical Devices in the Management of Sudden Cardiac Death

Raymond Yee, M.D., F.R.C.P.(C), F.A.C.C., **Arjun D. Sharma**, M.D., **and George J. Klein**, M.D., F.R.C.P.(C), F.A.C.C.

Department of Medicine, University of Western Ontario, London, Ontario N6A 5A5, Canada

INTRODUCTION

Sudden cardiac death frequently results from the precipitous onset of electrical instability, with development of a catastrophic cardiac arrhythmia. Studies have shown that the most frequent arrhythmia recorded by emergency medical response teams early after onset is ventricular fibrillation [1], although a bradyarrhythmia may also precipitate sudden death [2,3]. One approach to the reduction in the incidence of this major public health problem has been an attempt to identify those patients who are at highest risk of developing a lethal cardiac arrhythmia and intervening before they suffer an initial episode (primary prevention). The second approach has been to prevent the recurrence of sudden cardiac death in those individuals surviving a lethal or potentially lethal cardiac arrhythmia (secondary prevention).

The cornerstone of secondary prevention of malignant ventricular tachyarrhythmias is suppression by antiarrhythmic drugs, but, despite the introduction of newer, more potent drugs, there remain patients who are refractory to prophylactic drug therapy. Some of these patients may be candidates for a curative surgical or nonsurgical ablation of the arrhythmogenic substrate, but a large number of unfortunate patients are not. Under these cir-

The Prevention of Sudden Cardiac Death, pages 197–220

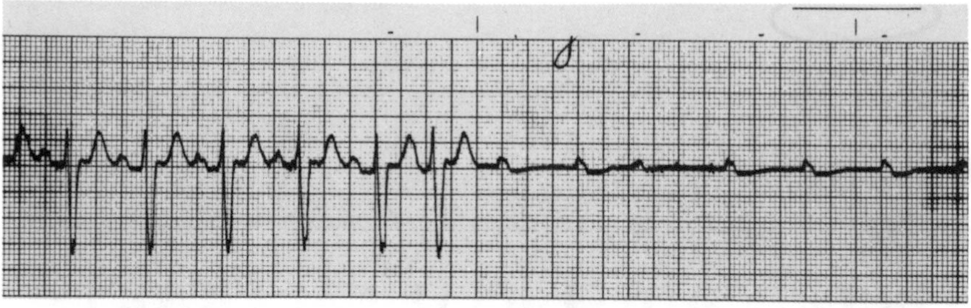

Fig. 9–1. This single-lead recording was obtained from a 65-year-old woman admitted to hospital for an acute anterolateral myocardial infarction associated with congestive heart failure. Several days later, she precipitously developed complete heart block, with ventricular asystole that was not preceded by any evidence of acute myocardial ischemia or AV block. The patient subsequently died despite temporary pacing (see text for discussion).

cumstances, devices that deliver electrical therapy for the suppression or termination of malignant cardiac arrhythmias are of value for long-term palliative management in combination with drugs.

This report focuses almost exclusively upon the available implantable device systems for electrical management of ventricular tachycardia (VT) or fibrillation but also encompasses the management of bradycardia-related sudden death and the future directions of research and development in this rapidly maturing field. These electrical device systems fall into two categories: 1) cardiac pacemakers providing bradycardia or antitachycardia pacing therapy and 2) electrical devices that deliver current for synchronized cardioversion or defibrillation (countershock).

SUDDEN CARDIAC DEATH SECONDARY TO BRADYARRHYTHMIAS

Whereas ventricular fibrillation appears to be the most frequent cardiac arrhythmia leading to sudden cardiac death, the importance of bradyarrhythmias must not be overlooked. Between 15% and 25% of out-of-hospital cardiac arrest victims when reached by emergency medical response teams are found to have a significant bradycardia. Continuous ambulatory recordings of cardiac arrest victims have revealed that the terminal arrhythmic event is sinus node arrest, high grade atrioventricular (AV) block, or asystole in up to 25% of cases [4,5]. An example of this is provided in Figure 9–1. The recording was taken from a 64-year-old woman who suffered an extensive anterolateral myocardial infarction. Several days following her admission, she developed sudden complete heart block that was not heralded by any preceding AV conduction abnormalities. Despite the immediate institution of resuscitative procedures that included temporary pacing, which was effective in achieving electrical systole, there was no effective mechanical systole and the patient died.

Although bradyarrhythmias account for a minority of sudden death events they are associated with a high mortality [3]. This suggests that bradycardia in many victims is another marker of severe underlying cardiac disease leading to death but is not causally related to sudden death. If so, the implantation of a permanent pacemaker would not be expected to have an appreciable effect on outcome. Nonetheless, survival following a bradyarrhythmic event warrants permanent pacing.

Because the development of a life-threatening bradycardia is often not preceded by intermediate changes in the electrocardiogram (ECG), the challenge has been to identify those patients at highest risk. Patients manifesting persistent AV or intraventricular conduction abnormalities following acute myocardial infarction have a higher risk of sudden death [6,7]. Frequently, the mechanism of sudden death is ventricular fibrillation, and the presence of conduction disturbances merely reflects the severity of cardiac disease [6]. There are no prospective studies demonstrating improvement in long-term survival in this subset of patients. Persistent high-grade AV block following myocardial infarction would warrant permanent pacing, but the need for pacing in patients with bundle branch block abnormalities is uncertain. At present, the guidelines for permanent pacing of patients who acquire AV or intraventricular conduction defects following myocardial infarction are left to the discretion of the individual physician. Patients with persistent high-grade AV block are the most likely candidates for permanent pacing.

VENTRICULAR TACHYARRHYTHMIAS AND SUDDEN CARDIAC DEATH

Ventricular tachyarrhythmias represent a major cause of sudden death in patients with left ventricular dysfunction secondary to myocardial infarction or primary myocardial disease. Ventricular fibrillation is the usual arrhythmia found at cardiac resuscitation, but ambulatory monitoring of sudden death victims frequently demonstrates that ventricular fibrillation is preceded by VT or flutter [5]. Studies have consistently shown that the outcome and prognosis of cardiac arrest victims is dependent primarily on the duration of the arrest [8]. The ultimate goal of electrical device systems has been to prevent recurrence or to minimize the time from the onset of the arrhythmia to restoration of normal rhythm. The electrical device systems available to date include 1) pacemakers with antitachycardia pacing capability, 2) the implantable cardioverter-defibrillator, and 3) the implantable transvenous cardioverter. Soon to become available will be the newer generation devices, which combine antitachycardia pacing, cardioversion, and defibrillation in a single, compact delivery system. In addition, some investigators have focused on improving technology related to conventional transthoracic countershock. Each of these devices is discussed in detail separately.

ANTITACHYCARDIA PACING

Implantable pacemakers serve two general purposes in the management of patients suffering from malignant ventricular arrhythmias: for the suppression or prevention of malignant ventricular tachyarrhythmias and for the termination of VT that does develop.

Prevention

Permanent pacemakers were first used in the 1950s for the suppression of VT or ventricular fibrillation [9–12], but experience over the past 3 decades has shown it to be useful in a limited number of circumstances only. The mechanism by which overdrive pacing achieves its benefit is undoubtedly multifactorial. Pacing at higher rates shortens diastole, which may reduce the opportunity for ectopic beats to appear or may directly suppress automaticity of ectopic tissue [13]. Tachyarrhythmias due to a reentrant mechanism may be facilitated by the greater dispersion in refractoriness of ventricular myocardium resulting from a slower rate. An increase in heart rate by pacing would tend to diminish this dispersion. Moreover, changes in the pattern of ventricular activation by pacing may impede engagement of the reentry circuit.

Patients whose manifest VT or ventricular fibrillation occurs secondary to a significant bradycardia would obviously benefit from permanent pacing. An example of this is the patient who develops QT prolongation and repeated episodes of polymorphous VT (torsades de pointes) in the setting of heart block. Antibradycardia pacing at normal rates would successfully prevent the reappearance of these tachyarrhythmias. However, the more commonly encountered situation is the development of VT in the setting of a normal heart rate. In these circumstances, a few patients may benefit from pacing the heart at somewhat faster rates (100–110 beats per minute), a method referred to as suppressive overdrive pacing. Temporary overdrive pacing for suppression may sometimes be of value in the acute care setting, such as following myocardial infarction or with drug-induced torsades de pointes, but the efficacy of permanent pacing for chronic management of these patients is low [9–12]. Temporary overdrive pacing is of value in patients with acquired reversible causes of long QT syndrome (drug toxicity, hypokalemia), but the role of permanent pacing in patients with congenital long QT syndrome and torsades de pointes is uncertain. A pacemaker is of value when the use of beta-blockers causes bradycardia, but a more definitive statement of the role of permanent pacing in patients with the congenital QT prolongation will likely require pooled data from a number of centers such as might be available through an international registry [14]. Regardless of the underlying

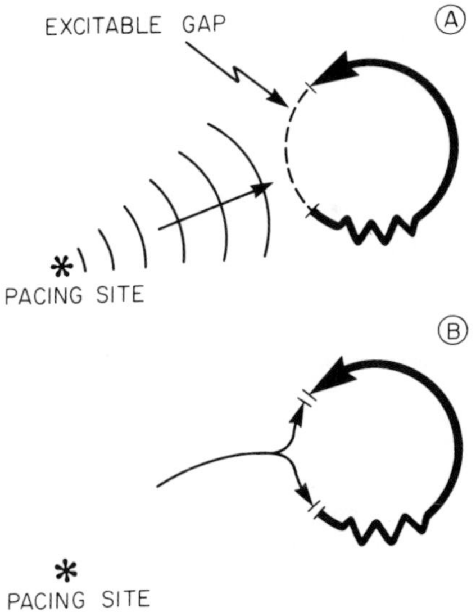

Fig. 9–2. This diagram depicts a reentrant tachycardia, with an anatomically or functionally defined reentrant circuit (see text for discussion).

cause, implantation of a permanent pacemaker to suppress VT should be undertaken only after temporary transvenous pacing has convincingly demonstrated suppression.

Termination

The other major role of permanent pacemakers is in the termination of spontaneous episodes of VT. The first reports of successful VT termination by pacing stimuli involved asynchronous pacing with fortuitous ventricular capture at a critical time during the cardiac cycle [15–17]. The interest in pacing as a therapeutic modality for VT increased following the important studies by Wellens and Dürrer as well as at other centers [18–21] demonstrating the usefulness of programmed ventricular stimulation for the initiation and termination of VT. The knowledge gained using these temporary pacing techniques was gradually incorporated into permanent pacemakers.

Pacing techniques are useful only for VTs that are the result of a reentrant mechanism (Fig. 9–2). A stable reentrant tachycardia is characterized by a wavefront of depolarization that traverses an anatomically or functionally defined circuit of any size. As the circuit is cyclically depolarized and repolarizes, there may exist a period of time between cycles when the circuit is no longer refractory and may be depolarized prematurely. The duration of that time interval (also called "excitable gap") is dependent on a balance between the conduction velocity of the wavefront and the refractory

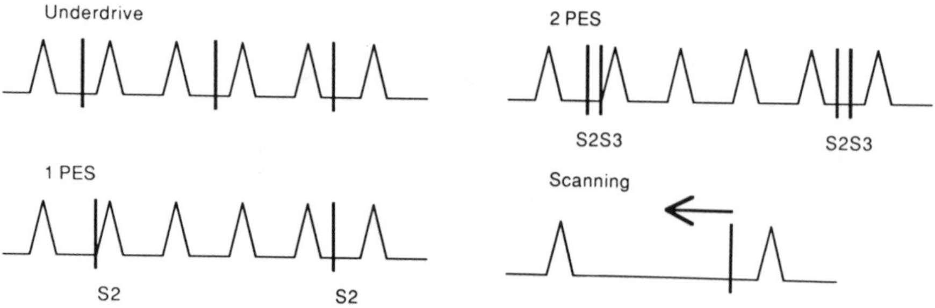

Fig. 9–3. Various pacing modalities are displayed in this diagram. PES, premature extrastimuli (see text for discussion).

period of the tissue. A paced beat that propagates from the site of stimulation into the reentrant circuit during this excitable gap depolarizes and renders the tissue refractory to the advancing tachycardia wavefront, and the tachycardia is extinguished.

The effectiveness of pacing stimuli in terminating any reentrant tachyarrhythmia is governed by a number of interrelated factors [22]. The majority of VT seen in the clinical setting appear to be due to a reentrant mechanism and are amendable to pacing termination, but VT secondary to enhanced automaticity responds only temporarily to pacing therapy by overdrive suppression, and the arrhythmia reappears when pacing is terminated. A tachycardia characterized by a very small anatomic circuit or a narrow excitable gap either as a result of the rapid rate of the tachycardia or prolonged refractoriness of tissue would encounter greater difficulty in penetrating the circuit. The distance from the pacing site to the reentrant circuit and the conduction properties of the intervening tissue dictate the likelihood that the paced beat will be able to penetrate the circuit during the excitable gap as does the rate of pacing or timing of the paced beat(s). Pacing from the atrium is ineffective in terminating all but the slowest VTs because of the conduction delay in the AV node [23,24]. Finally, metabolic and neurohumoral changes that develop secondary to the tachycardia may modulate conduction properties of the myocardium, affecting the response to and efficacy of pacing stimuli.

As a result of the application of programmed ventricular stimulation to the study of VT, a number of pacing modalities or ''stimulation protocols'' have been developed and incorporated into permanent pacing therapy. They can be simply classified into asynchronous underdrive pacing, programmed ventricular extrastimuli, trains of pacing stimuli, ultrarapid or subthreshold pacing, and combinations of these methods (see Figs. 9–3, 9–4).

Asynchronous underdrive pacing. This was the earliest technique used because permanent pacemakers initially had very limited features and programmability. Application of a magnet converted a demand pacemaker to

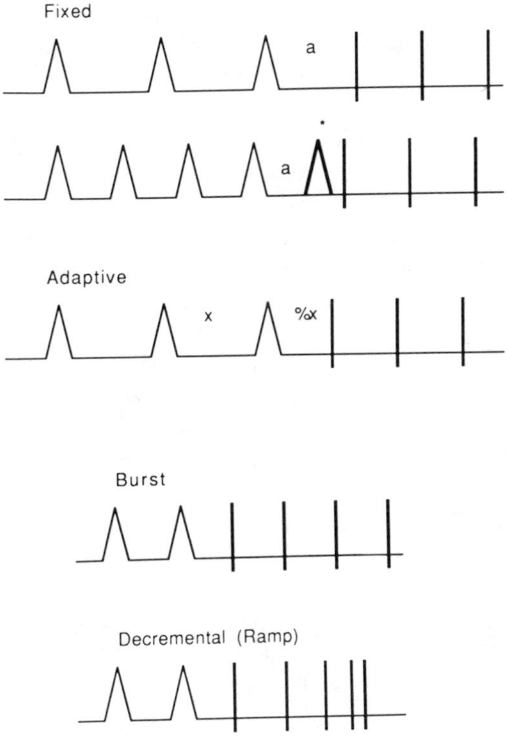

Fig. 9–4. Top panel illustrates VT, with the introduction of a train of pacing stimuli at a set coupling interval during the cardiac cycle. Middle panel shows what might occur if the same pacing train were delivered during a faster VT if no change in the coupling interval of the pacing train was instituted in response to the different VT rate. Bottom panel illustrates the advantages of adaptive pacing wherein the coupling interval of a pacing train is a percentage of the cycle length of the tachycardia.

the asynchronous mode. Pacing stimuli that are randomly introduced might fall outside the refractory period of the tissue at a critical time and fortuitously terminate the tachycardia. This technique is obviously unreliable since there is no control over the timing of stimuli, and it is infrequently employed.

Single or multiple extrastimuli. Similar in principle to underdrive pacing, this method entails controlled delivery of one or more pacing beats at a coupling interval following a tachycardia beat that can be programmed into the pacemaker unit. Some available devices deliver extrastimuli only at the coupling interval programmed; others scan the diastolic period, introducing stimuli repeatedly at earlier coupling intervals until termination is achieved.

Pacing trains. Single paced beats may fail to reach the reentrant circuit because of refractoriness of myocardium between the pacing site and the circuit. The delivery of a train of pacing stimuli may gradually "peel back" tissue refractoriness, and eventually the paced beats may penetrate the reentrant circuit. Trains of paced beats can be delivered in a number of ways, differing primarily in the timing of the stimuli. Overdrive pacing for termination of tachycardia (not to be confused with overdrive suppression) refers to pacing stimuli with equal interstimulus intervals delivered at a rate faster than the tachycardia. Fisher et al. [25] have arbitrarily defined it as pacing at less than 30 beats per minute faster than the tachycardia; stimulus trains greater than 30 beats per minute above the tachycardia are referred to as burst pacing. When the interval between successive beats is reduced, this is referred to as decremental pacing [26], whereas incremental pacing involves an increase in the interval between pacing stimuli.

Normally, pacing trains or extrastimuli are delivered at a preprogrammed coupling interval from the tachycardia beat, regardless of the rate of the tachycardia. This leads to the possibility that the same pacing train or stimulus may be effective in terminating a slow VT yet ineffective for a more rapid VT in the same patient (see Fig. 9–4). To improve the efficacy of pacing termination, pacing may be instituted at a coupling interval and rate that is a percentage of the particular episode of VT recognized, referred to as adaptive pacing. This is advantageous in patients with multiple VT rates or in whom the VT rate may change in response to antiarrhythmic drugs or other factors.

Ultrarapid and subthreshold pacing. This involves pacing stimuli that do not capture the ventricles because the very rapid burst of stimuli of low-current amplitude is delivered during the refractory period [27], yet these are of sufficient intensity to prolong refractoriness. This technique is still of an experimental nature and is not yet in the domain of clinical application.

Efficacy of Antitachycardia Pacing

As was stated above, the efficacy of pacing techniques is dependent on many variables. Using temporary pacing techniques, a number of studies have shown that termination of VT and rates of complications are critically dependent on the rate of the tachycardia. Fisher et al. [25] evaluated the efficacy of burst right ventricular (RV) pacing in 23 patients undergoing electrophysiology studies with repeated induction of VT. In total, 521 of 573 (89%) VT episodes were successfully terminated. When the tachycardia rate was >250 bpm or the patient was hypotensive, only 17% were terminated compared to 93% when VT rate was <250 bpm. Roy et al. [28] reported that 25 of 50 (50%) VT at a rate >200 bpm could not be terminated by programmed extrastimuli or burst pacing and required synchronized cardioversion, whereas 85 of 89 (95%) VT episodes <200 bpm were terminated by pacing.

Efficacy is also governed by the number of pacing stimuli, rate of pacing trains, and mode of pacing utilized. For instance, a single extrastimulus may terminate 18–57% [28–30] of VT episodes, whereas double extrastimuli (S_2S_3) were effective in up to 42% of episodes [29]. When overdrive pacing trains have been delivered, the success rate has been reported to range from 55% to 90%. The reason for this variability in reported efficacy rates is likely related to differences in tachycardia rate studied. Experience with newer pacing modalities is rather limited, but there is a suggestion that decremental pacing is more efficacious than standard burst pacing and is associated with less risk [26].

The greatest risk and disadvantage of antitachycardia pacing rests in the potential for VT acceleration or degeneration to ventricular fibrillation by pacing sequences. Fisher et al. [25] reported an incidence of 4%, but, since each patient had more than one induced episode of VT tested, almost one of every two patients showed such an adverse response. Other studies have reported an overall incidence of 18–35% using various pacing modalities [28,29]. The risk appears to be greatest in rapid VT necessitating the use of aggressive pacing techniques, such as longer trains and more rapid burst pacing. Naccarelli et al. [29] reported no episodes of acceleration using single premature extrastimuli but a 18% incidence with burst pacing. Roy et al. [28] found a 4% incidence with one, two, or three extrastimuli but a 35% incidence with burst pacing. There is some data to suggest that decremental pacing sequences are safer than burst pacing [26]. Thus, even though single and double extrastimuli are safer than pacing trains, the likelihood of successful VT termination is similarly low. It is this concern over the potential for acceleration or degeneration to ventricular fibrillation that has been the prime impediment to a more widespread employment of pacing techniques as a long-term therapeutic modality.

Permanent Pacing

Permanent pacemakers with antitachycardia pacing capacity can be divided into those that deliver therapy when manually activated and those that will automatically deliver preprogrammed therapy when VT is recognized. The first pacemakers that were designed specifically for management of tachyarrhythmias were the radiofrequency pacemakers [31,32]. The pacemaker was activated by a hand-held programmer, which required that the patient remain hemodynamically stable and conscious during the tachycardia or be able to reach medical care so that trained personnel could activate the device. Since then, increasingly sophisticated implantable devices capable of manual or automatic function and delivering a variety of pacing modes have been introduced. Many pacemakers are equipped with memory capacity to remember the effective pacing sequence of the previous episode(s) and deliver it first in future attacks, thereby reducing the time taken to achieve termination. Counters may also be available to allow the clinician to evaluate the number of tachycardia episodes treated, their characteristics, and the effective pacing mode.

The ideal candidate for antitachycardia pacing is the patient who has recurrent monomorphic VT that is relatively slow and hemodynamically well tolerated. Consistent VT termination by antitachycardia pacing must be demonstrated before implantation of this device, and such testing should be performed with the patient on the antiarrhythmic drug regimen he or she is expected to take chronically. The minimum number of episodes of VT that should be subjected to repeated antitachycardia pacing, to ensure safety and efficacy, is arbitrary, but Fisher et al. [33,34] have suggested that 100 episodes is a reasonable number. Once the device is implanted, testing should again be repeated to confirm the most effective and safe pacing regimen for each patient.

Permanent pacemakers with antitachycardia pacing capability have most frequently been used in patients with supraventricular tachycardias and their application to VT is much less. Fisher et al. [33] reported 20 patients with VT in whom a permanent pacemaker was implanted for purposes of termination. After a mean follow-up of 37 months, actuarial efficacy was reported as 78% and 55% at 1 and 5 years, respectively. The incidence of sudden death was 20% (four patients), but apparently none could clearly be related to pacing failure.

More widespread use of antitachycardia pacing for the long-term management of patient with VT has been impeded by the ever-present risk of VT acceleration or degeneration to ventricular fibrillation. Some patients are required to activate their devices only in the presence of medical personnel who can deliver emergency care including defibrillation in the event of an adverse response. The future of antitachycardia pacing in the management of malignant ventricular arrhythmias rests on two possible directions in research. The first is the development of other pacing modalities, such as subthreshold or ultrarapid trains of pacing stimuli, or combinations of various pacing modalities. The second is to combine antitachycardia pacing with devices capable of automatic defibrillation (see below).

AUTOMATIC IMPLANTABLE CARDIOVERTER AND DEFIBRILLATOR (AICD) (Fig. 9–5)

Although antitachycardia pacing may be of value in some patients with slower, well tolerated VT that can be reliably and safely terminated by pacing techniques following careful assessment, it plays no role in the management of the patient with rapid, poorly tolerated VT, nor in those patients with the propensity for developing ventricular fibrillation. Synchronized cardioversion and defibrillation [35] are the most effective means of terminating these malignant arrhythmias.

Previous studies have shown that the outcome following an episode of sudden cardiac death is closely related to the time required to terminate the arrhythmia [8]. Until this decade, the only available method of delivering countershock utilized manually activated devices that delivered transthoracic current. Several investigators recognized the need for a more rapidly responsive, effective, and safe method of delivering electrical countershock to patients at high risk of sudden death. A logical proposal was to develop an implantable device that could automatically detect and deliver countershock. In the 1960s and 1970s, at least two laboratories were actively engaged in developing such a system [36,37]. Ultimately, Mirowski and his colleagues [38–40] were able to develop the first automatic implantable defibrillator for clinical use. It was their enormous effort that resulted in the development and implantation of the first automatic implantable defibrillator, tested first in animals [38,39] and finally implanted in humans in 1980 [40]. Since then, there have been a total of over 3,000 worldwide implants of this device, with a cumulative implant time exceeding 39,000 implant-months [41]. There is no doubt that the technological achievements have had a measurable and profound influence on our approach to the management of patients with malignant ventricular arrhythmias, and the results indicate a significant improvement in short-term survival of this group of patients.

The initial device (AID, Intec Systems, Inc.) weighed 250 g and was powered by a lithium battery [40,42,43]. This unit was interfaced to the heart by a spring coil electrode positioned in the superior vena cava near the junction with the right atrium and a second patch electrode over the left ventricular (LV) apex. The device delivered a truncated, exponential, unsynchronized pulse of approximately 25 J and could recycle three further times to deliver up to 30 J if the first and second shocks were unsuccessful. Tachyarrhythmia detection was based only on monitoring of the probability density function (PDF) through the lead system. The PDF is a measure of the time that sensed ventricular activity spends within preset limits of the isoelectric potential. Ventricular fibrillation and other tachycardias characterized by sinusoidal waveforms demonstrate minimal isoelectric potential activity. Activation and deactivation of the device as well as measurement of capacitor charge time are conducted using a ring magnet. A noninvasive analyzer permits interrogation of the device to determine the number of discharges and the capacitor charge time, which are used to determine the optimal time for generator replacement.

The first series of implantations were performed only in patients in whom ventricular fibrillation was documented at least once. The spring electrode was inserted through the internal jugular vein and tunneled down along the chest wall to be connected to the generator. The apical patch was sutured to the epicardium through a left thoracotomy. There was no assessment of defibrillation efficacy during the implant procedure.

The fundamental components of the system have remained unchanged, but a number of significant modifications have been made. These include the addition of a higher-energy device (theoretically up to 35–40 J), incorporation of synchronized cardioversion for VT, and employment of a second patch electrode in lieu of the spring electrode to improve defibrillation efficacy [44]. To accommodate cardioversion capability, heart rate was added to the tachycardia detection algorithm, since slower VT would not be recognized by the PDF criteria alone. For rate sensing and synchronization, an endocardial bipolar ventricular lead or two epimyocardial screw-in electrodes were provided. One model provided both heart rate-sensing and PDF criteria (AID-B); a second utilized only heart rate (AID-BR) [44–46]. The PDF criterion reduces but does not eliminate the misdetection of a supraventricular tachycardia and may allow somewhat slower VT that are less sinusoidal in morphology to escape detection. Rate sensing, on the other hand, would aid in detection of slower tachycardia episodes. The present generation of the device remains nonprogrammable, with an actual lifespan of less than 24 months [47,48].

Several alternative surgical approaches have been developed [44]. A median sternotomy has been employed, particularly in the patient undergoing concomitant procedures such as coronary bypass grafting. A subxiphoid and subcostal approach that avoids a thoracotomy has also been described. Initially, there was no device to measure defibrillation efficacy during the implantation procedure, and defibrillation efficacy as defined by the measurement of the defibrillation threshold (DFT) was not routinely measured until 1982 [49], with the development of an external defibrillation unit that could be connected to the electrodes. Routine measurement of the DFT at implant revealed that some patients could not be defibrillated using the existing leads. The replacement of the spring electrode by a second patch (patch-patch configuration) and larger-surface-area patches have improved defibrillation efficacy. Cannom and Winkle [50] have stated that a 10 J margin of safety (the difference between the energy output of the device and the minimum energy required to defibrillate as measured using the external defibrillation unit) was optimal. Whether a value <10 is sufficient and safe to proceed with implantation has not been delineated. A disturbing finding has been the effect of amiodarone loading on the intraoperative DFT reported by several centers [48,51]. Such findings reinforce the need for careful evaluation of candidates and their adjunctive drug therapy prior to and following defibrillator implantations. No similar effects have been reported with other antiarrhythmics. Whether a similar interaction occurs with amiodarone and other discharge waveforms such as sequential and bidirectional simultaneous shocks is not known at this time.

The initial report concerning the first 52 patients in whom the AID and AICD were implanted suggested an improvement in overall mortality of 48% at 1 year [52]. These data were derived by comparing actual mortality with the predicted mortality assuming that death would have occurred at the time of the first device discharge had it not been implanted. Although the assumptions made and the conclusions drawn from these early studies were viewed in some quarters with concern, subsequent reports from various implanting centers seem to have confirmed the efficacy of the device in preventing sudden death [47,48,53–55]. Echt et al. [54] reported the Stanford Group experience with the first 70 patients receiving the first- and second-generation devices. After a follow-up of 1–33 months (mean 8.9 months) sudden death mortality was 1.8%, and total cardiac mortality was 10.1% at 1 year. Over the follow-up period, over one-half the patients had received shocks, and most were on adjunctive antiarrhythmic drug therapy. Complications related to the operative procedure (infection, death) and problems with the AICD system (lead fracture causing inappropriate shocks, shocks delivered to sinus rhythm or supraventricular tachycardia, and excessively high defibrillation threshold) were reported. More recent reports from other U.S. centers involving comparable numbers of patients have mirrored these results, with life table mortality estimates of up to 6.6% at 1 year [48,53,55] and similar profiles of complications.

A report based on information collected by the AICD manufacturers registry concerning 949 patients receiving an implantable defibrillator to August, 1986, was recently published. The patient population ranged in age from 11 to 80 years (mean 58 years). Males outnumbered females by more than 3:1, and 72% suffered from coronary artery disease; two-thirds were concomitantly on antiarrhythmic drugs, principally amiodarone. Slightly over 50% had received shocks, with an average of 7.1 shocks per patient for that subset of patients who did receive shocks. The overall 1 year sudden death rate was only 2.0%, with a nonsudden cardiac death rate of 6.7%. An interesting study by Fogoros et al. [56] compared three groups of patients with ventricular tachyarrhythmias treated by implantation of a defibrillator or amiodarone. The study involved a small number of patients, and they were not randomized for therapy received. The authors showed that the actuarial risk of sudden death was 31% greater if patients received amiodarone alone compared to patients who received a defibrillator. There have been no studies involving a randomized, prospective trial of implantable defibrillators vs. empiric amiodarone or other antiarrhythmic drug therapy. In the absence of such information, these data have been compared with previously published studies. The consistently lower 1 year sudden cardiac death rates reported so far argues persuasively that the use of an implantable defibrillator indeed significantly reduces sudden death.

Many of the complications that occurred during the early experience with the first- and second-generation device (lead fracture, high defibrillation threshold, lead migration, misdirected pulses, and premature pulse generator failure) were related to faults in hardware design or manufacture and were overcome through improvements in the entire system. Others, such as inappropriate shocks for supraventricular rhythms [54,57] and adverse interaction with implanted pacemakers are to a large extent inherent limitations of existing technology. Unipolar pacemaker stimulus artifacts may cause oversensing and be mistaken for VT, whereas the same pacing spikes may result in failure to detect ventricular fibrillation [54,58]. This can be circumvented by using a bipolar pacemaker and locating the catheter far from the rate sensing leads of the defibrillator [54,59]. The risks of surgery must be borne by the patient and include death and pocket infection. As with all electrical devices, regular follow-up is required. Shocks are associated with physical discomfort and psychological stress that may become a major difficulty in some patients [54]. Some of the fear of subsequent shocks that patients express can be traced back to the psychological trauma that patients experience when shocked while completely conscious [60].

At the present time, the implantable cardioverter-defibrillator is a good therapeutic choice for the patient with infrequent episodes of drug-refractory VT or ventricular fibrillation who is not a candidate for a definitive cure by surgical or catheter ablation of the arrhythmogenic substrate and in the patient in whom complete suppression or cure cannot be ensured. Patients with frequent episodes of nonsustained VT are less suited for the AICD because the device may be triggered by the tachycardia and discharged after normal sinus rhythm has resumed (Fig. 5).

There is no doubt that the achievement of a fully implantable, reliable, and safe automatic cardioverter-defibrillator was an extremely important landmark in cardiovascular management. Nonetheless, the present generation of devices has well recognized limitations that significantly limit their usefulness in the clinical setting. The cardioverter-defibrillator is a nonprogrammable device. The heart rate criteria for tachycardia detection are fixed at manufacture and must be specified for each individual patient prior to implantation. More importantly, temporal changes in VT or ventricular fibrillation characteristics such as those resulting from the addition of antiarrhythmic drugs may adversely affect optimal functioning of the device. For instance, the addition of an antiarrhythmic drug such as procainamide or amiodarone to the patient's therapy regimen may slow the rate of VT below the rate cut-off of an implanted device.

It would also be advantageous for the energy deliverable by the AICD to be programmable to lower values so that there could possibly be energy savings and improvements in the life span of the device in patients who are demonstrated to have a low defibrillation threshold. Other limitations include the size of the present device, cost, longevity, and need for a surgical procedure. One of the clear goals is the development of a device that, like modern pacemakers, may be implanted without the need for general anesthesia or access to the chest cavity. Recent developments of the AICD system that overcome the need for a thoracotomy for lead placement appear to be an important step in that direction [61]. The new lead electrode system employs a tripolar endocardial catheter that is inserted percutaneously through the

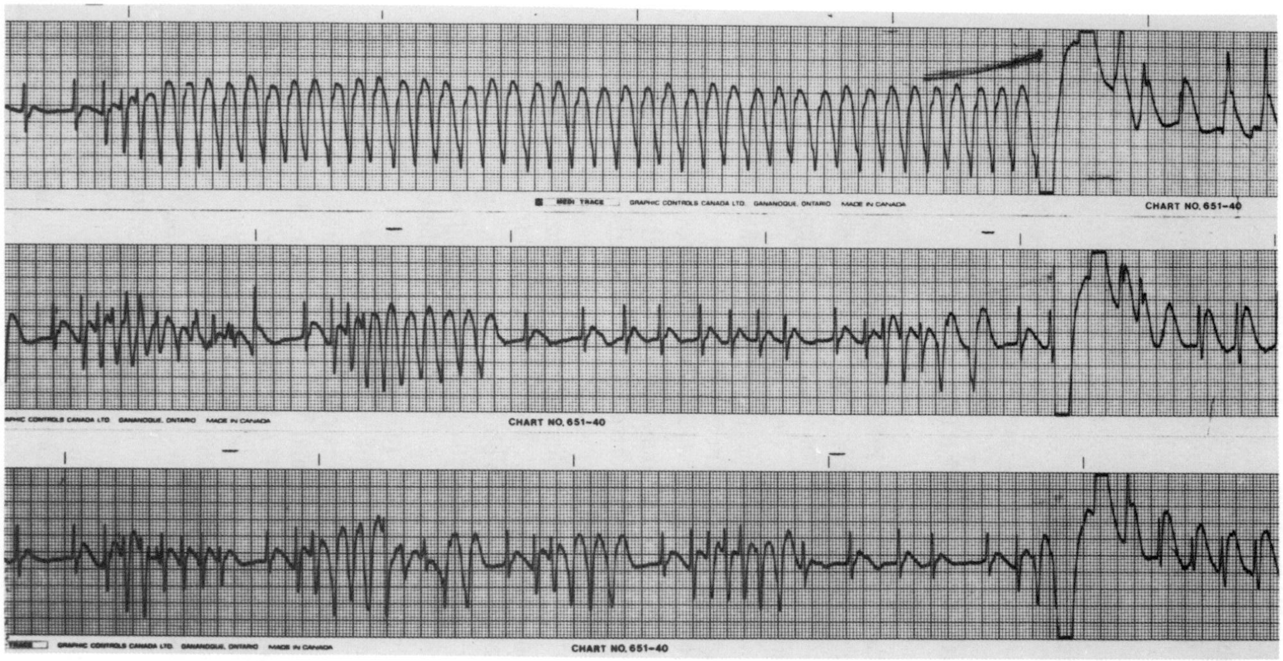

Fig. 9–5. Three separate rhythm strips taken following implantation of an AICD. Rhythm strip 1 shows appropriate sensing of rapid VT, with restoration of a normal rhythm following the first discharge. Rhythm strips 2 and 3 show bursts of nonsustained VT that spontaneously terminated but are sufficiently long that they trigger tachycardia detection by the device, with obligatory discharge during normal rhythm.

subclavian vein, with the tip lodged in the right ventricle. There are also two defibrillating electrodes on the catheter, one resting within the RV cavity, the second located at the right atrial/superior vena cava junction. A submuscular patch electrode is implanted in the chest wall at the midaxillary line. Defibrillating current is delivered simultaneously over the two current pathways. Exciting developments and steady progress such as this no doubt, will continue to improve significantly the safety, efficacy, and usefulness of this system in the clinical setting.

THE TRANSVENOUS CARDIOVERTER

The transvenous cardioverter (model 7210, Medtronic, Inc.) was introduced for clinical evaluation in 1984 for treatment of VT but has been implanted in only a limited number of patients [62–65]. The generator weighed 95 g and delivered synchronized shocks of truncated exponential waveform at programmable energy from 0.06 to 2.0 J for the first three shocks. Two further shocks at the maximum output of the device were then delivered if tachycardia persisted. Therapy could be delivered automatically or only upon telemetry command if desired. The unit also provided ventricular demand pacing and could be manually commanded to serve as a programmable stimulator, delivering drive trains and extrastimuli for tachycardia induction and pacing termination of episodes. As with conventional pacemakers, it had bidirectional telemetry that transmitted marker pulses, electrograms, programmed settings, and generator replacement indicators. The lead system consisted of a bipolar tined catheter, with one pair of cardioversion electrodes at the catheter tip and the second pair located 100–150 mm proximally. Shocks were delivered between these electrodes; the distal electrodes also served as the rate-sensing and pacing electrode. The entire device could be implanted without thoracotomy.

Initial reports on the first series of patients appeared promising [62]. Seven patients received the device, and the mean cardioversion threshold was 0.43 J and ranged from 0.07 to 1.7 J. On short-term follow-up of 1–6 months, most tachycardia episodes were terminated by the device, but inappropriate shocks for rapid atrial fibrillation and VT acceleration were also reported as adverse responses. A more recent report from 1987 [65] summarized the cumulative experience of the device implanted in 29 patients. Follow-up ranged from 1 to 40 months, with a mean of 24 months. There were a total of 12 deaths, six in the first year of follow-up. Of the 12 patients, five died with the device in the automatic therapy mode, and four of these deaths were judged to be related to an arrhythmia. Of the remaining 17, VT acceleration by shocks was documented in two patients. There have been no further implants of this system.

COMBINATION ANTITACHYCARDIA PACING AND COUNTERSHOCK THERAPY

A brief review of the advantages and limitations of antitachycardia pacing in comparison with cardioversion-defibrillation quickly reveals that these two methods of therapy are not mutually exclusive but, rather, provide complimentary therapy. Indeed, the "ideal" tachycardia management device should offer graded therapy for VT, with antitachycardia pacing for slower, well tolerated VT and synchronized, low-energy cardioversion for more rapid, poorly tolerated VT. Because of the risk of VT acceleration or degeneration to ventricular fibrillation, back-up defibrillation should also be provided. Some patients might have concomitant bradyarrhythmias or develop bradycardia following therapy for VT or ventricular fibrillation. Therefore, bradycardia pacing would also be an advantageous addition, removing the need for a separate, permanent pacemaker implant.

Although the benefits of such a system were recognized rather early, no such single device offering all these features was available until 1987. As an alternative, some centers have implanted both an antitachycardia pacemaker and an automatic implantable cardioverter-defibrillator in selected patients [66–68]. Because of careful patient selection, the outcome has been positive, but there is a clear recognition of the potential dangers of implanting two separate antitachycardia devices that are not capable of communicating together [58,59,66], and a single device combining all these therapies is more desirable.

THE IMPLANTABLE PACEMAKER CARDIOVERTER DEFIBRILLATOR

The first implantable pacemaker cardioverter defibrillator (PCD) that provided comprehensive antitachycardia therapy in a single compact system was introduced for human implant in 1987 [69]. The PCD 7215 (Medtronic, Inc) weighs 180 g, is powered by two lithium batteries and delivers programmable pacing therapy or shocks of truncated exponential waveform (Fig. 9–6). Tachycardia detection is based on cycle length-related criteria that are programmed individually for VT and ventricular fibrillation detection. If VT is recognized, the device can deliver up to four therapies per episode of tachycardia. For VT, that therapy may consist of a series of adaptive burst or adaptive autodecremental pacing sequences or, alternatively, synchronized cardioversion from 0.2 to 15 J. For ventricular fibrillation, up to four defibrillating shocks can be delivered for each episode, with energy programmable from 1 to 15 J. In the event of bradycardia, the device offers ventricular demand pacing.

There are four epicardial leads in this system; three are epicardial

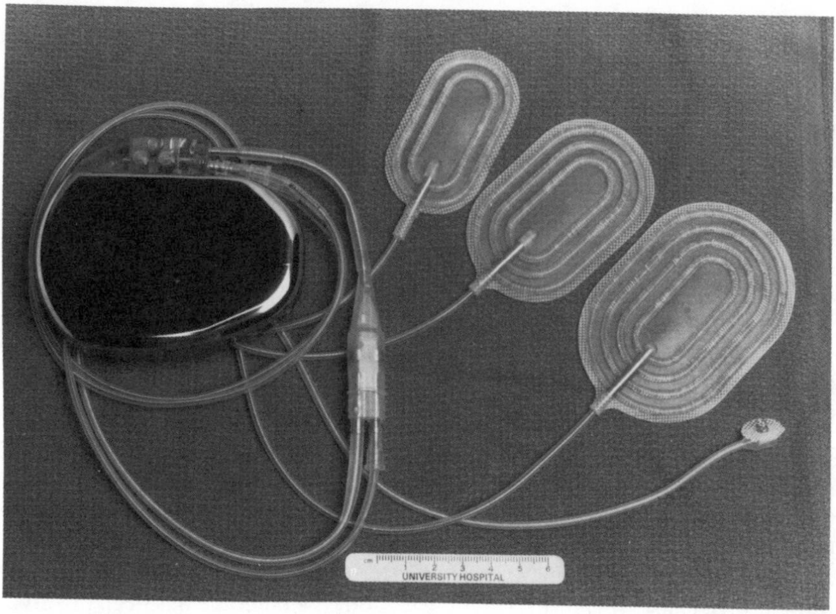

Fig. 9–6. PCD 7215 generator displayed along with the countershock patch electrodes (available in three sizes) and the epimyocardial screw-in lead.

countershock patch electrodes and one is an epimyocardial screw-in lead for modified bipolar rate sensing and pacing. The three-patch-electrode array allows for single- or dual-current-pathway countershock. Dual-pathway countershock may be delivered using simultaneous or sequential pulses.

The first four patients to receive this device were men ranging in age from 45 to 75 years. Each patient had drug-refractory VT and one had had one episode of ventricular fibrillation prior to implantation of the device. The underlying cause of these malignant ventricular arrhythmias was ischemic heart disease with previous myocardial infarction in two patients and valvular heart disease and dilated cardiomyopathy in the other two patients.

At surgical implantation, electrodes were applied through a median sternotomy. Ventricular fibrillation was induced with AC current on three separate occasions, and a single 7.5 J sequential pulse shock was delivered using an external defibrillator each time. Successful defibrillation with three consecutive attempts indicated that the true defibrillation threshold would be less than 7.5 J, thereby ensuring that the maximum output of the device (15 J) allowed at least a 100% margin of safety (2 × DFT) for ventricular defibrillation. All four patients met these criteria, and the generator was implanted. The final test involved induction of ventricular fibrillation and allowing the pacemaker-cardioverter-defibrillator automatically to sense and deliver one defibrillating shock at 15 J.

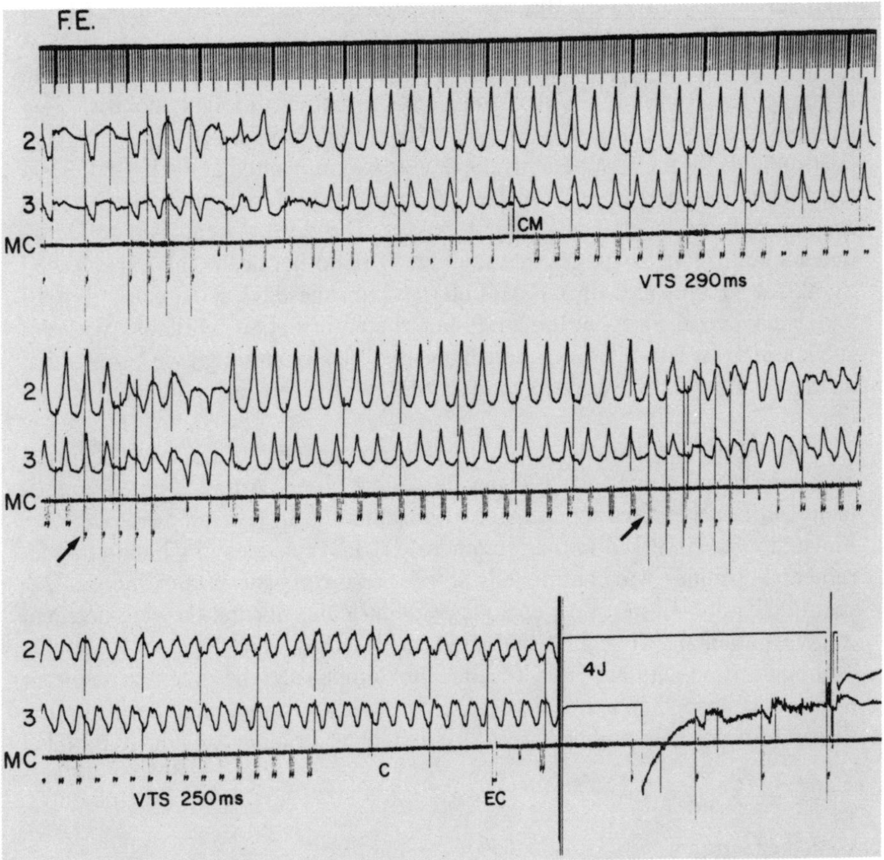

Fig. 9–7. Recording taken during PCD evaluation prior to patient discharge. Surface ECG leads 2 and 3 and the marker channel of the PCD are displayed in each panel. Automatic therapy delivery was initiated at the cancel magnet command (CM), and pacing therapy was delivered (arrow). When pacing therapy accelerated the VT, the PCD charged the capacitor (C) and delivered a 4 J shock (see text for explanation).

An example of the PCD's capabilities is shown in Figure 9–7. At the time of postoperative testing of the device, VT was induced using the PCD as a programmable stimulator. Sustained VT at a cycle length of 290 msec was induced by three ventricular extrastimuli. The PCD was then allowed automatically to detect and deliver programmed therapy. VT was detected as indicated by the marker pulses and two sequences of ramp (autodecremental) pacing therapy were delivered, but these failed to terminate the tachycardia, and the second sequence accelerated the VT to a cycle length of 250 msec. This caused the PCD to advance to the next programmed therapy, which was a 4 J synchronized shock. The tachycardia was terminated, followed by a brief period of bradycardia that was interrupted by ventricular demand pacing from the PCD.

Recent data [70] are available on follow-up of these patients ranging from 1.5 to 16 months, with a total of 30.5 patient implant months. Two patients (patients 2 and 4) continue to carry the device (16 and 9 months postimplant). In the first patient, the device was explanted at the time of heart transplantation performed for hemodynamic and functional deterioration secondary to poor left ventricular function. The third patient died suddenly under circumstances suggesting suicide. Prior to his death, he experienced a total of 11 episodes of VT. Counters within the device indicated that all had been successfully terminated, but the information available was not sufficient to ascertain the exact mechanism of death, although we believe that death was likely the result of a bradycardia, with electromechanical dissociation.

In these four patients, a total of 145 spontaneous VT episodes occurred over the follow-up period, 126 in one patient alone. Autodecremental antitachycardia pacing was successful in terminating 83% of all episodes; cardioversion was utilized in the remainder. Of 120 episodes in which autodecremental pacing was attempted before resorting to cardioversion, 7% required cardioversion. Five episodes of ventricular fibrillation were detected in two patients. All were terminated successfully by 10 or 15 J shocks. Although these data are early results, they emphasize the potential value of a single device that can deliver pacing, cardioversion, and defibrillation therapy for patients with recurrent malignant ventricular tachyarrhythmias.

CONCLUSIONS

The field of implantable device therapy for the long-term management of patients with sudden cardiac death due to malignant arrhythmias is rapidly expanding and maturing in a manner that parallels that seen in previous decades with permanent pacemakers for bradyarrhythmias. Improvements in understanding of the factors that determine the efficacy and complications of pacing and countershock therapies as well as technological advancements will have a major impact on the reliability, safety, and efficacy of such devices. There is active research into better methods of detecting and distinguishing ventricular arrhythmias from supraventricular arrhythmias and different methods of delivering countershock energy and different pulse waveforms that hold the potential for improving therapeutic efficacy. However, the increasing flexibility and features of future programmable devices raises the problem of increased complexity, with its attendant risk to the patient and difficulties for the implanting physician. The challenges for the future are not only to develop better and more efficacious therapeutic devices but also to manage this complexity.

REFERENCES

1. Adgey AAJ, Scott ME, Allen JD, et al.: Management of ventricular fibrillation outside hospital. Lancet 1:1169, 1969.
2. Iseri LT, Humphrey SB, Siner EJ: Prehospital bradyasystolic cardiac arrest. Ann Intern Med 88:741–745, 1978.
3. Myerburg RJ, Zaman L, Luceri R, et al.: Prehospital cardiac arrest with idioventricular rhythm (abstract). Circulation 68:356, 1983.
4. Panidis IP, Morganroth J: Sudden death in hospitalized patients: Cardiac rhythm disturbances detected by ambulatory electrocardiographic monitoring. J Am Coll Cardiol 2:798–805, 1983.
5. Kempf FC Jr, Josephson ME: Cardiac arrest recorded on ambulatory electrocardiograms. Am J Cardiol 53:1577–1582, 1984.
6. Lie KI, Leim KL, Schuilenberg RM, Davd GK, Dürrer D: Early identification of patients developing late in-hospital ventricular fibrillation after discharge from the coronary care unit. Am J Cardiol 41:674–677, 1978.
7. Hauer RNW, Lie KI, Leim KL, Dürrer D: Long-term prognosis in patients with bundle branch block complicating acute anteroseptal infarction. Am J Cardiol 49:1581–1585, 1982.
8. Kerber RE, Jensen SR, Gascho JA, Grayzel J, Hoyt R, Kennedy J: Determinants of defibrillation: Prospective analysis of 183 patients. Am J Cardiol 52:739–745, 1983.
9. Swedberg J, Malm A. Pacemaker stimulation in ventricular paroxysmal tachycardia. Acta Chir Scand 128:610–615, 1964.
10. DeSanctis RW, Kastor JA: Rapid intracardiac pacing for treatment of recurrent ventricular tachyarrhythmias in the absence of heart block. Am Heart J 76:168–171, 1968.
11. Escher DJW: The treatment of tachyarrhythmias by artificial cardiac pacing. Am Heart J 78:829–832, 1969.
12. Escher DJW, Furman S: Emergency treatment of cardiac arrhythmias. JAMA 214:2028–2034, 1970.
13. Vassalle M: Electrogenic suppression of automaticity in sheep and dog Purkinje fibers. Circ Res 27:361, 1970.
14. Moss AJ, Schwartz PJ, Crampton RS, Locati E, Carleen E: The long QT syndrome: A prospective international study. Circulation 71:17–21, 1985.
15. Bürchell HB, Merideth J: Management of cardiac tachyarrhythmias with cardiac pacemakers. Ann NY Acad Sci 167:546–556, 1969.
16. Bennett MA, Pentecost BL: Reversion of ventricular tachycarida by pacemaker stimulation. Br Heart J 33:922–927, 1971.
17. Moss AJ, Rivers RJ: Termination and inhibition of recurrent tachycardias by implanted pervenous pacemakers. Circulation 50:942–947, 1974.
18. Wellens HJ, Schuilenburg RM, Dürrer D: Electrical stimulation of the heart in patients with ventricular tachycardia. Circulation 46:216–226, 1972.
19. Wellens HJ, Lie KI, Dürrer D: Further observations on ventricular tachycardia as studied by electrical stimulation of the heart. Circulation 49:647–653, 1974.
20. Josephson ME, Horowitz N, Farshidi A, Kastor JA: Recurrent sustained ventricular tachycardia. Circulation 57:431–440, 1978.
21. Mason JW, Winkle RA: Electrode-catheter arrhythmia induction in the selection and assessment of antiarrhythmic drug therapy for recurrent ventricular tachycardia. Circulation 58:971–985, 1978.
22. Wellens JHH: Value and limitations of programmed electrical stimulation of the heart in the study and treatment of tachycardias. Circulation 57:845–853, 1978.
23. Waxman MB, Bonet JF, Wald RW: Self-conversion of drug resistant ventricular tachycardia by rapid atrial pacing. PACE 6:900–907, 1983.
24. Wellens HJJ, Bar FW, Farre J, et al.: Initiation and termination of ventricular tachycardia

by supraventricular stimuli: Incidence and electrophysiologic determinants as observed during programmed stimulation of the heart. Am J Cardiol 46:576, 1980.
25. Fisher JD, Mehra R, Furman S: Termination of ventricular tachycardia with bursts of rapid ventricular pacing. Am J Cardiol 41:94–102, 1978.
26. Charos GS, Haffajee CI, Gold RL, Bishop RL, Berkovitis VB, Alpert JS: A theoretically and practically more effective method for interruption of ventricular tachycardia: Self-adapting autodecremental overdrive pacing. Circulation 73:309–315, 1986.
27. Swerdlow CD, Liem LB, Franz MR: Summation and inhibition by ultrarapid train pacing in the human ventricle. Circulation 76:1101–1109, 1987.
28. Roy D, Waxman HL, Buxton AE, et al.: Termination of ventricular tachycardia: Role of tachycardia cycle length. Am J Cardiol 50:1346–1350, 1982.
29. Naccarelli GV, Zipes DP, Rahilly GT, Heger JJ, Prystowsky EN: Influence of tachycardia cycle length and antiarrhythmic drugs on pacing termination and acceleration of ventricular tachycardia. Am Heart J 105:1–5, 1983.
30. Fisher JD, Kim SG, Matos JA, Ostrow E: Comparative effectiveness of pacing techniques for termination of well-tolerated sustained ventricular tachycardia. PACE 6:915–922, 1983.
31. Kahn A, Morris JJ, Citron P: Patient-initiated rapid atrial pacing to manage supraventricular tachycardia. Am J Cardiol 38:200–204, 1976.
32. Peters RW, Shafton E, Frank S, Thomas AN, Scheinman MM: Radiofrequency triggered pacemaker: Uses and limitations. Ann Intern Med 88:17–22, 1978.
33. Fisher JD, Johnston DR, Kim SG, Furman S, Mercando AM: Implantable pacers for tachycardia termination: Stimulation techniques and long-term efficacy. PACE 9:1325–1333, 1986.
34. Fisher JD, Johnston DR, Furman S, Mercando AD, Kim SG: Long-term efficacy of antitachycardia pacing for supraventricular and ventricular tachycardias. Am J Cardiol 60:1311–1316, 1987.
35. Lown B, Axelrod P: Implanted standby defibrillators. Circulation 46:637–639, 1972.
36. Mirowski M, Mower MM, Staewer WS, Tabatznik B, Mendeloff AI: Standby automatic defibrillator. Arch Intern Med 126:158–161, 1970.
37. Schuder JC, Stoeckle H, Gold JH, West JA, Keskar PY: Experimental ventricular defibrillation with an automatic and completely implanted system. Trans Am Soc Artif Int Organs 16:207–212, 1970.
38. Mirowski M, Mower MM, Langer A, Heilman MS, Schreibman J: A chronically implanted system for automatic defibrillation in active conscious dogs. Circulation 58: 90–94, 1978.
39. Mirowski M, Mower MM, Bhagavan BS, et al.: Chronic animal and bench testing of the implantable automatic defibrillator. Paper presented at VIth World Symposium on Cardiac Pacing, October 2–5, 1979, Montreal.
40. Mirowski M, Reid PR, Mower MM, et al.: Termination of malignant ventricular arrhythmias with an implanted automatic defibrillator in human beings. N Engl J Med 303: 322–324, 1980.
41. Mirowski M: Worldwide clinical experience with the use of the automatic implantable cardioverter-defibrillator. In Furlanello F, Betini R, Disertori M, et al. (eds): "The New Frontiers of Arrhythmias." Rome: CIC-Edizioni Internazionali s.r.l., 1988, pp 509–513.
42. Mirowski M, Reid PR, Watkins L, Weisfeldt ML, Mower MM: Clinical treatment of life-threatening ventricular tachyarrhythmias with the automatic implantable defibrillator. Am Heart J 102:265–270, 1981.
43. Watkins L Jr, Mower MM, Reid PR, Platia EV, Griffith LSC, Mirowski M: Trials of the automatic implantable defibrillator in man. J Thorac Cardiovasc Surg 86:381–387, 1983.

44. Mirowski M, Mower MM, Veltri EP, Juanteguy JM, Reid PR: Recent clinical experience with the automatic implantable cardioverter-defibrillator. Med Instrument 20:285–291, 1986.
45. Reid PR, Mirowski M, Mower MM, et al.: Clinical evaluation of the internal automatic cardioverter-defibrillator in survivors of sudden cardiac death. Am J Cardiol 51:1608–1613, 1983.
46. Mirowski M: The automatic implantable cardioverter-defibrillator: An overview. J Am Coll Cardiol 6:461–466, 1985.
47. Gabry MD, Brodman R, Johnston D, et al.: Automatic implantable cardioverter-defibrillator: Patient survival, battery longevity and shock delivery analysis. J Am Coll Cardiol 9:1349–1356, 1987.
48. Kelly PA, Cannom DS, Garan H, et al.: The automatic implantable cardioverter-defibrillator: Efficacy, complications and survival in patients with malignant ventricular arrhythmias. J Am Coll Cardiol 11:1278–1286, 1988.
49. Winkle RA, Stinson EB, Bach SM Jr, Echt DS, Oyer P, Armstrong K: Measurement of cardioversion/defibrillation thresholds in man by a truncated exponential waveform and an apical patch-superior vena caval spring electrode configuration. Circulation 69:766–771, 1984.
50. Cannom DS, Winkle RA: Implantation of the automatic implantable cardioverter defibrillator (AICD): Practical aspects. PACE 9:793–809, 1986.
51. Troup PJ, Chapman PD, Olinger GN, Kleinman LH: The implanted defibrillator: Relation of defibrillating lead configuration and clinical variables to defibrillation threshold. J Am Coll Cardiol 6:1315–1321, 1985.
52. Mirowski M, Reid PR, Winkle RA, et al.: Mortality in patients with implanted automatic defibrillators. Ann Intern Med 98:585–588, 1983.
53. Winkle RA, Thomas A: The automatic implantable cardioverter defibrillator: The U.S. experience. In Brugada P, Wellens HJJ (eds): ''Cardiac Arrhythmias: Where To Go From Here?'' Mount Kisco, NY: Futura Publishing Company, Inc., 1987, pp 663–680.
54. Echt DS, Armstrong K, Schmidt P, Oyer PE, Stinson EB, Winkle RA: Clinical experience, complications, and survival in 70 patients with the automatic implantable cardioverter/defibrillator. Circulation 71:289–296, 1985.
55. Tchou PJ, Kadri N, Anderson J, Caceres JA, Jazayeri M, Akhtar M: Automatic implantable cardioverter defibrillators and survival of patients with left ventricular dysfunction and malignant ventricular arrhythmias. Ann Intern Med 109:529–534, 1988.
56. Fogoros RN, Fiedler SB, Elson JJ: The automatic implantable cardioverter-defibrillator in drug-refractory ventricular tachyarrhythmias. Ann Intern Med 107:635–641, 1987.
57. Poole JE, Troutman CL, Anderson J, Bardy GH, Greene HL: Inappropriate and appropriate discharges of the automatic implantable cardioverter defibrillator (abstract). J Am Coll Cardiol 11:210A, 1988.
58. Kim SG, Furman S, Waspe LE, Brodman R, Fisher JD: Unipolar pacer artifacts induced failure of an automatic implantable cardioverter/defibrillator to detect ventricular fibrillation. Am J Cardiol 57:880–884, 1986.
59. Ruffy R, Lal R, Kouchoukos NT, Kim SS: Combined bipolar dual chamber pacing and automatic implantable cardioverter/defibrillator. J Am Coll Cardial 7:933–937, 1986.
60. Kowey PR: The calamity of cardioversion of conscious patients. Am J Cardiol 61:1106–1107, 1988.
61. Saksena S, Parsonnet V: Implantation of a cardioverter/defibrillator without thoracotomy using a triple electrode system. JAMA 259:69–72, 1988.
62. Zipes DP, Heger JJ, Miles WM, et al.: Early experience with an implantable cardioverter. N Engl J Med 311:485–490, 1984.
63. Miles WM, Prystowsky EN, Heger JJ, Zipes DP: The implantable transvenous cardio-

verter: Long-term efficacy and reproducible induction of ventricular tachycardia. Circulation 74:518–524, 1986.

64. Zipes DP, Prystowsky EN, Browne KF, Chilson DA, Heger JJ: Additional observations of transvenous cardioversion of recurrent ventricular tachycardia. Am Heart J 104: 163–164, 1982.
65. Zipes DP: Electrical treatment of tachycardia. Circulation 75:190–193, 1987.
66. Manz M, Gerckens U, Funke HD, Kirchhoff PG, Lüderitz B: Combination of antitachycardia pacemaker and automatic implantable cardioverter/defibrillator for ventricular tachycardia. PACE 9:676–684, 1986.
67. Lüderitz B, Gerckens U, Manz M: Automatic implantable cardioverter/defibrillator (AICD) and antitachycardia pacemaker (Tachylog): Combined use in ventricular tachyarrhythmias. PACE 9:1356–1360, 1986.
68. Masterson M, Maloney JD, Wilkoff B, Morant V, Golding L, Castle LW: Automatic anti-tachycardia pacemaker (Orthocor 11 284A) and automatic implantable cardioverter defibrillator as therapy for recurrent ventricular tachycardia (abstract). PACE 10:416, 1987.
69. Yee R, Guiraudon GM, Jones DL, Sharma AD, Kallok MJ, Norris C, Klein GJ: Implantation of a pacemaker/cardioverter/defibrillator in man: Initial results of a new generation device (abstract). J Am Coll Cardiol 11:208A, 1988.
70. Yee R, Guiraudon GM, Klein GJ, Jones DL, Sharma AD, Norris C, Kallok MJ: The pacemaker-cardioverter-defibrillator: Clinical experience at implant and on short term follow-up. PACE (in press).

Chapter 10

The Role of Cardiac Surgery in the Prevention of Sudden Death

Ross Brooks, M.D., M.Sc., **Hasan Garan,** M.D., **Peter N. Smith,** M.D., **and Jeremy N. Ruskin,** M.D.

Cardiac Unit, Massachusetts General Hospital, Harvard Medical School, Boston, Massachusetts 02104

INTRODUCTION

Each year in the United States, more than 350,000 lives are lost as a result of sudden death [1,2]. Although both cardiac and noncardiac causes may be responsible [3], in the vast majority of cases, sudden death is caused by the development of a ventricular arrhythmia, such as sustained ventricular tachycardia (VT) or ventricular fibrillation [4]. Since most patients with life-threatening ventricular arrhythmias have underlying cardiac abnormalities (Table 10–1), interventions aimed at preventing sudden death may be directed at both the causal disease process as well as the involved arrhythmia. Because of the frequent existence of potentially correctable anatomic cardiac abnormalities, surgical procedures are often indicated in these patients.

Over the past decade, surgical procedures for treating cardiac arrhythmias have evolved substantially such that they now must be considered as viable alternatives to other therapy in selected patients (e.g., antiarrhythmic drugs or the automatic implantable cardioverter-defibrillator [AICD]) [5]. The development of these techniques has paralleled both an increased recognition of conditions associated with arrhythmias as well as a better under-

The Prevention of Sudden Cardiac Death, pages 221–260

TABLE 10–1. Major Causes of Ventricular Tachycardia and Sudden Cardiac Death

Coronary artery disease	Inflammatory or infiltrative conditions
Congenital	Primary cardiac tumors
Anomalous coronary vessels	Myocarditis
Acquired	Sarcoid heart disease
Atherosclerotic	Amyloid heart disease
Preinfarction (no myocardiac scar)	Myocardial contusion
Periinfarction	Postinflammatory fibrosis from a number of causes
Postinfarction (scar ± aneurysm)[a]	
Coronary artery vasospasm	Long QT syndrome
Cardiomyopathy	Congenital (idiopathic)
Hypertrophic cardiomyopathy[a]	Acquired (mainly drug-induced)
Nonischemic dilated cardiomyopathy[a]	Ventricular preexcitation (W-P-W) syndrome
Arrthythmogenic right ventricular dysplasia or dilated cardiomyopathy	Drug-induced
	Antiarrhythmics (proarrhythmic effects)
Hypertensive cardiomyopathy	Digitalis toxicity
Congential cardiac anomalies	Cocaine, tricyclic antidepressant toxicity
Repaired tetralogy of Fallot	Ethanol
Repaired transposition of the great arteries	Electrolyte derangements
Repaired ventricular septal defects	Severe hypokalemia
Valvular abnormalities	Severe hypomagnesemia
Aortic stenosis	Miscellaneous
Mitral valve prolapse	Ventricular aneurysms (congenital, postinfarction, posttrauma)
	Idiopathic (no identifiable structural abnormality or predisposing condition)

[a]Most common predisposing causes of ventricular arrhythmias and cardiac arrest.

standing of the mechanisms of arrhythmias in these conditions. Surgical procedures designed to prevent sudden death may be directed primarily at the underlying disease process (e.g., coronary artery bypass grafting) or the involved arrhythmogenic substrate (i.e., ventricular antiarrhythmia surgery), although combined approaches are often used. In certain patients with life-threatening arrhythmias, a surgical approach may be the preferred treatment. When successfully performed, surgical intervention, unlike other treatment modalities, provides the possibility of an arrhythmia cure. This outcome is the most desirable treatment option for a patient, since, in eliminating the arrhythmogenic substrate, it may also reduce the need for chronic adjuvant drug therapy or back-up electrical devices.

This chapter reviews the current role of cardiac surgery in the management of patients at risk for sudden cardiac death. Since the majority of sudden deaths are arrhythmogenic in nature and accounted for by ventricular arrhythmias in patients with coronary artery disease, this syndrome will receive particular emphasis.

SPECTRUM OF HEART DISEASE IN PATIENTS WITH SUDDEN ARRHYTHMIC DEATH

Although diverse conditions are associated with ventricular arrhythmias, relatively few account for the majority of sudden cardiac deaths (Table 10–1). To gain insight into the type and prevalence of various conditions associated with sudden cardiac death, patients from cardiac arrest series may be examined [4,6–10]. Clinical findings in patients successfully resuscitated from sudden death as well as pathology data obtained through postmortem examination in nonsurvivors of cardiac arrest show that there are important differences in the diseases afflicting younger and older patient subsets [11–12a]. In younger patients (<40 years), who often have cardiac arrest in the setting of physical exertion, ischemic heart disease is rarely the cause [12,12a], whereas the dominant disease processes are cardiomyopathies, particularly the hypertrophic form [13–15]. Anomalous coronary vessels (e.g., an origin of the left coronary artery from the right sinus of valsalva and course between the great arteries) [16], or an intramural location of the left anterior descending coronary artery (so-called "myocardial bridge") [17], are also occasionally found in young victims of sudden death. In these patients, ischemically mediated ventricular arrhythmias are the presumed cause of exertional sudden death. Congenital coronary artery anomalies are important to recognize, since they are potentially amenable to specific surgical treatment, usually coronary artery reimplantation or bypass grafting procedures, as a means of arrhythmia and sudden death prevention [18]. In most series, up to 10% of patients studied have no structural heart disease identified [4,6–10]. Conditions such as coronary artery vasospasm or the long QT and Wolff-Parkinson-White (W-P-W) syndromes may explain arrhythmias in patients with structurally normal hearts, whereas in others the tachycardias are "idiopathic" in origin (Table 10–1) [19].

Older persons (>40 years), who account for the majority of patients in series of out-of-hospital cardiac arrest, show a preponderence of acquired atherosclerotic coronary artery disease and, to a lesser extent, nonischemic dilated cardiomyopathy [4,6–10,20]. Indeed, more than 90% of current surgical procedures for VT are performed in patients with coronary artery disease [21], and up to three-fourths of patients undergoing AICD implantation have this predisposing condition [22]. In most patients with ventricular arrhythmias in the setting of ischemic heart disease, a previous transmural myocardial infarction and associated left ventricular dysfunction are the rule [20,23–25]. A variety of noncoronary-related cardiac diseases, such as cardiomyopathy and aortic and mitral valve disease, account for the remainder of structural abnormalities in patients in these series [4,6–10].

Although the relationship between arrhythmias and underlying disease processes is usually well defined, the recognition of patients at risk for potentially life-threatening events is less than satisfactory. Consequently,

TABLE 10–2. Conditions in Which Surgery May Successfully Reduce or Eliminate the Potential Risk for Sudden Death[a]

Cardiac condition	Surgical procedure
Anomalous coronary vessels	CABG
W-P-W syndrome	Bypass tract division
LQTS, refractory to β-blockers	Left cervicothoracic sympathectomy
Left main stem or three-vessel CAD, with reduced left ventricular function	CABG (±AICD)
CAD, with preserved left ventricular function and inducible VF	CABG (±AICD)
CAD, with localized ventricular scar/aneurysm, and a mappable VT	Map-directed endocardial resection ± aneurysmectomy ± CABG
Localized ventricular aneurysms or tumors	Map-directed myocardial resection
Severe dilated cardiomyopathy	Cardiac transplantation
Critical valvular aortic stenosis	AVR

[a]Abbreviations: AVR, aortic valve replacement; CABG, coronary artery bypass grafting; CAD, coronary artery disease; LQTS, long QT syndrome; W-P-W, Wolff-Parkinson-White Syndrome; VF, ventricular fibrillation; VT, ventricular tachycardia.

therapeutic interventions are commonly performed in patients after, rather than before, cardiac arrest occurs. Primary prevention of the underlying disease processes themselves (e.g., atherosclerosis) and timely secondary intervention before cardiac arrest occurs (e.g., postmyocardial infarction) are measures that will ultimately have the greatest impact on reducing sudden cardiac death mortality.

CARDIAC SURGICAL PROCEDURES FOR SPECIFIC DISEASES

Surgery for the Long QT Syndrome (LQTS)

The LQTS represents a condition in which a primary abnormality of ventricular repolarization predisposes to development of polymorphic VT called "torsade de pointes" [26]. In the vast majority of patients, no associated structural cardiac abnormalities are found [27]. Prolongation of the electrocardiographic QT interval may be congenital (idiopathic LQTS) or acquired in various disease states, principally as a consequence of antiarrhythmic drug toxicity or severe electrolyte derangement. The latter causes are important to recognize, since they are reversible. Recently, Jackman et al. [28] proposed a classification for the idiopathic LQTS that has therapeutic implications. Accordingly, most arrhythmias exhibit either "pause-dependent" or "adrenergic-dependent" triggering mechanisms, although some patients may show intermediate characteristics [28]. With the idiopathic LQTS, a neurogenic basis for the disorder has been proposed, which appears to involve an imbalance in left- and right-sided cardiac sympathetic innervation [27,29]. Accordingly, left stellate ganglion overactivity or underactivity of the right stellate ganglion is proposed as the triggering mechanism for adrenergic-dependent arrhythmias [29]. Such an asymmetry of sympathetic cardiac stimulation is thought to lead to heterogeneity or "dispersion" of ventricular refractoriness as evidenced by prolongation of the QT interval. Torsade de pointes in this setting may be provoked by stress-induced changes in sympathetic tone, which can occur as a result of emotional excitement or physical exertion [28]. In untreated patients with the LQTS, mortality rates are high, and these may be reduced considerably by antiadrenergic measures [27,30]. β-Adrenergic-blocking drugs, such as propranolol, are considered the mainstay of treatment for this condition [30]. Institution of effective β-blocker therapy has been shown to prevent recurrent arrhythmias and to reduce the incidence of sudden death [27,30]. Following experimental studies in which unilateral left stellate ganglionectomy are observed to increase the threshold for ventricular fibrillation and to decrease the incidence of ventricular arrhythmias [31], high cervicothoracic left sympathectomy evolved as a specific surgical therapy for the LQTS [32]. This procedure can be performed extrapleurally and involves removal of the lower portion of the left stellate ganglion and the first three to five thoracic sympathetic ganglia [30]. Patients not controlled by β-blockers alone may be considered for this form of surgery. In a series of 52 patients described by Schwartz and colleagues [29,30] who underwent stellectomy for arrhythmias refractory to maximal doses of β-blockers, the incidence of recurrent syncope and sudden death was reportedly lower in comparison to patients with arrhythmias persisting after treatment with β-blockers alone. However, some late deaths in this series were also reported [29,30]. Others have reported the failure of this operation to control arrhythmias, and its precise role in the management of patients with this disorder is not clearly established [33]. Recently, chronic atrial pacing for the bradycardia-dependent LQTS and AICD implantation have been gaining acceptance as alternatives to pharmacological and surgical therapy [34].

Surgery in the W-P-W Syndrome

Programmed electrical stimulation of the heart as described by Durrer and Wellens in 1967 [35] was first used to initiate atrioventricular reentrant supraventricular tachycardia associated with the W-P-W syndrome. The presence of accessory atrioventricular pathways was subsequently demonstrated by epicardial mapping studies, and this technique was advocated to guide the surgical division of these pathways. The first successful operation for W-P-W was performed in 1968 by Sealy and colleagues at Duke University [36]. Epicardial mapping localized the site of preexcitation to the right lateral base of the heart [36]. Subsequently, endocardial mapping techniques using electrode catheters placed into the atrium, coronary sinus, and ventricle were developed by Gallagher and colleagues [37] to determine the location of bypass tracts preoperatively and thus simplify the procedures necessary at the time of surgery. After the report in 1979 by the Duke University group who established that rapidly conducted atrial fibrillation with degeneration into ventricular fibrillation was the cause of cardiac arrest in patients with the W-P-W syndrome, an awareness of this potential complication led to an expanded use of electrophysiologic testing as a means of identifying high-risk patient subsets [38]. Stratification of patients into high- and low-risk subsets for sudden death is based on the properties of the accessory pathway, particularly its capacity for rapid conduction during atrial fibrillation [38]. The potential for rapid anterograde accessory pathway conduction is the main reason for recommending surgery to patients, although some groups consider surgery as the treatment of choice for symptomatic patients with reciprocating tachycardias.

Surgery for the W-P-W syndrome is rather unique, in that accessory pathways can neither be seen nor palpated by the operating surgeon. The operative procedure as originally described by Sealy, Gallagher, and colleagues [39] includes epicardial mapping during normothermic perfusion to localize the atrial and ventricular insertions of the accessory pathway(s), followed by total body hypothermia to 28°C, cross-clamping of the ascending aorta, and the use of cold cardioplegia. Surgery has led to the practical classification of accessory pathways into four main anatomic locations, left (most common)- and right-sided free-wall, and anterior (least common) and posterior septal positions. Multiple tracts are found in 15–20% of patients [40,41]. Surgery is technically simpler for free-wall than for septal tracts and is potentially simplest for right-sided free-wall tracts, since the latter may not require extracorpeal circulation [39]. The surgical approach is initiated by median sternotomy, and exposure for the purpose of surgical dissection is obtained by opening the atrium [39]. The surgical approach to septal tracts is more difficult, particularly in the case of posterior septal pathways. Surgery for these pathways involves meticulous dissection of the pyramidal space that lies on top of the interventricular septum posteriorly and is associated with an increased risk of heart block from inadvertent damage to the normal conduction system [42]. More recently, Guiraudon, Klein, and colleagues [43] have reported the successful use of an external closed-heart approach in conjunction with cryoablation for the ablation of left-free wall accessory pathways. This approach is feasible, since most free-wall bypass tracts are located epicardially [44]. This procedure also overcomes the need for cardiopulmonary bypass and aortic cross-clamping and can be performed under normothermic conditions where continuous monitoring of atrioventricular conduction is possible [43].

In a review by Gallagher et al. [40] of the first 267 patients undergoing operation for W-P-W at Duke University, the success rate was 98% for right free-wall pathways, 94% for left free-wall pathways, 85% for anterior septal pathways, and 81% for posterior septal pathways. The overall mortality was 4.1% and was largely accounted for by patients with associated congenital anomalies (e.g., Ebstein's anomaly). Mortality in patients with normal heart function was 1.1%. Heart block occurred in 16 of 81 (20%) posterior septal pathways and one of 27 (0.04%) anterior septal pathways [40]. Cox et al. [47] have recently reported that his modifications of Sealy's original surgical technique have resulted in the successful division of 100% of accessory pathways in 118 patients. Overall mortality in this series was 5% but was 0.8% for patients without associated cardiac anomalies undergoing elective operation [41]. There were no reoperations, and an 0.8% incidence of complete heart block was reported.

Surgery to interrupt the bundle of His has also been performed in patients with rapidly conducting supraventricular tachyarrhythmias unrelated to the W-P-W syndrome [45]. Cryosurgical treatment of atrioventricular nodal reentrant tachycardia is an alternative to surgical dissection [46]. More recently, percutaneous electrode catheter ablation of the bundle of His has been successfully performed in patients, and this has largely supplanted intracardiac surgery for this purpose [47]. In conjunction with these procedures, a permanently implanted dual-chamber or ventricular pacemaker is usually necessary. Similarly, successful electrode catheter ablation of posterior septal accessory pathways has been reported by some workers [48].

It is difficult to know the impact that surgery has had on the prevention of sudden cardiac death in patients with the W-P-W syndrome. Clearly, patients at high risk for potentially malignant arrhythmias can be identified before morbid events occur. In the vast majority of cases, a successful surgical outcome is the rule, and the involved procedures can be performed with a very low incidence of morbidity and mortality. In these patients, successful surgery eliminates the substrate for sudden cardiac death and is, therefore, a curative procedure.

Surgery for Ventricular Arrhythmias in Coronary Artery Disease

Sympathectomy. Sympathectomy was one of the first "indirect" surgical methods used to treat patients with ventricular arrhythmias unrelated to the LQTS. The rationale for this approach was the observation that enhanced sympathetic activity predisposed the heart to ventricular arrhythmias, whereas reduced activity decreased this tendency [49]. In 1961, Estes and Izlar [50] described a patient with recurrent VT who underwent cardiac sympathectomy. Unilateral left posterior sympathectomy alone failed to control VT, but the arrhythmia was abolished after a subsequent right dorsal procedure was performed (i.e., bilateral sympathectomy). Subsequently, Sealy and Oldham [51] tested this procedure in six patients with coronary artery disease and ventricular arrhythmias. Although sympathectomy abolished arrhythmias in three patients, the remaining patients were not helped by the procedure. In a collective review of 15 patients undergoing this procedure for refractory ventricular arrhythmias, the operative mortality was stated to be 10%, with an overall success rate of 67% [52]. This technique was largely abandoned with the introduction of cardiopulmonary bypass and initiation of coronary artery bypass grafting and related surgical procedures [53]. The basis for the results in successful cases were not clear. Recent work in animals has shown that transmural myocardial infarction may interrupt epicardial neural pathways and thus create a heterogeneous zone of sympathetic innervation distal to the area of infarction [54]. Such an assymetry of ventricular innervation may be a factor predisposing to arrhythmogensis. The rationale for sympathectomy is to eliminate areas of heterogeneous innervation in a manner analogous to the LQTS. This therapy was recently tested in a randomized trial in Europe [55]. In the Italian multicenter study, 144 patients with anterior myocardial infarction complicated by early VT or ventricular fibrillation were randomized to three treatment subgroups: placebo, β-blocker treatment with oxprenolol, and high thoracic left sympathectomy [55]. Over a mean follow-up of 20 months, the placebo group had a 22% incidence of sudden death compared to 5.2% for 869 patients without periinfarction ventricular tachycardia/fibrillation. Both antiadrenergic interventions proved effective, although sudden death rate was lower in patients treated with β-blockers than sympathectomy (2.7% vs. 3.6%) [29,55]. Sympathetic denervation is primarily advocated as an alternative to β-blocker therapy for patients with contraindications to the latter agents.

Finally, cardiac denervation has also been proposed as a treatment for patients with coronary artery vasospasm. In this setting, patients with ischemically mediated arrhythmias resulting from vasospasm may benefit from such a procedure [56]. Currently, an AICD represents the preferred treatment for high-risk patients.

Coronary artery bypass grafting. Among the first cardiac procedures used to treat ventricular arrhythmias in patients with ischemic heart disease was coronary artery bypass grafting, alone or in combination with aneurysmectomy [57–59]. The rationale for this approach was the observation that multivessel coronary artery disease and accompanying angina were frequently present in such patients. By virtue of its ability to increase blood flow to areas of ischemia, coronary artery bypass grafting was advocated as a means of correcting factors predisposing to arrhythmias. The success of "empiric" coronary artery bypass grafting has not been uniform, and results have been difficult to interpret for a number of reasons. Most such studies were also performed before programmed ventricular stimulation was systematically used in patients to evaluate arrhythmia vulnerability [58]. Relatively poor overall results have been observed in patients treated with bypass grafting alone, suggesting that ischemia is not a common inciting mechanism of most arrhythmias [60]. As a result of attempts to control postinfarction arrhythmias using bypass grafting, it also became apparent that the procedure is associated with an extremely high mortality when performed early (<30 days) after acute myocardial infarction [61]. Elective revascularization to relieve chronic ischemia can be safely performed with a low perioperative mortality, but does not appear to have a major impact on overall mortality. When whole group analysis was performed, two of the three major randomized revascularization trials (Coronary Artery Surgery [62] and Veterans Administration Cooperative Study [63]) showed no overall mortality differences between the groups of patients randomized to medical and surgical therapy. Analysis of the Coronary Artery Surgery Study Registry data, however, revealed a significantly lower sudden death rate in patients assigned to surgery [63a]. This reduction was most pronounced in patients with a three-vessel disease and a history of congestive failure [63a]. In the European Coronary Surgery Study, 5 year survival rates were significantly higher in the group of patients assigned to surgical treatment [64–64a], although differences after 12 years of follow-up were less apparent [65]. The principal explanation for the discordance in results between the Veterans Administration and Coronary Artery Surgery Studies and the European Study are important differences in baseline variables related to survival in the two groups (e.g., inclusion of patients with left main coronary artery disease, resting ischemia, and markedly positive exercise stress test results) [66]. However, in the European Study, surgical therapy was also associated with a reduction in sudden cardiac deaths [64,65].

Other data are also consistent with the hypothesis that ischemia is not a frequent inciting factor for ventricular arrhythmias in patients with coronary artery disease. Evidence for acute myocardial infarction is present in less than 20% of patients with out-of-hospital ventricular fibrillation [67]. Symptoms such as angina are also similarly lacking in the majority of these patients to invoke as a precipitating event [67a]. With currently available methods, patients with spontaneous arrhythmias reproduced by electrophysiologic testing also do not manifest subjective or objective ischemic endpoints antecedent to arrhythmia induction [68]. This finding suggests that ischemia is not a requirement for arrhythmia development in the laboratory setting and therefore need not be invoked to explain spontaneous events. Indeed, the apparent infrequency with which ischemia is implicated in arrhythmogenesis is consistent with the concept that a fixed substrate is responsible for most cases of recurrent monomorphic VT and some cases of ventricular fibrillation.

In some patients, however, symptomatic or "silent" ischemia is recognized as an important contributor to arrhythmia development [69]. These cases include many patients with spontaneous ventricular fibrillation as well as patients with reproducible exercise-induced ventricular arrhythmias and those with VT during angina with accompanying objective ischemic changes [70–73]. In such patients, therapy for the arrhythmia is aimed primarily at preventing recurrent ischemia. Successful antiischemic therapy, particularly surgical revascularization, is generally associated with long-term arrhythmia suppression [70–73]. The superiority of surgical revascularization over medical treatment in prolonging survival in patients with left main stem coronary artery disease [64,74] as well as in patients with three-vessel coronary artery disease and impaired left ventricular function is also well established [75].

The value of revascularization as a primary intervention for some ventricular arrhythmias is currently being reexamined [76,77]. Recent data have demonstrated the effectiveness of revascularization alone in highly selected patients with severe coronary artery disease and ventricular fibrillation. In one study, all ten patients with inducible ventricular fibrillation during preoperative electrophysiologic testing no longer had inducible arrhythmias when testing was repeated after coronary artery bypass grafting [77]. In contrast, only 20% of patients with sustained monomorphic VT had arrhythmias suppressed by bypass grafting alone [77]. Another recent study [77a] has shown a less than 100% success rate of this procedure in patients with ventricular fibrillation and emphasizes the need for postoperative electrophysiologic testing in all patients. The explanation for the apparent differential effect of revascularization in the suppression of ventricular fibrillation vs. VT is not known but may be related to the relief of chronic ischemia. Another possible explanation may relate to improvement in mechanical left ventricular function, with secondary effects on arrhythmogenesis. It has been recognized that patients with poor left ventricular function manifest a higher incidence of electrically inducible arrhythmias [78] and a lower response rate to antiarrhythmic drugs than patients with well preserved ventricular function [79]. Ventricular dysfunction is also recognized as a powerful independent predictor of both overall and sudden death mortality in diverse groups such as postmyocardial infarction patients [80], cardiac arrest survivors [23], and patients with chronic ischemic heart disease [10] or congestive cardiomyopathy [81]. Patients with poor left ventricular function and three-vessel coronary artery disease have an improved survival with bypass surgery, whereas patients with normal ventricular function do not seem to benefit as much from these procedures [75] unless angina is severe, (i.e., class III–IV) [75a]. Similarly, coronary artery revascularization is an independent predictor of survival in postcardiac arrest patients [82], and may be of most benefit in those with reduced left ventricular function. Surgical revascularization in some patients may improve survival by restoring coronary blood flow, thereby improving both contractility and electrophysiologic properties in areas of chronically ischemic myocardium [83]. The relationship between mechanical cardiac function and the electrophysiologic milieu responsible for arrhythmogenesis in ischemic heart disease is complex and merits further study.

Simple aneurysmectomy. Although the association between ventricular aneurysms and ventricular arrhythmias was first recognized by Sir Thomas Lewis in 1909 [84], successful resection of a ventricular aneurysm with cure of the associated tachycardia was not undertaken until 1956, as reported by Couch in 1959 [85]. Subsequently, aneurysmectomy, or infarctectomy, alone or in combination with coronary artery bypass grafting, was employed to treat intractable arrhythmias. When analyzed critically, these indirect procedures were associated with in-hospital death rates of 10–45%, spontaneous VT recurrence rates of 5–80%, and an overall success rate of approximately 50% [86]. The long-term results were generally poor, with 5 year actuarial survival rates of approximately 30% [86]. These unsatisfactory results led to renewed interest in more direct surgical procedures for refractory VT in patients with ischemic heart disease.

A more sophisticated approach to surgery for VT was possible only after major advances in the understanding of the mechanisms responsible for these arrhythmias. The pioneering work of Wellens et al. [87] using techniques of programmed electrical stimulation demonstrated that the mechanism of chronic recurrent VT following myocardial infarction was reentry. On the basis of experimental data generated by Wittig and Boineau [88], and by Boineau and Cox [86], it was recognized that the site of reentry was frequently localized to the border zone between infarcted aneurysmal tissue and normal myocardium, often along the interventricular septum. The poor results of simple aneurysmectomy were ascribed to a failure to excise the border zone of the aneurysm, particularly when it involved the septum. Conversely, successful cases were attributed to fortuitous removal of arrhythmogenic tissue [89,90]. Based on these observations, a variety of novel operations for VT began to emerge in the late 1970s. Surgical antiarrhythmia techniques may be subdivided into generalized and localized procedures. The initial operations developed were "visually guided" generalized procedures (encircling endocardial ventriculotomy, extensive endocardial resection). Subsequently, modified procedures (e.g., "focal" subendocardial resection) were developed using electrophysiologic mapping techniques to localize these arrhythmias to specific regions of the ventricle ("map-guided" arrhythmia surgery).

Non map ("visually")-guided ventricular arrhythmia surgery. In 1978, Guiraudon, Fontaine, and coworkers [91] introduced a new procedure, the encircling endocardial ventriculotomy, as a specific surgical technique for the treatment of VT. This technique followed from the initial success of a simple ventriculotomy used to interrupt VT in a small number of patients with nonischemic and cardiomyopathy [92,93]. The encircling procedure was developed principally for patients with ischemic heart disease and previous myocardial infarction as a means of anatomically excluding the area responsible for VT from the rest of the heart. Since experimental animal and human data suggested that areas responsible for the arrhythmias were located along the border of the infarct or aneurysm [94,95], these workers believed that a circular ventriculotomy performed outside the limits of the border zone would isolate the VT from the normal working myocardium. Accordingly, it was postulated that the incision itself and/or the subsequent scar that formed would either interrupt the reentrant pathways or contain them within an area from which there was exit block to the functioning myocardium [91]. However, clinical experience with this technique has demonstrated that the encircled area not infrequently continues to beat synchronously with the rest of the heart, indicating that denervation is incomplete, and ''isolation'' of the arrhythmia may not represent the explanation for success of the procedure. More recent data show that both complete and partial encircling incisions interrupt coronary blood flow to the encompassed area, thus transferring the heterogeneously damaged arrhythmogenic substrate to a homogeneous fibrotic scar without electrical activity [96,97].

The encircling procedure is carried out after entrance into the ventricular cavity by a standard ventriculotomy through the aneurysm or infarction. A transmural ventriculotomy is performed around the border of subendocardial fibrosis, sparing the epicardium and coronary arteries. The ventriculotomy is then repaired with running sutures. As originally described, this procedure did not require intraoperative mapping, since the incision was directed at anatomical landmarks [91]. In the initial series of five patients with refractory VT who underwent the procedure, there were no perioperative deaths, or VT recurrences, over a follow-up period of 6–24 months in the absence of antiarrhythmic drugs [91]. To reduce the risk of papillary muscle damage and of long-term ventricular dysfunction secondary to the extensive myotomy incision, a modification of the original Guiraudon procedure was described—the partial or limited encircling endocardial ventriculotomy—which encompassed exclusively a map-identified arrhythmogenic area [98]. In a 1984 report, Ostermeyer et al. [98] compared complete and partial endocardial ventriculotomy in 40 patients and found comparable results in terms of VT suppression but a significantly greater incidence of late ventricular dysfunction in patients undergoing the complete procedure. Similar results were also described in a more recent series of 93 consecutive patients reported by these workers [98a]. In an updated series involving 23 patients undergoing complete or partial encircling procedures, Guiraudon et al. [99] reported a 9% operative mortality, and an additional two patients died during follow-up unrelated to arrhythmias. Among 21 patients surviving the operation, 95% had no further ventricular tachycardia, although 23% required concommitant drugs for arrhythmia suppression. Guiruadon et al. [100] have also described the results of encircling endocardidal cryoablation in 16 patients. In this procedure, a cryolesion rather than a surgical incision is used to isolate damaged from normal myocardium. In this series, one patient died postoperatively, and 14 patients remained drug- and arrhythmia-free over a mean follow-up of 16 months. Postoperative left ventricular function was also preserved with this procedure [100].

In 1982, Moran et al. [101] reported the use of visually directed "extended" endocardial resection. This technique was a modification of the "focal," map-guided myocardial resection procedure introduced earlier by Josephson, Harken, and colleagues [102,103]. With the extended endocardial resection procedure, all areas of visible scar are resected from the underlying myocardium. Forty patients in the Moran et al. series underwent the procedure in conjunction with aneurysmectomy and/or coronary artery bypass grafting [101]. Epicardial and endocardial mapping was attempted intraoperatively in 36 patients, although in 15 patients these procedures could not be successfully completed. Operative mortality was 10%. Of the surviving patients, 7.6% had VT induced during a postoperative electrophysiologic study (one patient with map-guided surgery and two patients with visually guided surgery). These results showed that removal of all visible endocardial scar tissue may produce satisfactory results in patients in whom intraoperative mapping is not possible or cannot be completed. As shown by this study [101] and by other studies [104], however, the origin of the VT occasionally lies outside the limits of a visible endocardial scar, accounting for the failure of nonmap-guided procedures in some patients to control arrhythmias. Other groups have successfully utilized nonmap-guided extensive endocardial resection or encircling endocardial resection procedures alone or in combination with aneurysmectomy and coronary artery bypass grafting in small series of patients to control ventricular arrhythmias in coronary artery disease [105,105a,106]. As judged by the inability to induce VT postoperatively, these procedures were considered successful in the short term. However, the long-term outcome of the patients remains uncertain.

As recently reviewed by Cox [5], the postoperative arrhythmia inducibility rate is slightly, but not significantly, lower with generalized compared to localized arrhythmia procedures. These data suggest that the former may be the preferred technique. One concern with visually-guided generalized ventricular surgical procedures is whether excess amounts of myocardium are being sacrificed that may adversely affect short- and long-term mechanical ventricular function. With the encircling endocardial ventriculotomy, a marked decrease in regional blood flow and concomitant depression of regional myocardial function of any nonfibrosed tissue that is encircled has been shown experimentally [97], and ventricular function may worsen after this procedure. In some series, this procedure is also associated with a high perioperative mortality [106,107]. For these reasons, the procedure has largely been abandoned as a primary surgical technique for ventricular arrhythmias. Aneurysmectomy has become a standard cardiac procedure and has been shown to produce improvements in both left ventricular function [107,108], as well as functional class, in patients with preserved nonaneurysmal cardiac segments [109]. Focal or extensive endocardial resection and partial encircling ventriculotomy procedures also do not appear to cause significant hemodynamic impairment [107,110]. Accordingly, endocardial resection, usually in conjunction with aneurysmectomy, has become the preferred surgical procedure at many institutions for the treatment of drug-resistant sustained ventricular arrhythmias [21]. An advantage of encircling endocardial ventriculotomy over resection procedures is that the posterior papillary muscle, where scar tissue is commonly located, may be safely encircled without compromising mitral valve function. However, the ventriculotomy cannot be safely extended to the mitral or aortic annulus to complete the encirclement. Completion of the encirclement or ablation in surgically inaccessible areas (e.g., septal and posterior scars) may be accomplished with techniques such as cryoablation [111].

Map-guided ventricular arrhythmia surgery. The rationale for a "direct" antiarrhythmic surgical approach is the observation that the region of origin of most ventricular arrhythmias, or areas essential to arrhythmia propogation can be precisely located using map-guided electrophysiologic procedures. Electrically guided operations use preoperative and intraoperative electrical recordings in conjunction with visual landmarks to direct the surgeon to specific areas of interest within the ventricle, potentially limiting the extent of myocardium ablated, isolated, or removed.

Ventricular mapping techniques. A number of different electrical mapping techniques have been developed that may be used alone or in combination. These include, "activation sequence mapping" [112], "fragmentation mapping" [113], "pace mapping" [114,115], and newer techniques involving "cryotermination mapping" [111]. Activation sequence mapping involves the analysis of recordings taken at a number of different epicardial and/or endocardial sites during VT. The electrograms obtained either simultaneously or sequentially at various sites are compared to those of reference surface ECG leads and fixed electrograms from normal regions of the right and left ventricles [112]. Sites of early (presystolic) ventricular electrical activation are identified. The "earliest site of activation" (usually ≥25 msec before the surface QRS complex) relative to the reference electrodes is taken to represent the region of origin of the tachycardia (see below) [112,116,117]. In fragmentation mapping, endocardial recordings are obtained during sinus rhythm rather than during tachycardia [113]. The electrograms obtained at various sites are examined for the presence of low-amplitude "fractionated" or fragmented electrical activity, which coincides with the QRS complex, but frequently outlasts its duration. This activity appears to represent areas of slow, disorganized, and asynchronous myocardial activation, thought to correspond to "late potentials" detected by high-resolution surface ECG techniques [117,117a]. The occurrence of fractionated electrograms during sinus rhythm is often a nonspecific finding since the correlation between these sites and the site of origin of VT is poor [118,119]. In some patients, however, an area containing the longest fractionated electrogram during sinus rhythm is correlated with the earliest site of activation during VT [120]. In occasional patients, an area showing fractionated activity during sinus rhythm becomes continuous during VT (i.e., ''continuous electrical activity'') [121]. This activity appears to identify a critical element of the reentrant circuit [121]. Pace mapping is a crude technique for localizing the origin of a tachycardia in which the surface ECG morphology of a tachycardia is mimicked by pacing at various ventricular sites [115]. Endocardial pacing is superior to epicardial pacing for this purpose, but the former technique is limited as an intraoperative procedure because fewer surface leads are available for recording and comparison. The procedure is generally performed preoperatively and is most useful in patients in whom the spontaneous tachycardia has been documented but cannot be reproduced by programmed cardiac stimulation or in whom catheter mapping is not feasible. In cryothermal mapping, a cryoprobe cooled to 0°C is applied to various ventricular sites during tachycardia induced intraoperatively [111]. A cryothermal termination site is an area at which the application of the cryoprobe causes reproducible termination of the tachycardia. Since interruption of electrical activity by cooling is reversible, the tachycardia can be restarted and the procedure repeated to ensure that cessation of the tachycardia was not accidental. As was shown by Gallagher et al. [111], the cryotermination site is often remote from the site of earliest activation and may coincide with critical segments of reentry pathways. Cryoablation at −60°C alone or in conjunction with subendocardial resection may be performed. Myocardial cryolesions are discrete and sharply demarcated from undamaged myocardium. These areas contain a homogeneous area of electrical inactivity and are not arrhythmogenic [122]. This technique is very useful for ablating tachycardias in areas that are inaccessible to surgical ablation (e.g., base of a papillary muscle).

Epicardial vs. endocardial mapping. Epicardial mapping was the initial intraoperative technique used for localizing sites of origin of VT. Endocardial mapping is currently judged to provide a more accurate anatomical localization in most patients with ischemic heart disease but is technically more difficult to perform in the intraoperative setting [116,117]. Endocardial catheter mapping can be performed preoperatively, and the data obtained by various techniques generally correlate well with the results of intraoperative testing [117,123]. In experienced hands, catheter endocardial mapping is able to predict the origin of VT within 4 cm^2 of that determined by intraoperative endocardial mapping [117]. The technique of focal subendocardial resection as originally described by Harken and Josephson, was based on experimental and clinical findings showing that arrhythmogenic regions often appeared to reside in islands of viable myocardial cells and Purkinje tissue that survive beneath the immediate endocardial layers of infarcted tissue [123a]. The earliest site of activation as determined by endocardial mapping is taken to represent the region of origin of the tachycardia. As was shown by Spielman et al. [124], the site of epicardial breakthrough may differ anatomically from the endocardial site of activation by a varying extent (5 mm to 6 cm). Using intramural needle electrodes, these workers further showed that, in the setting of healed infarction, activation of the endocardium during VT is always recorded earlier than that of the epicardium [116]. These data are consistent with an endocardial site of origin during VT, with secondary epicardial activation [116]. Inasmuch as the myocardium may be inhomogeneously damaged, deeper (intramural) sites of tachycardia origin may also exist [125]. Because of the potential complexity of the involved reentrant pathways, the sequence of epicardial activation from any given endocardial site is not always predictible, and the earliest site of epicardial breakthrough may not correspond to the origin of the tachycardia [126]. For these reasons, activation sequence, fragmentation, or pace mapping of the endocardium are considered superior to the corresponding epicardial techniques for precise tachycardia localization in patients with VT occurring in the setting of healed myocardial infarction [116,124].

Results of map-directed ventricular arrhythmia surgery. Josephson and coworkers [127] have reported the largest series of patients undergoing map-guided localized subendocardial resection for drug-refractory VT. The amount of tissue excised during this surgical procedure ranges between 4 and 12 cm^2 [127]. In a 1985 report, 119 patients had undergone this procedure for drug-refractory VT 3 weeks to 10 years after acute myocardial infarction [127]. One hundred five patients (88%) underwent aneurysmectomy, and 72 patients (61%) had concomitant coronary artery bypass surgery. Operative mortality was higher in patients undergoing the procedure within 4 months of myocardial infarction (group 1) and 1 year after infarction (group 2), 12% vs. 7%, respectively. In 21% of group 1 and in 34% of group 2 patients, surgery alone was considered a primary failure as judged by postoperative inducible VT, late spontaneous recurrences, or sudden deaths in the absence of antiarrhythmic drugs. Five year actuarial survival curves for group 1 and group 2 patients were 66% and 59%, respectively, after a mean follow-up of 23 months. This series has been recently updated and now includes more than 269 patients [128]. Operative mortality is cited at 15% and overall surgical success is 68%; clinical success (no antiarrhythmia epiodes or sudden death during a mean follow-up of 5 years with or without antiarrhythmic drugs) is 90%. Smaller series of patients undergoing this approach combined with supplementary cryothermy show similarly high success rates over the short term [31]. Some workers have also advocated the use of a ''regional'' map-directed approach. In this approach, all areas of ventricle activated before the QRS complex are ablated, rather than limiting the procedure to the earliest site of activation [129].

Report of the surgical ablation registry. In 1985, an international registry was established to collect information on patients with ventricular arrhythmias undergoing electrophysiologically guided operations. In a 1987 report of the registry from eight participating centers, data on a total of 665 patients with a mean age of 55 years were presented [21]. Ninety percent of patients had coronary artery disease with a previous myocardial infarction. Anterior infarctions were predominant (57%). In 62% of patients a left ventricular aneurysm was present. The mean ejection fraction for the group was 30.6%, and more than 60% of patients were in NYHA functional class III or IV at the time of surgery. Sixty-six percent of patients had chronic recurrent VT, whereas 24% had chronic recurrent VT and episodes of ventricular fibrillation. Three percent of patients had primary ventricular fibrillation [21].

The most commonly used procedure was localized endocardial resection (33.2%). In 16.1% of patients, combined endocardial resection and cryosurgery were performed. In 9.3%, the approach was complete encircling ventriculotomy; another 16.8% were treated using partial encircling ventriculotomy. Cryosurgery alone was carried out in 7.4%. In 12.5%, techniques such as extended endocardial resection or combinations of various procedures were used. In addition, aneurysmectomy was carried out in 73% and coronary artery bypass grafting was performed in 55% of patients [21].

Overall surgical mortality was 12% and was highly dependent on the preoperative functional status. Mortality was lower for patients undergoing localized procedures, i.e., limited endocardial resection, cryosurgery, or partial encircling endocardial ventriculotomy, as opposed to generalized procedures. Actuarial survival curves showed that 72% of patients were alive 2 years after surgery, and 57% were alive at 5 years. Survival was highly dependent on left ventricular function. Ninety percent of patients with an ejection fraction >40% were alive at 5 years, compared to 65% with ejection fractions between 20.1% and 40%, and 55% for patients with ejection fractions below 20%. Fifty-one patients (8%) had an early relapse of VT occurring a median of 2.5 days after operation. Over a follow-up period of 27 ± 27.4 months, 68 patients (10.5%) had a recurrence of VT. The overall (early and late) out-of-hospital recurrence rate of arrhythmic events was 16% (105 of 648 patients), with sudden death occurring in 5.7% of patients. Of 330 patients undergoing a postoperative electrophysiologic study, clinical VT was induced in 17%, whereas 73% had no inducible arrhythmias or nonsustained VT. A "nonclinical" VT was induced in a further 9%. During follow-up, 12% of patients with no inducible VT and 13% of patients with inducible, nonclinical VT had an arrhythmic event compared to 41% of patients with inducible clinical VT. Clinical VT could be induced in only 2.9% of patients undergoing complete encircling endocardial ventriculotomy, whereas, with other types of antitachycardia operations, postoperative inducibility was higher (partial endocardial encircling ventriculotomy 12.5%, localized endocardial resection 22.9%) [21].

Factors associated with surgical failure. According to univariate analysis of the registry data, multiple sites of VT origin, multiple distinct morphologies of VT, and inferior and lateral ventricular sites of origin were predictive of surgical failure [21]. As well, patients with no previous myocardial infarction, or inferior myocardial infarction as opposed to anterior infarction, had a significantly higher postoperative recurrence rate of VT (39% and 40% vs. 16%, respectively $P < 0.01$) [21]. Global ejection fraction was not a predictor of surgical failure and did not predict perioperative mortality. Another predictor of surgical failure is a short time (<3 months) between surgery and myocardial infarction [129a]. Such patients have been noted to have a higher mean number of VT morphologies than patients undergoing surgery after 3 months. Failures in cases of apparently successful endocardial resection may be due to the fact that earliest sites of activation were not mapped, critical components of the reentrant circuit were not removed [130], a second VT site was not excised [131], or the VT involved a macroreentry mechanism that the excisional process failed to modify [132].

An important consideration in assessing postoperative inducibility is the manner in which the surgical procedure is performed. Many surgeons initially map the tachycardia under normothermic conditions and then, after identifying the site(s) of origin, cross-clamp the aorta and arrest the heart with cold cardioplegia. The ablative surgical procedure is then performed with the heart in the arrested state. After completion of the surgical procedure, the aortic cross clamp is released, and the heart is allowed to rewarm. This is followed by attempts to reinduce the VT to document the efficacy of the procedure. However, the effects of cardiopolegic arrest per se on arrhythmia inducibility are not known, and some uncertainty exists regarding the significance of a noninducible arrhythmia at the time of intraoperative testing under these conditions. Cox [5] argues that the performance of VT surgery in this manner is associated with a higher incidence of false-positive results, as indicated by the 20–30% inducibility rate of VT noted at the time of postoperative electrophysiologic testing, in comparison to results obtained in patients with procedures performed under normothermic bypass conditions. The avoidance of cardioplegia and performance of VT surgery in the normothermic, beating heart is one factor cited in the low (2%) postoperative inducibility rate in the Duke-Barnes series [5]. In this series, noninducibility at the completion of the intraoperative procedure was associated with noninducibility at the time of postoperative electrophysiologic testing 7–10 days later in 98% of 65 patients undergoing this procedure [5]. However, a negative postoperative electrophysiologic study does not uniformly confer long-term protection against recurrent arrhythmias, since small numbers of patients in various series have experienced sudden death despite the negative postoperative results [127]. In the Duke-Barnes series, despite a negative postoperative electrophysiologic test result, recurrent arrhythmias and/or sudden death occurred in 13% of patients over a mean follow-up period of 5 years [5]. The occurrence of new ischemic events or other causes of sudden death in these patients cannot be excluded.

In summary, a comparison of available data indicates that the results obtained from map-directed VT surgical procedures are generally superior to those obtained from nonmap-guided procedures [105a,133,134]. The question has been raised whether extensive mapping may paradoxically increase the operative mortality rate because of the extra time required to perform these procedures. Although direct comparative data are lacking, Cox [5] concluded from an analysis of data from various sources that operative mortalities for map-guided and blind procedures were the same. Currently, map-directed subendocardial resection is considered the standard surgical procedure for VT in most institutions.

Newer mapping systems. The first intraoperative mapping system used consisted of one fixed (reference) and one roving bipolar electrode [135]. Mapping was performed by moving the hand-held roving electrode to a number of preselected epicardial and endocardial positions. When surgery for VT became an accepted therapy, it became apparent that the single-point mapping system was suboptimal. Arrhythmias often lasted only a few cycles intraoperatively and occasionally were multifocal in origin. As well, sustained arrhythmias often became hemodynamically unstable, necessitating their termination before all data were collected. For these reasons, multielectrode systems capable of simultaneous recordings became necessary to facilitate VT surgery. The first multielectrode array to become clinically feasible for mapping VT intraoperatively was the so-called "sock" electrode developed at Duke University [136]. This sock consisted of 32 bipolar electrodes embedded in silastic buttons that were held in place on the epicardial surface of the heart by an elastic mesh stocking material. Simultaneous electrograms were recorded on a 32-channel analog recorder. Subsequently, these and other workers developed computerized mapping systems capable of rapid data aquisition and analysis of more than 100 epicardial/endocardial sites [137]. The simultaneously recorded electrograms may be displayed in various ways such as an "isochrone" map, which shows the relative activation sequence of the ventricle. The major limitation of the sock electrode was that only epicardial data could be obtained. However, data from this electrode were used to guide the subsequent placement of "plunge" needle electrodes inserted through the wall of the myocardium in selected sites to further delineate the earliest sites of endocardial activation [136]. A multipoint plunge electrode and a so-called "egg" electrode were among the first attempts to record simultaneous electrograms from multiple endocardial points [136].

The ideal intraoperative mapping system would incorporate the ability to record data from multiple sites simultaneously and record endocardial data without opening the ventricle. A promising new approach to VT mapping has been developed at the University of Toronto [138]. In this procedure, an electrode-studded endocardial balloon is inserted into the ventricle via the atrium across the mitral valve or tricuspid valve. Mapping with this system thus avoids the necessity of first performing a ventriculotomy. Recordings from up to 112 endocardial sites are simultaneously obtained using a computerized mapping system. In a preliminary report of this technique, 15 patients undergoing the transatrial balloon approach were compared with 15 patients mapped with a standard approach using a hand-held endocardial probe through a left ventriculotomy [138]. Mapping was described as being more complete with the balloon approach and led to more extensive ablation. During electrophysiologic studies performed 2 weeks after operation, 36% (5/14) of patients in the standard approach group compared to 8% (1/12) of patients in the transatrial balloon group still had inducible VT. There were no late VT recurrences or sudden deaths in the transatrial balloon group over a mean follow-up period of 12 months, compared to a 36% incidence of recurrent VT in the standard approach group (mean follow-up 31 months). This system can also be used therapeutically since an ablative electric shock can be delivered at the earliest site(s) of activation without removal of the balloon. Preliminary results with this technique appear promising [139].

Surgery vs. the AICD for Patients With Ischemic VT

In the last decade, the AICD has emerged as the most important new modality for the treatment of life-threatening ventricular arrhythmias [140]. Because it has proved highly effective in preventing sudden death, the implantable defibrillator must be considered the standard for assessing the efficacy of other methods. Implantation of the defibrillator is also a relatively simple surgical procedure in comparison to ventricular arrhythmia surgery, so this technology is potentially available for a far greater number of patients. The manufacturer of the currently available AICD (CPI) has recently reported on 6,041 patients undergoing primary device implantation through February, 1989 [22]. Seventy-four percent of devices are currently implanted in patients with coronary artery disease, and 13% of patients receiving AICDs have nonischemic cardiomyopathy. The perioperative death rate among 800 patients reported in six series was 2.3% [141–146]. Using life-table (Kaplan-Meier) analysis, the 5 year sudden-death-free survival rate approaches 95%, with an overall cardiac survival rate of 82.6%. However, the average length of follow-up for these patients is still very short (12 months) [22]. The mean age (60 years) and left ventricular ejection fraction (32%) of patients in AICD and surgical series are similar [22].

Comparative results of surgery and the AICD. Based on an analysis of the data presented in the preceding paragraphs, the AICD would appear to represent the preferred nonpharmacologic treatment option for patients with drug-resistant ventricular arrythmias. In comparing the results between current surgical and AICD series, it should be noted that the patients making up these series may differ in important respects (e.g., presenting arrhythmia, type of underlying heart disease, preoperative condition, etc.). These factors may account for differences in patient outcome and must be borne in mind when interpretating the results of various interventions. Most patients who are considered for nonpharmacologic therapy have undergone an initial trial of electrophysiologically guided serial drug testing [142]. Patients with drug-

TABLE 10–3. "Ideal" Surgical Candidate for Map-Directed VT Ablation Procedure

Inducible, hemodynamically well tolerated, sustained monomorphic VT refractory to medical therapy
Coronary artery disease with bypassable vessels
Discrete, anterior left ventricular aneurysm
Good overall left ventricular function, with preserved functional status (LVEF ≥30%, NYHA class ≤II)
Adequate preoperative endocardial map, with VT at an accessible site

resistant, life-threatening ventricular arrhythmias may be candidates for antiarrhythmia surgery or an AICD. It must be emphasized that, in the early phase, the main reason for attempting antitachycardia surgery was the lack of a viable alternative therapy in patients who often had advanced left ventricular dysfunction. If antiarrhythmic drugs alone were ineffective, there was often little choice but to proceed with surgery, despite the obvious risks in such patients. As was mentioned above, the high intraoperative mortality rates cited (12–15%) in part reflect the poor surgical candidacy of these patients [127,128]. The AICD now provides the previously missing therapeutic option for patients with medically refractory VT who are not optimal surgical candidates because of severe, diffuse left ventricular dysfunction. Currently, patients at prohibitively high operative risk are not subjected to ventricular surgery, so the operative mortality and long-term survival rates of patients in future surgical series should improve. It should be noted that patients with advanced left ventricular dysfunction (left ventricular ejection fraction <20%, NYHA functional class III or higher) do relatively poorly over the ensuing 2 years regardless of the intervention employed [127,147]. The outcome of surgery is also highly dependent on ventricular function, and patients with well preserved ventricular function do significantly better than those with poor ventricular function [127]. Thus "ideal" surgical candidates may be expected to compare favorably to similar patients receiving an AICD (Table 10–3).

The University of Pennsylvania group has recently compared the results obtained in patients undergoing subendocardial resection (n = 269) and those receiving an AICD (n = 77) [128]. The overall mean age and left ventricular ejection fractions were similar for the two groups [128]. These groups differed, however, in terms of presenting and induced arrhythmias. All patients receiving an AICD had previous cardiac arrest compared to 50% of patients undergoing subendocardial resection. One hundred percent of patients undergoing subendocardial resection had sustained monomorphic VT in contrast to 55% of patients in the AICD group. Twenty-six percent of patients in the AICD group had no inducible ventricular arrhythmias; 19% had inducible polymorphic VT or ventricular fibrillation. Operative mortality was 3% for the AICD patients vs. 15% for the subendocardial resection group. The 4 year actuarial survival rate (including operative mortality) in both groups was approximately 60%. Death in the two groups was mainly from congestive failure. Sudden-death-free survival at 3 years was approximately 95% for the subendocardial resection group vs. 90% for the AICD group. As expected, at 3 years, the subendocardial resection group had significantly fewer recurrent arrhythmias than the AICD group (5% vs. 56%), and were receiving fewer antiarrhythmic drugs on a long-term basis (33% vs. 66%). Finally, at least one complication related to the AICD or implantation was reported in 60% of AICD patients [128].

Current recommendations. Therapy for patients at high risk for sudden death must be individualized, and the most appropriate intervention depends on a number of factors, including the type and severity of underlying heart disease, coronary anatomy, left ventricular ejection fraction, NYHA functional status, preoperative electrophysiologic findings, and other comorbid factors (Fig. 10–1). Patients who are considered poor surgical candidates based on hemodynamic and/or coronary anatomic considerations should receive an AICD, particularly if preoperative electrophysiologic testing reveals ventricular fibrillation or hemodynamically compromising sustained VT (Table 10–4). Similarly, patients with documented out-of-hospital ventricular fibrillation in the absence of a reversible predisposing factor (e.g., acute myocardial infarction) or inducible arrythmias should receive an AICD (Fig. 10–1). For patients with inducible sustained monomorphic VT in whom all morphologies can be induced and satisfactorily mapped preoperatively, map-guided extended endocardial resection represents an excellent therapeutic option (Table 10–3). As a corollary, patients with slow, well tolerated, or frequently recurring VTs are not well suited to receive currently available AICDs. A surgical option may be the ideal solution for a patient with a previous anterior infarction, discrete aneurysm, and otherwise preserved ventricular function in whom coronary revascularization is also indicated. These patients may benefit from combined map-directed endocardial resection, aneurysmectomy, and coronary revascularization (Fig. 10–1). If at the time of surgery all arrhythmogenic tissue cannot be removed, cryoablation and/or a localized encircling procedure may be used to complete the ablation in surgically inaccessible sites. If intraoperative mapping cannot be successfully completed, a visually guided procedure may be used in conjunction with the placement of one or both epicardial AICD patches in patients who remain inducible after normothermic bypass or when surgery is performed

Fig. 10–1. Management strategy for patients with drug-refractory, life-threatening ventricular arrhythmias. Abbreviations: AICD, automatic implantable cardioverter-defibrillator; CABG, coronary artery bypass grafting; CAD, coronary artery disease; EP, electrophysiologic; LV, left ventricular; MVT, monomorphic ventricular tachycardia; VA, ventricular arrhythmia; VF, ventricular fibrillation; VT, ventricular tachycardia. (See text for details.)

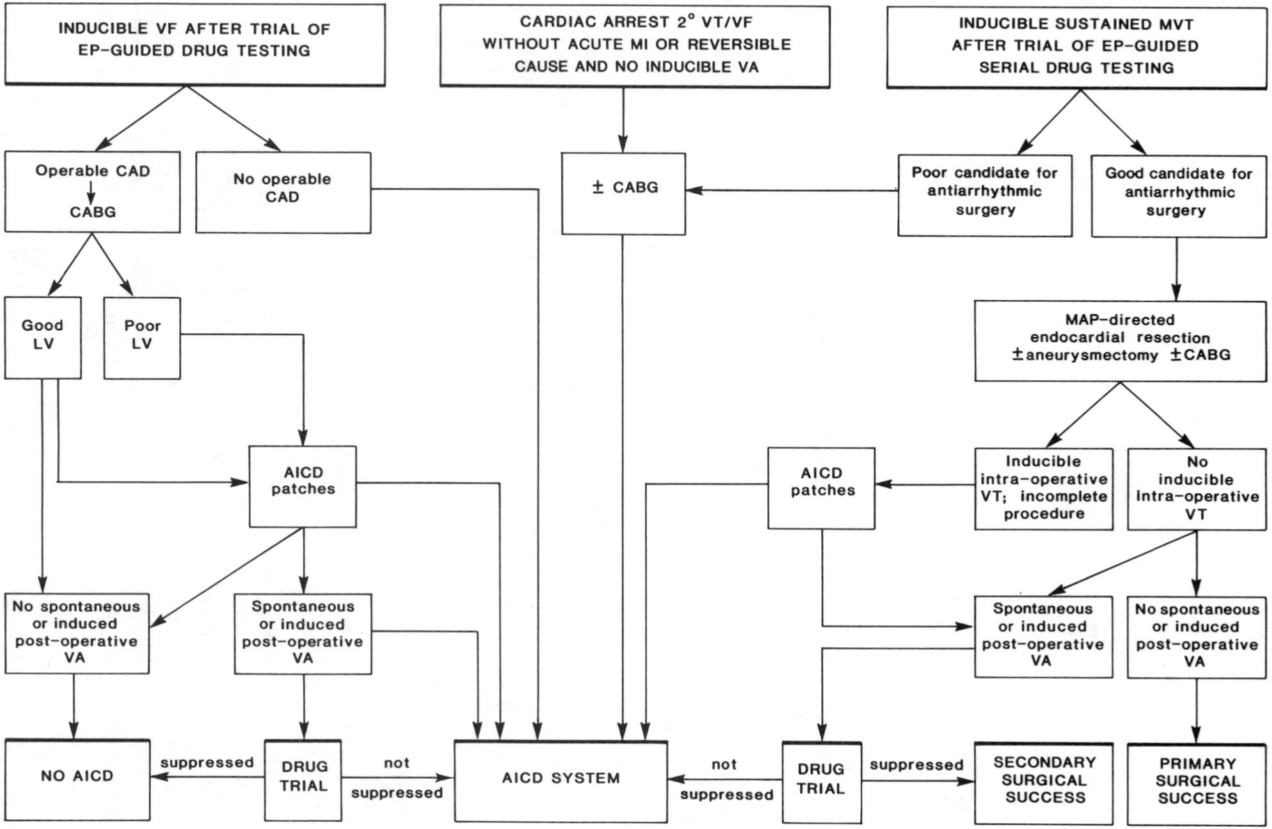
INDUCIBLE VF AFTER TRIAL OF EP-GUIDED DRUG TESTING
CARDIAC ARREST 2° VT/VF WITHOUT ACUTE MI OR REVERSIBLE CAUSE AND NO INDUCIBLE VA
INDUCIBLE SUSTAINED MVT AFTER TRIAL OF EP-GUIDED SERIAL DRUG TESTING
Operable CAD → CABG
No operable CAD
± CABG
Poor candidate for antiarrhythmic surgery
Good candidate for antiarrhythmic surgery
Good LV
Poor LV
MAP-directed endocardial resection ±aneurysmectomy ±CABG
AICD patches
AICD patches
Inducible intra-operative VT; incomplete procedure
No inducible Intra-operative VT
No spontaneous or induced post-operative VA
Spontaneous or induced post-operative VA
Spontaneous or induced post-operative VA
No spontaneous or induced post-operative VA
NO AICD
suppressed
DRUG TRIAL
not suppressed
AICD SYSTEM
not suppressed
DRUG TRIAL
suppressed
SECONDARY SURGICAL SUCCESS
PRIMARY SURGICAL SUCCESS

TABLE 10–4. Situations in Which an AICD Is Preferred Over Surgery for Treatment of Drug-Refractory, Life-Threatening Ventricular Arrhythmias

Patients with inducible ventricular fibrillation or hemodynamically unstable polymorphic ventricular tachycardia
Patients with sustained monomorphic ventricular tachycardia in whom map-guided procedures cannot be adequately performed
Patients with cardiac arrest due to ventricular fibrillation, with no inducible ventricular arrhythmias
Patients with attempted map-directed surgery who remain inducible intra- or postoperatively
Most patients with ventricular arrhythmias on the basis of nonischemic cardiomyopathies
Patients with poor overall ventricular function (LVEF $\leq$ 20%, NYHA class $\geq$ III).

under cardioplegic arrest (Fig. 10–1). The placement of one or more patches at the time of the initial surgery will avoid the necessity of performing a second thoracotomy should an AICD later become necessary. Coronary artery bypass grafting occasionally constitutes the only treatment necessary in patients with inducible ventricular fibrillation, particularly if preoperative ventricular function is good [76,77]. Conversely, in patients with primary ventricular fibrillation in the setting of poor ventricular function, one or both AICD patches should also be placed at the time of bypass grafting. Most patients with inducible sustained ventricular arrhythmias at postoperative electrophysiologic testing should subsequently undergo placement of an AICD system, although some arrhythmias may be suppressed by antiarrhythmic drugs. Finally, most patients with malignant ventricular arrhythmias occurring in association with nonischemic cardiomyopathies and/or poor ventricular function should receive an AICD rather than an attempted ablative surgical procedure (Table 10–4).

Surgery for Patients With Cardiomyopathies Unrelated to Ischemic Heart Disease

The relationship between ventricular arrhythmias and sudden death in patients with nonischemic (dilated), isolated right ventricular and hypertrophic cardiomyopathies has become better established in recent years [148]. Experience with the surgical treatment of these arrhythmias is much more limited [149], whereas AICD implantation has now become the preferred nonpharmacologic modality for the prevention of sudden death in most patients.

Right ventricular cardiomyopathy (dysplasia). This entity, as first described in depth by a French group in 1982 [150], has recently been identified as a rare condition associated with sudden death in young people [151]. The mechanism of sudden death is VT (hence the name arrhythmogenic right ventricular dysplasia; ARVD). Intraoperative mapping studies have shown that VT in these patients originates in the right ventricle [152]. Fontaine and coworkers [149] were the first to describe the use of a surgical approach to treat arrhythmias associated with this condition. These investigations used intraoperative epicardial mapping techniques to localize the arrhythmia to specific regions of the right ventricle. Mapping was followed by a simple ventriculotomy, sometimes with excision of tissue at the site of origin of VT. Among 15 patients undergoing operative procedures for this condition, no perioperative deaths were reported, although one-third of patients had a late relapse of VT occurring between the fifth and forty-fifth postoperative months [152]. The poor overall results of surgery for this condition compared to coronary artery disease are ascribed to the diffuse nature of the disease and a multifocal VT origin. The persistence of late potentials after surgery is performed is also consistent with the existence of an ongoing substrate for arrhythmogenesis [152], whereas their abolition has been associated with arrhythmia suppression [153]. Because of the poor outcome observed with map-guided surgery, Sealy and coworkers with the Duke University group developed a different surgical approach for treating this condition. Their procedure consisted of anatomically disconnecting the right ventricle from the left heart through a transmural encircling ventriculotomy in conjunction with cryosurgery [60]. This procedure successfully abolished intractable VT in the three patients reported. Guiraudon and coworkers [154] have also successfully employed this approach in a small number of patients.

Nonischemic (dilated) cardiomyopathy. Although most patients with nonischemic (idiopathic) dilated cardiomyopathy ultimately die from progressive left ventricular pump dysfunction and congestive heart failure, accumulating data indicate that many patients succumb prematurely to sudden death from ventricular arrhythmias [155–157]. The pathogenesis of ventricular arrhythmias in this condition is also less clearly established than for coronary artery disease. Since this disease involves diffuse myocardial damage, a single focal reentrant arrhythmogenic substrate may not underlie these arrhythmias, and map-guided surgical procedures are therefore less likely to be of long-term benefit to these patients. Since patients with nonischemic dilated cardiomyopathy do not have additional indications for surgery (e.g., coronary artery bypass grafting), there is reluctance to submit such patients to cardiac surgery solely for the purpose of an attempted surgical ablation [157]. The performance of surgery, particularly in patients with advanced left ventricular dysfunction, is associated with high perioperative mortality. Avoiding unnecessary surgery is also an important consideration for potential cardiac transplant candidates. For these reasons, arrhythmia surgery in patients with dilated cardiomyopathy has not evolved as an important antiarrhythmic therapy. Currently, most patients with dilated cardiomyopathies and life-threatening ventricular arrhythmias should receive an AICD as the primary treatment to prevent sudden cardiac death [158], and the AICD may now provide a "bridge" for high-risk patients with arrhythmias awaiting transplantation [159]. Orthotropic heart transplantation has become the definitive surgical procedure for prolonging survival in patients with end-stage ventricular dysfunction [160]. At one time this procedure was also advocated for the treatment of malignant ventricular arrhythmias [161].

One of the first patients to undergo a map-directed VT surgical procedure was a 33–year-old man with dilated cardiomyopathy. During epicardial mapping, this patient demonstrated two distinct VT morphologies [92]. A transmural ventriculotomy was performed at each site of origin. The patient subsequently remained arrhythmia-free but died 9 months later from congestive failure [93]. Because of their ineffectiveness, there have been few attempted surgical procedures for arrhythmias in patients with idiopathic dilated cardiomyopathy.

Hypertrophic cardiomyopathy. Patients with hypertrophic cardiomyopathy are also at significant risk for sudden death, although the mechanism of sudden death remains less clearly established [148,162]. Ventricular arrhythmias are recognized as a potential cause, although in patients with severe obstructive hypertrophic cardiomyopathy a primary hemodynamic event may be the mechanism in many cases [148]. The role of surgery in the prevention of sudden death in this condition remains to be defined. At present, surgical intervention is reserved for symptomatic patients with features of severe left ventricular outflow tract obstruction. Myotomy/myomectomy improves symptoms, but whether it prevents sudden death or improves prognosis is controversial [163]. Furthermore, map-directed surgery is not indicated in patients with hypertrophic cardiomyopathy since the mechanism and sites of origin of ventricular arrhythmias in this setting are poorly understood [164].

Surgery for Valvular Heart Disease

Aortic stenosis. Critical valvular aortic stenosis is a recognized risk factor for sudden cardiac death [165,166]. Classically, patients with severe aortic stenosis develop symptoms during exertion, implying that a primary hemodynamic event may be causal. Because of myocardial hypertrophy and secondary fibrosis resulting from chronic pressure overload [167], patients with aortic stenosis may also be at increased risk of sudden death from primary ventricular arrhythmias [168–170], as are patients with hypertensive left ventricular hypertrophy [171,172]. Another arrythmic cause of death may involve heart block due to coexistant conduction system disease. In patients with hemodynamically significant valvular disease and well preserved ventricular function, surgical replacement of the aortic valve is associated with relief of symptoms and improved prognosis [173–175]. Patients with concomitant aortic valve and coronary artery disease with events presumed secondary to valvular stenosis require careful evaluation to exclude associated ischemically mediated arrhythmias. In patients with associated coronary artery disease, concomitant surgical revascularization is associated with a significant reduction in the occurrence of late sudden deaths compared to patients receiving valve replacement alone [176].

Mitral valve prolapse. Another valvular abnormality occasionally associated with sudden cardiac death is mitral valve prolapse. Although ventricular ectopic activity is frequently described, only a minority of patients with this condition develop malignant arrhythmias, and sudden death is a rare complication of the disorder [177,178]. Among patients with this disorder, there are few reported attempts to correlate anatomic and electrophysiologic findings. Such studies are needed to establish definitively a cause and effect relationship between the valvular dysfunction and documented arrhythmias. Ventricular mapping studies during tachycardia have been performed in a limited number of patients, but in some cases the apparent site of origin of VT as determined by these techniques was remote from the area of the mitral valve [179–183]. This finding suggests that the valvular abnormality may not be the causal factor for arrhythmogenesis in all patients. Such data also imply that surgical replacement of the mitral valve, per se, may not represent a useful procedure for suppressing arrhythmias or improving prognosis. In a few instances, the origin of the tachycardia has apparently been localized to the mitral valve area, with improved control of ventricular tachycardia following mitral valve replacement [184–186]. Most notably, Cobbs and King [185] described a patient who underwent intraoperative epicardial mapping at the time of mitral valve replacement. In this patient, the earliest site of activation during VT was apparently localized to the posterior papillary muscle. Following mitral valve replacement, the arrhythmia, atlhough not completely abolished, was far easier to control. Similarly, Ross et al. [184] described a patient with mitral valve prolapse and drug-refractory VT in whom improved arrhythmia control was observed following valve replacement. These cases imply a causal relationship between the valvular disease and arrhythmogenesis, although both patients suffered from severe degrees of valvular regurgitation sufficient to cause secondary left ventricular dysfunction. In the absence of hemodynamically significant mitral regurgitation, or proved origin of VT within the mitral valve apparatus, replacement of the mitral valve is not indicated for patients with mitral valve disease and ventricular arrhythmias.

Repaired Congenital Heart Defects

Complex congenital heart defects such as tetralogy of Fallot and transposition of the great vessels may now be successfully repaired in infancy and childhood, and, as a result of early intracardiac surgery, the prognosis for prolonged survival in these patients has steadily improved [187]. Sudden death is a recognized late complication of repaired tetralogy and in most instances is due to the development of a ventricular arrhythmia [188]. High-risk patients for arrhythmic events are mainly those with poor postoperative hemodynamic results and residual anatomic abnormalities [187,189]. A nidus for ventricular arrhythmias may reside at the right ventriculotomy site or may be associated with the myocardial patch used to repair the ventricular septal defect [190]. However, patients with myopathic ventricles may also harbor a diffuse substrate for arrhythmogenesis [191]. Small numbers of patients with repaired tetralogy have undergone successful map-guided surgical VT ablation [190]. Ventricular arrythmias may also be causal in some instances of sudden death associated with Ebstein's anomaly of the tricuspid valve.

Surgery for Miscellaneous Cardiac Conditions Associated With Ventricular Arrhythmias

A number of miscellaneous cardiac conditions such as localized left and right ventricular aneurysms [192,193], ventricular tumors [194–197], and other focal diseases [198] may be associated with intractable and/or life-threatening ventricular arrhythmias. In some instances, endocardial mapping has been used to localize otherwise inapparent abnormalities. The relationship between focal ventricular abnormalities and ventricular tachycardia is particularly well illustrated by the reports of Garson et al. [194–196]. These workers have described findings in 21 infants, 3.5–31 months old, who underwent surgical exploration for incessant VTs. In 12 patients, a visible discrete abnormality <1 cm^2 was identified. Nine patients had myocardial hamartomas (Purkinjie cell tumors), and one patient each had a rhabdomyoma and focal myocarditis. In two patients, the results of biopsy were normal. In the remaining nine patients, diffuse ventricular abnormalities were found. In most patients, preoperative echocardiography and angiocardiography disclosed no focal defects, although some ventricular enlargement was described. In all patients, endocardial mapping of the VT was possible, and, in those patients who had a discrete lesion identified at the earliest site of activation, the tachycardia was abolished after surgical excision of the involved area. In 14 of 15 patients with impaired left ventricular function, ventricular function improved after VT was suppressed [194–196]. Map-directed VT surgery has also been performed in small numbers of patients without apparent structural abnormalities and presumed ''idiopathic'' VT [152]. However, since the vast majority of patients with monomorphic VT in the setting of normal ventricular function and absent cardiac disease are at low risk for sudden death, map-directed surgery is indicated only for intractable cases [19]. The arrhythmias in most of these patients are usually satisfactorily controlled by antiarrhythmic drug therapy alone.

SUMMARY

Many congenital and acquired structural cardiac diseases may predispose to ventricular arrhythmias and thus place the patient at an increased risk for premature death. Patients at high risk for life-threatening arrhythmia development and sudden cardiac death may be candidates for a variety of currently available surgical interventions (Table 10–2). Some procedures (e.g., coronary artery bypass grafting) may reduce the risk of arrhythmia development by preventing inciting events (e.g., myocardial ischemia); others (e.g., accessory pathway ablation, map-directed endocardial resection) may eliminate the arrhythmogenic potential by removing the underlying anatomic substrate. The accumulated experience over the first decade of antiarrhythmia surgery indicates that these procedures may be effectively and safely performed in appropriately selected patients. In future years, ventricular arrhythmia surgery should be associated with lower intraoperative mortality rates because of better patient selection. As established procedures continue to be further modified, and as newer procedures (e.g., balloon mapping and electrical ablation, laser fulguration [199,200]) are developed and tested, the outcome of patients undergoing surgical treatment to prevent sudden cardiac death should improve further in the years to come. It should be remembered, however, that, although these procedures may prevent premature arrhythmic death, they cannot be expected to alter the natural history of the underlying heart disease (e.g., pump failure). Primary intervention for the underlying disease processes themselves (e.g., atherosclerosis) will ultimately be necessary to eliminate the problem of sudden cardiac death [201].

ACKNOWLEDGMENT

We thank Diane Bachiri for her assistance in the preparation of the manuscript.

REFERENCES

1. Kuller L, Lillenfeld A, Fisher R: Epidemiologic study of sudden and unexpected deaths due to arteriosclerotic heart disease. Circulation 34:1056–1068, 1966.
2. WHO Scientific Group: Sudden cardiac death. WHO Tech Rev Ser 726:5–25, 1985.
3. Myerburg R, Castellanos A: Cardiac arrest and sudden cardiac death. In Braunwald E (ed): ''Heart Disease, A Textbook of Cardiovascular Medicine.'' Philadelphia: W.B. Saunders Co., 1988; pp 742–777.
4. Wilber DJ, Garan H, Finkelstein D, et al.: Out-of-hospital cardiac arrest. Use of electrophysiologic testing in the prediction of long-term outcome. N Engl J Med 318:19–24, 1988.
5. Cox JL: Patient selection criteria and results of surgery for refractory ischemic ventricular tachycardia. Circulation 79 [Suppl I]:I-163–I-177, 1989.
6. Roy D, Waxman HL, Kienzie MG, Buxton AE, Marchlinski FE, Josephson ME: Clinical characteristics and long-term follow-up in 119 survivors of cardiac arrest: Relation to inducibility at electrophysiologic testing. Am J Cardiol 52:969–974, 1983.
7. Morady F, Scheinman MM, Hess DS, Sung RJ, Shen E, Shapiro W: Electrophysiologic testing in the management of survivors of out-of-hospital cardiac arrest. Am J Cardiol 51:85–89, 1983.

8. Baum RS, Alvarez H III, Cobb LA: Survival after resuscitation of out-of-hospital ventricular fibrillation. Circulation 50:1231–1235, 1974.
9. Goldstein S, Landis JR, Leighton R, et al.: Characteristics of the resuscitated out-of-hospital caridac arrest victim with coronary heart disease. Circulation 64:977–984, 1981.
10. Swerdlow CD, Winkle RA, Mason JW: Determinants of survival in patients with ventricular arrhythmias. N Engl J Med 308:1436–1442, 1983.
11. Davis MJ: Pathological view of sudden cardiac death. Br Heart J 45:88–96, 1981.
12. Topaz O, Edwards JE: Pathologic features of sudden death in children, adults, and young adults. Chest 87:476–482, 1985.
12a. Topaz O, Perin E, Cox M, et al.: Young adult survivors of sudden cardiac arrest: Analysis of invasive evaluation in 22 subjects. Am Heart J 118:281–287, 1989.
13. Maron BJ, Roberts WC, Epstein SE: Sudden death in hypertrophic cardiomyopathy: A profile of 78 patients. Circulation 65:1388–1394, 1982.
14. Maron BJ, Epstein SE, Roberts WC: Causes of sudden death in competitive athletes. J Am Coll Cardiol 7:204–214, 1986.
15. Maron BJ, Roberts WC, Edwards JE, McAllister HA, Foley DD, Epstein SE: Sudden death in patients with hypertrophic cardiomyopathy: Characterization of 26 patients without functional limitation. Am J Cardiol 41:803–810, 1978.
16. Roberts WC: Congenital coronary arterial anomalies unassociated with major anomalies of the heart or great vessels. In Roberts WC (ed): ''Adult Congenital Heart Disease.'' Philadelphia: F.A. Davis, 1987, pp 583–629.
17. Moroles AR, Romanelli R, Boucek RJ: The mural left anterior descending coronary artery, strenuous exercise and sudden death. Circulation 62:230–237, 1980.
18. Liberthson RR, Dinsmore RE, Fallon JT: Aberrant coronary artery origin from the aorta: Report of 18 patients, review of the literature and delineation of natural history and management. Circulation 59:748–754, 1979.
19. Brooks R, Burgess JH: Idiopathic ventricular tachycardia: A review. Medicine 67:271–294, 1988.
20. Weaver WD, Lorch GS, Alvarez HA, et al.: Angiographic findings and prognostic indicators in patients resuscitated from sudden cardiac death. Circulation 54:895–900, 1976.
21. Borggrefe M, Podczeck A, Ostermyer J, Briethardt G, and the Surgical Ablation Registry: In Breithardt G, Borggrefe M, Zipes DP (eds): ''Nonpharmacologic Therapy of Tachyarrhythmias.'' Mount Kisco, NY: Futura Publishing Co., 1987, pp 109–132.
22. Cardiac Pacemakers Incorporated (CPI). Data on file. (Courtesy, Matt O'Neal).
23. Ritchie JL, Hallstrom AP, Troubaugh GB, Caldwell JH, Cobb LA: Out-of-hospital sudden coronary death: Rest and exercise radionuclide left ventricular function in survivors. Am J Cardiol 55:645, 1985.
24. Myerburg RJ, Conde CA, Sung RJ, et al.: Clinical electrophysiologic and hemodynamic profile of patients resuscitated from prehospital cardiac arrest. Am J Med 68:568–576, 1980.
25. Freedman RA, Swerdlow CD, Soderholm-Difatce, et al.: Clinical predictors of cardiac arrest: Importance of gender and prior myocardial infarction. J Am Coll Cardiol 12: 973–978, 1988.
26. Moss AJ: Prolonged QT-interval syndromes. JAMA 256:2985–2987, 1986.
27. Moss AJ, Schwartz PJ, Crampton RS, Locati E, Carleen MA: The long QT syndrome: A prospective international study. Circulation 71:17–21, 1985.
28. Jackman WM, Friony KJ, Anderson JL, et al.: The long QT syndrome: a critical review, new clinical observations, and a unifying hypothesis. Prog Cardiovasc Dis 31:115–172, 1988.
29. Schwartz PJ, Vanoli F: Indirect approaches in the treatment of malignant ventricular

arrhythmias: The role of left stellectomy. In Breithardt G, Borggrefe, Zipes DP (eds): ''Nonpharmacologic Therapy of Arrhythmias.'' Mount Kisco, NY: Futura Publishing Company, 1987, pp 143–158.
30. Schwartz PJ: Prevention of arrhythmias in the long QT syndrome. In Kulbertus HE (ed): ''Medical Management of Arrhythmias.'' Edinburgh: Churchill Livingston, 1986, pp 153–161.
31. Schwartz PJ, Snebold NG, Brown AM: Effects of unilateral cardiac sympathetic denervation on ventricular fibrillation threshold. Am J Cardiol 37:1034, 1976.
32. Moss AJ, McDonald J: Unilateral cervicothoracic sympathetic ganglionectomy for treatment of the long QT interval syndrome. N Engl J Med 285:903–904, 1971.
33. Bhandari AK, Morady F, Shen EN, Schwartz A, Mason J, Schienman M: Is left cervicothoracic sympathectomy effective treatment for patients with the prolonged QT syndrome? Circulation 68(III):1707, 1983.
34. Eldar M, Griffin JC, Abbott, et al.: Permanent cardiac pacing in patients with the long QT syndrome. J Am Coll Cardiol 10:600–607, 1987.
35. Durrer D, Schoo L, Schulenburg RM, Wellens HJJ: The role of premature beats in the initiation and termination of supraventricular tachycardia in the WPW syndrome. Circulation 36:644–662, 1967.
36. Cobb FR, Blumenschein SD, Sealy WC, Boineau JP, Wagner GS, Wallace AG: Successful surgical interruption of the bundle of kent in a patient with Wolff-Parkinson-White Syndrome. Circulation 38:1018–1029, 1968.
37. Gallagher JJ, Sealy WC, Wallace AG, Kassel J: Correlation between catheter electrophysiologic studies and findings on mapping of ventricular excitation in the WPW syndrome. In Wellens HJJ, Lie H, Janse MJ (eds): ''Conduction System of the Heart.'' Philadelphia: Lea and Febiger, 1976, pp 588–612.
38. Klein GJ, Bashore TM, Sellers TD, Pritchett EL, Smith WM, Gallagher JJ: Ventricular fibrillation in the Wolff-Parkinson-White syndrome. N Engl J Med 301:1080–1085, 1979.
39. Sealy WC, Gallagher JJ, Wallace AG: The surgical treatment of the Wolff-Parkinson-White syndrome. Evolution of improved methods for identification and interruption of the Kent bundle. Ann Thoracic Surg 22:443–457, 1975.
40. Gallagher JJ, Sealy WC, Cox JL, German LD, Ksell JH, Bardy GH, Packer DL: Results of surgery for preexcitation caused by Accessory atrioventricular pathways in 267 consecutive cases. In Josephson ME, Wellens HJJ (eds): ''Tachycardias: Mechanisms, Diagnosis, Management.'' Philadelphia: Lea and Febiger, 1984, pp 259–270.
41. Cox JL, Gallagher JJ, Cain ME: Experience with 118 consecutive patients undergoing operation for the Wolff-Parkinson-White syndrome. J Thorac Cardiovasc Surg 90:490–501, 1985.
42. Sealy WC, Mikat EM: Anatomical problems with identification and interruption of posterior septal kent bundles. Ann Thorac Surg 36:584–595, 1983.
43. Guiraudon GC, Klein GC, Gulamhusein S, et al.: Surgical repair of Wolff-Parkinson-White syndrome: A new closed-heart technique. Ann Thorac Surg 37:67–71, 1984.
44. Anderson RH, Becker AE: Stanley Kent and accessory atrio-ventricular connections. J Thorac Cardiovasc Surg 81:649–658, 1981.
45. Sealy WC, Gallagher JJ, Kasell J: His bundle interruption for control of inappropriate responses to atrial arrhythmias. Ann Thorac Surg 32:429–437, 1981.
46. Cox JL, Holman WL, Cain ME: Cryosurgical treatment of atrioventricular node reentrant tachycardia. Circulation 76:1329–1336, 1987.
47. Scheinman MM, Evans-Bell GT, and the Executive Committee of the Percutaneous Mapping and Ablation Registry. In Fontaine G, Scheinman MM (eds): ''Ablation in Cardiac Arrhythmias.'' Mount Kisco, NY: Futura Publishing Co., 1987, pp 161–169.
48. Morady F, Scheinman MM, Kou WH: Long-term results of catheter ablation of a pos-

teroseptal accessory atrioventricular conduction in 48 patients. Circulation 79:1160–1170, 1989.
49. Lown B, Verrier RL: Neural activity and ventricular fibrillation. N Engl J Med 294: 1165–1170, 1976.
50. Estes EH, Izlar HL: Recurrent ventricular tachycardia. A case successfully treated by bilateral cardiac sympathectomy. Am J Med 31:493–497, 1961.
51. Sealy WC, Oldham NH: Surgical treatment of malignant ventricular arrhythmias by sympathectomy, coronary artery bypass grafts, and heart wall resection. Proceedings of an International Symposium on Electrophysiology, Sydney, Australia, October, 1977.
52. Kadowaki MH, Levett JM: Sympathectomy in the treatment of angina and arrhythmias. Ann Thorac Surg 41:572–578, 1986.
53. Favaloro R: Saphenous vein autograft replacement of severe segmental coronary artery occlusion. Ann Thorac Surg 5:335–339, 1968.
54. Minardo JD, Tuli MM, Mock BH, Weiner RE, Pride HP, Wellman HN, Zipes DP: Scintigraphic and electrophysiological evidence of canine myocardial sympathetic denervation and produced by myocardial infarction or phenol application. Circulation 78: 1008–1019, 1988.
55. Schwartz PJ, Motolese M, Pollavinni G, et al., and the Sudden Death Italian Prevention Group: Surgical and pharmacological antiadrenergic interventions in the prevention of sudden death after a first myocardial infarction. Circulation 72:III-358, 1985.
56. Grondin CM, Limet R: Sympathetic denervation in association with coronary artery bypass grafting in patients with prinzmetal's angina. Ann Thorac Surg 23:111, 1977.
57. Tilkian AG, Pfeifer JF, Barry WH, et al.: Evaluation of aortocoronary venous bypass grafting for prevention of cardiac arrhythmias. Am Heart J 98:15–19, 1979.
58. Gallagher JJ: Surgical treatment of arrhythmias: Current status and future directions. Am J Cardiol 41:1035–1044, 1978.
59. Graham AF, Miller DC, Stinson EP, et al.: Surgical treatment of refractory life-threatening ventricular tachycardia. Am J Cardiol 32:909–912, 1973.
60. Cox JL: Surgery for cardiac arrhythmias. Curr Prob Cardiol 8:1–60, 1983.
61. Ricks WB, Winkle RA, Shumway NE, et al.: Surgical management of life-threatening ventricular arrhythmias in patients with coronary artery disease. Circulation 56:38–42, 1977.
62. CASS Principal Investigators: Coronary Artery Surgery Study (CASS). A randomized trial of coronary artery bypass surgery: survival data. Circulation 68:939–950, 1983.
63. The Veterans Administration Coronary Artery Bypass Surgery Cooperative Study: Eleven-year survival in the Veterans Administration randomized trial of coronary bypass surgery for stable angina. N Engl J Med 311:1333–1339, 1984.
63a. Holmes DR, Davis KB, Mock MB, et al.: The effect of medical and surgical treatment on subsequent sudden death in patients with coronary artery disease: A report from the Coronary Artery Surgery Study. Circulation 73:1254–1263, 1986.
64. European Coronary Surgery Study Group: Coronary bypass surgery in stable angina pectoris: Survival at two years. Lancet 1:889–893, 1979.
64a. European Coronary Surgery Group: Long-term results of prospective randomized study of coronary artery bypass surgery in stable angina pectoris. Lancet II:1173–1180, 1982.
65. Varnauskas E, and the European Coronary Surgery Study Group: Twelve year follow-up of survival in the randomized European Coronary Surgery Study. N Engl J Med 319: 332–337, 1988.
66. Killip T, Ryan TJ: Randomized trials in coronary artery bypass surgery. Circulation 71:418–421, 1985.
67. Cobb LA, Baum RS, Alvarez H, Schaffer WA: Resuscitation from out-of-hospital ventricular fibrillation: Four year follow-up. Circulation 51 [Suppl III]:223, 1975.

67a. Goldstein S, Medendorf SV, Landis JR, et al.: Analysis of cardiac symptoms preceding cardiac arrest. Am J Cardiol 58:1195–1198, 1986.

68. Sellers TD, Beller GA, Gibson RS, Watson DD, Di Marco JP: Prevalence of ischemia by quantitative thallium-201 scintigraphy in patients with ventricular tachycardia of fibrillation inducible by programmed stimulation. Am J Cardiol 59:828–832, 1987.

69. Sharma B, Asinger R, Francis GS, Hodges M, Wyeth RP: Painless ischemia in out-of-hospital ventricular fibrillation. Am J Crdiol 59:740–745, 1987.

70. Weiner DA, Levine SR, Klein MD, Ryan TJ: Ventricular arrhythmias during exercise testing: Mechanism, response to coronary bypass surgery and prognostic significance. Am J Cardiol 53:1553–1557, 1984.

71. Lehrman KL, Tilkian AG, Hultgren HN, Fowler RE: Effect of coronary arterial bypass surgery on exercise-induced ventricular arrythmias. Am J Cardiol 44:1056–1061, 1979.

72. Bryson AL, Parisi AF, Schechter E, et al.: Life-threatening ventricular arrhythmias induced by exercise. Cessation after coronary bypass surgery. Am J Cardiol 32:995–999, 1973.

73. Morady F, DiCarlo L, Winston S, et al.: Clinical features and prognosis of patients with out-of-hospital cardiac arrest and a normal electrophysiologic study. J Am Coll Cardiol 4:39–44, 1984.

74. Takaro T, Hultgren H, Lipton M, Detere K, and participants in the Veterans Administration Cooperative Study Group: VA cooperative randomized study for coronary arterial occlusive disease. II. Left main disease. Circulation 54:III-107, 1976.

75. Killiip T, Assamani E, Davis K, and the CASS Principal Investigators and their associates: Coronary Artery Surgery Study: a randomized trial of coronary bypass surgery. Eight years follow-up and survival in patients with reduced ejection fraction. Circulation 72:V-102–V-109, 1985.

75a. Myers WO, Schaff HV, Gersh BJ, et al.: Improved survival of surgically-treated patients with triple vessel coronary artery disease and severe angina pectoris. J Thorac Cardiovasc Surg 97:487–495, 1989.

76. Kelly PA, Freeman CS, Ruskin JN, et al.: Effect of myocardial revascularization on inducible ventricular arrhythmias (abstract). J Am Coll Cardiol 13:174A, 1989.

77. Kelly P, Ruskin JN, Vlahakes G, Buckley MJ, Freman CS, Garan H. Surgical coronary revascularization in survivors of prehospital cardiac arrest: Its effect on inducible ventriculars and long-term survival. J Am Coll Cardiol (in press).

77a. Kron IL, Lerman BB, Haines DE, Flanagon TL, DiMarco JP: Coronary artery bypass grafting in patients with ventricular fibrillation. Ann Thorac Surg 48:85–89, 1989.

78. Meissner MD, Kay HR, Horowitz L, et al.: Relation of acute antiarrhythmic drug efficacy of left ventricular function in coronary artery disease. Am J Cardiol 61:1050–1055, 1988.

79. Kuchar DL, Rottman J, Berger E, et al.: Prediction of successful suppression of sustained ventricular tachyarrhythmias by serial drug testing from data derived at the initial electrophysiologic study. J Am Coll Cardiol 12:982–988, 1988.

80. Bigger JT, Fleiss JL, Kleiger R, et al.: The relationships among ventricular arrhythmias, left ventricular dysfunction, and mortality in the 2 years after myocardial infarction. Circulation 69:250, 1984.

81. Fuster V, Gersh BJ, Giuliani ER, et al.: The natural history of idiopathic dilated cardiomyopathy. Am J Cardiol 47:525–531, 1981.

82. Kaiser GA, Ghahramani A, Golooki H, et al.: Role of coronary artery surgery in patients surviving unexpected cardiac arrest. Surgery 787:749–754, 1975.

83. Braunwald E, Rutherford JD: Reversible ischemic left ventricular dysfunction evidence for "hibernating" myocardium. J Am Coll Cardiol 8:1467–1470, 1986.

84. Lewis T: The experimental production of paroxysmal tachycardia and the effects of ligation of the coronary arteries. Heart 1:98, 1909.

85. Couch OA: Cardiac aneurysm with ventricular tachycardia and subsequent excision of aneurysm. Circulation 20:251–253, 1959.
86. Boineau JP, Cox JL: Rationale for a direct surgical approach to control ventricular arrhythmias. Am J Cardiol 49:381–396, 1982.
87. Wellens HJ, Schullenberg RM, Durrer D: Electrical stimulation of the heart in patients with ventricular tachycardia. Circulation 46:216–230, 1972.
88. Wittig JH, Boineau JP: Surgical treatment of ventricular arrhythmias using epicardial, transmural and endocardial mapping. Ann Thorac Surg 20:117–126, 1975.
89. Harken AH, Horowitz LN, Josephson ME: Comparison of standard aneurysmectomy with directed endocardial resection for treatment of recurrent sustained ventricular tachycardia. J Thorac Cardiovasc Surg 80:527–534, 1980.
90. Mason JW, Stinson EB: Comparison of efficacy of map-guided to blind myocardial resection for recurrent ventricular arrhythmia. Circulation 62[Suppl III]:263, 1980.
91. Guiraudon G, Fontaine G, Frank R, et al.: Encircling endocardial ventriculotomy: A new surgical treatment for life-threatening ventricular arrhythmias resistant to medical treatment following myocardial infarction. Ann Thorac Surg 26:438–444, 1978.
92. Guiraudon G, Frank R, Fontaine G: Interet des cartographies dans le traitment chirugical des tachycardias ventriculaires regelles recidivants. Nouv Presse Med 3:321, 1974.
93. Fontaine G, Guiraudon G, Frank R, et al.: La cartographie epicardique et le traitement chirurgical par simple ventriculotomie de par reentree. Certaines tachycardes ventriculaires rebelles. Arch Mal Coeur 68:113–124, 1975.
94. Scherlag BJ, El-Sherif N, Hopen RR, et al.: Characterization and localization of ventricular arrhythmias resulting from myocardial ischemia and infarction. Circ Res 35: 372–383, 1974.
95. El-Sherif N, Scherlag BJ, Lazzara R, et al.: Reentrant ventricular arrhythmias in the late myocardial infarction period: I. Conduction characteristics of the infarction zone. Circulation 55:686–702, 1977.
96. Ungerleider RM, Holman WL, Colcagno D, et al.: Encircling endocardial ventriculotomy for refractory ischemic ventricular tachycardia: III. Effects on regional left ventricular function. J Thorac Cardiovasc Surg 83:857–864, 1982.
97. Ungerleider RM, Holman WL, Stanley TE, et al.: Encircling endocardial ventriculotomy for refractory ischemic ventricular tachycardia. II: Effects on regional myocardial blood flow. J Thorac Cardiovasc Surg 83:850–856, 1982.
98. Ostermeyer J, Breithardt G, Borggrefe M, et al.: Complete versus partial encircling endocardial ventriculotomy. J Thorac Cardiovasc Surg 87:517–525, 1984.
98a. Ostermeyer J, Borggrefe M, Breithardt G, et al.: Direct operations for management of life-threatening ischemic ventricular tachycardia. J Thorac Cardiovasc Surg 94:848–865, 1987.
99. Guiraudon G, Fontaine G, Frank R, et al.: Encircling endocardial ventriculotomy. Late follow-up results. Circulation 62[Suppl III]:III-320, 1980.
100. Guiraudon GC, Klein G, Jones D, McLellan D: Encircling endocardial cryoablation for ventricular arrhythmias after myocardial infarction: further experience (abstract). Circulation 72:III-222, 1985.
101. Moran J, Kehoe R, Loeb J: Extended endocardial resection for the treatment of ventricular tachycardia. Ann Thorac Surg 34:538–552, 1982.
102. Josephson ME, Harken AH, Horowitz LN. Endocardial excision—A new surgical technique for the treatment of recurrent ventricular tachycardia. Circulation 60:1430–1439, 1979.
103. Harken AH, Josephson ME, Horowitz LN: Surgical endocardial resection for the treatment of malignant ventricular tachycardia. Ann Surg 190:456–460, 1979.
104. Krafehek J, Lawrie G, Roberts R, Magro S, Wyndham C: Surgical ablation of ventricular

tachycardia: Improved results with a map-directed regional approach. Circulation 73: 1239–1247, 1986.

105. Kron I, Lerman B, DiMarco J: Extended subendocardial resection: a surgical approach to ventricular tachyarrhythmias that cannot be mapped intraoperatively. J Thorac Cardiovasc Surg 90:586–591, 1985.

105a. Swerdlow CD, Mason JW, Stinson EB, Ayer PE, Winkle RA, Derby GC: Results of operations for ventricular tachycardia in 105 patients. J Thorac Cardiovasc Surg 92: 105–113, 1986.

106. Landymore RW, Kinley CE, Gardner M: Encircling endocardial resection with complete removal of endocardial scar without intraoperative mapping for the ablation of drug-resistant ventricular tachycardia. J Thorac Cardiovasc Surg 89:18–24, 1985.

107. Cox JL, Gallagher JJ, Ungerleider RM: Encircling endocardial ventriculotomy for refractory ischemic ventricular tachycardia: clinical indications, surgical technique, mechanism of action, and results. J Thorac Cardiovasc Surg 83:865–872, 1982.

108. Martin JL, Untereker WJ, Harken AH, Horowitz LN, Josephson ME: Aneurysmectomy and endocardial resection for ventricular tachycardia: Favourable hemodynamic and antiarrhythmic result in patients with global left ventricular dysfunction. Am Heart J 103:960–965, 1982.

109. Magovern GJ, Sakert T, Simpson K, et al.: Surgical therapy for left ventricular aneurysms. A ten year experience. Circulation 79[Suppl I]:I-102–I-107, 1989.

109a. Kienzle MG, Doherty JU, Roy D, Waxman HL, Harken AH, Josephson ME: Subendocardial resection for refractory ventricular tachycardia. Effects on ambulatory electrograms, programmed stimulation and ejection fraction, and relation to outcome. J Am Coll Cardiol 2:853–858, 1983.

110. Mickelborough LL, Wilson GJ, Weiser RD, et al.: Endocardial excision versus encircling endocardial ventriculotomy: A comparison of effects on ventricular structure and function. J Thorac Cardiovasc Surg 91:779–787, 1986.

111. Gallagher JJ, DelRossi AJ, Fernandez J, Maranhao V, Strong MD, White M, Gessman LJ: Cryothermal mapping of recurrent ventricular tachycardia in man. Circulation 71: 733–739, 1985.

112. Josephson ME, Horowitz LN, Farshidi A, et al.: Recurrent sustained ventricular tachycardia. 2. Endocardial mapping. Circulation 57:440–447, 1978.

113. Wiener I, Mindich B: Fragmented endocardial electrical activity in patients with ventricular tachycardia: A new guide to surgical therapy. Am Heart J 107:86–90, 1984.

114. Curry PVL, O'Keefe D, Pitcher E, Sowton E, Devarall PB, Yates AK: Localization of ventricular tachycardia by a new technique—Pace mapping. Circulation 60 [Suppl II] II–25, 1979.

115. Josephson ME, Waxman HL, Cain ME, et al.: Ventricular activation during ventricular endocardial pacing. II. Role of pace-mapping to localize origin of ventricular tachycardia. Am J Cardiol 50:11–22, 1982.

116. Horowitz LN, Josephson ME, Harken AH: Epicardial and endocardial activation during sustained ventricular tachycardia in man. Circulation 61:1227–1238, 1980.

117. Marchlinski FE, Almendral JM, Cassidy DM, et al.: Localization of endocardial site for catheter ablation of ventricular tachycardia. In Fontaine G, Scheinmann MM (eds): "Ablation in Cardiac Arrhythmias." Mount Kisco, NY: Futura, 1987, pp 289–309.

117a. Simson MB, Untereker WJ, Spielman SR, et al.: Relation between late potentials on the body surface and directly recorded fragmented electrograms in patients with ventricular tachycardia. Am J Cardiol 51:105–112, 1983.

118. Vassallo JA, Cassidy D, Simpson MB, et al.: The relationship of late potentials to the site of origin of ventricular tachycardia. Am J Cardiol, 55:985–989, 1985.

119. Kienzle MG, Miller J, Falcone R, et al.: Intraoperative endocardial mapping during sinus

rhythm: Relationship to site of origin of ventricular tachycardia. Circulation 70:957–965, 1984.

120. Speilman SR, Horowitz LN, Greenspan AM, et al.: Activation mapping in sinus rhythm in patients with ventricular tachycardia—Relationship to cycle length and site of origin (abstract). Am J Cardiol 47:497, 1981.

121. Josephson ME, Horowitz LN, Farshidi A, et al.: Continuous local electrical activity: A mechanism of recurrent ventricular tachycardia. Circulation 57:659–665, 1979.

122. Klein GJ, Harrison L, Ideker RF, Smith WM, Kosell J, Wallace AG, Gallagher JJ: Reaction of myocardium in cryosurgery: Electrophysiology and arrhythmogenic potential. Circulation 59:364–372, 1979.

123. Josephson ME, Horowitz LN, Spielman SR, et al.: Comparison of endocardial catheter mapping with intraoperative mapping of ventricular tachycardia. Circulation 61:395–404, 1980.

123a. Fenoglio JJ, Pham TD, Harken AH, et al.: Recurrent sustained ventricular tachycardia: Structure and ultrastructure of subendocardial regions in which tachycardia originates. Circulation 68:518–533, 1983.

124. Spielman SR, Michelson EL, Horowitz LN, et al.: The limitations of epicardial mapping as a guide to the surgical treatment of ventricular tachycardia. Circulation 57:666–671, 1978.

125. Garan H, Fallon JT, Rosenthal S, Ruskin JN: Endocardial, intramural and epicardial activation patterns during sustained monomorphic ventricular tachycardia in late canine myocardial infarction. Circ Res 60:879–896, 1987.

126. Josephson ME, Horowitz LN, Waxman HL, et al.: Sustained ventricular tachycardia: Role of the 12-lead electrocardiogram in localizing site of origin. Circulation 64:257–265, 1981.

127. Miller JM, Marchlinski FE, Harken AH, Hargrove WC, Josephson ME: Subendocardial resection for sustained ventricular tachycardia in the early period after acute myocardial infarction. Am J Cardiol 55:980–984, 1985.

128. Hargrove WC, Miller JM: Risk stratification and management of patients with recurrent ventricular tachycardia and other malignant ventricular arrhythmias. Circulation 79[Suppl I]:I-178–I-181, 1989.

129. Haines DE, Lerman BB, Kron IL, DiMarco JP: Surgical ablation of ventricular tachycardi with sequential map-guided subendocardial resection: Electrophysiological assessment and long-term follow-up. Circulation 77:131–141, 1988.

129a. Brondt B, Martins JB, Kienzle MG: Predictors of failure after endocardial resection for sustained ventricular tachycardia. J Thorac Cardiovasc Surg 95:495–500, 1988.

130. Miller JM, Kienzle dMG, Harken AH, Josephson ME: Subendocardial resection for ventricular tachycardia: Predictors of surgical success. Circulation 70:624–630, 1984.

131. Waspe LE, Brodman R, Kim SG, Matos JA, Johnston DR, Scavin GM, Fisher JD: Activation mapping in patients with coronary artery disease with multiple ventricular tachycardia origins: occurrence and therapeutic implications of widely separate apparent sites of origin. J Am Coll Cardiol 5:1075–1086, 1985.

132. Caceres J, Jazayeri M, McKinnie J, et al.: Sustained bundle branch reentry as a mechanism of clinical tachycardia. Circulation 79:256–270, 1989.

133. Mason JW, Stinson EB, Winkle RA, et al.: Relative efficacy of blind left ventricular aneurysm resection for the treatment of recurrent ventricular tachycardia. Am J Cardiol 49:241–248, 1982.

134. Miller JM, Gottlieb CD, Marchlinski FE, et al.: Does ventricular tachycardia mapping influence the success of antiarrhythmic therapy? J Am Coll Cardiol 11:112A, 1988.

135. Gallagher JJ, Kasell J, Sealy WC, Pritchett ELC, Wallace AG: Epicardial mapping in the Wolff-Parkinson-White syndrome. Circulation 57:854–866, 1978.

136. Cox JL: Intraoperative computerized mapping techniques: Do they help us to treat our

patients better surgically? In Brugada P, Wellens HJJ (eds): ''Cardiac Arrhythmias: Where Do We Go From Here?'' Mount Kisco, NY: Futura, 1987, pp 613–637.
137. Ideker RE, Smith WM, Wallace AG, et al.: A computerized method for the rapid display of ventricular activation during the intraoperative study of arrhythmias. Circulation 59:449–458, 1979.
138. Mickelborough LL, Harris L, Downer E, Parson I, Gray G: A new intraoperative approach for endocardial mapping of ventricular tachycardia. J Thorac Cardiovasc Surg 95:271–280, 1988.
139. Mickelborough LL, Wilson GJ, Harris L, Tashiro T, Parsons I, Gray G: Balloon electric shock ablation. J Thorac Cardiovasc Surg 97:135–146, 1989.
140. Brooks R, Garan H, McGovern BA, Ruskin JN: The automatic implantable cardioverter defibrillator (AICD): Historical perspective, current utilization, and future directions. In Braunwald E (ed): ''Heart Disease: Clinical Update.'' Philadelphia: W.B. Saunders Co., 1990.
141. Echt DS, Armstrong K, Schmidt P, et al.: Clinical experience, complications, and survival in 70 patients with the automatic implantable cardioverter defibrillator. Circulation 71:289–296, 1985.
142. Kelly PA, Cannom DS, Garan H, et al.: The automatic implantable cardioverter/defibrillator: Efficacy, complications and survival in patients with malignant ventricular arrhythmias. J Am Coll Cardiol 11:1278–1286, 1988.
143. Kulbertus HE, Nisam S. The implantable defibrillator AICD: European clinical experience. In Brugada D, Wellens HJJ (eds): ''Cardiac Arrhythmias: Where Do We Go From Here?'' Mount Kisco, NY: Futura, 1987, pp 681–686.
144. Reid PR, Griffith LSC, Platia EV, et al.: The automatic implantable cardioverter/defibrillator: Five-year clinical results. In Breithardt G, Borggrefe M, Zipes DP (eds): ''Nonpharmacologic Therapy of Tachyarrhythmias.'' Mount Kisco, NY: Futura Publishing Co., 1987, pp 447–486.
145. Tchou PJ, Kadri N, Anderson J, Caceres JA, Jazayeri M, Akhtar M: The automatic implantable cardioverter/defibrillators and survival of patients with left ventricular dysfunction and malignant ventricular arrhythmias. Ann Intern Med 109:529–534, 1988.
146. Winkle RA, Mead RH, Ruder MA, Gaudini VA, Smith NA, Bach WS, Schmidt P, Shipman T: Long-term outcome with the automatic implantable cardioverter/defibrillator. J Am Coll Cardiol 13:1353–1361, 1989.
147. Levine JH, Richards A, Mellits D, et al.: Does poor cardiac function preclude benefit from an automatic implantable cardioverter defibrillator? (abstract). J Am Coll Cardiol 13:65A, 1989.
148. McKenna WJ, Krikler DM, Goodwin JF: Arrhythmias in dilated and hypertrophic cardiomyopathy. Med Clin North Am 68:983–1000, 1984.
149. Fontaine G, Guiraudon G, Frank R, et al.: Surgical management of ventricular tachycardia unrelated to myocardial ischemia or infarction. Am J Cardiol 49:397–410, 1982.
150. Marcus FE, Fontaine GH, Guiraudon G, Frank R, Laurenceau JL, Malergue C, Grosgogeat Y: Right ventricular dysplasia: a report of 24 cases. Circulation 65:384–398, 1982.
151. Thiene G, Nava A, Corrado D, Rossi L, Pennelli N: Right ventricular cardiomyopathy and sudden death in young people. N Engl J Med 318:129–133, 1988.
152. Fontaine G, Guiraudon G, Freank R, et al.: Surgical management of ventricular tachycardia unrelated to myocardial infarction. In Josephson ME, Wellens HJJ (eds): ''Tachycardias: Mechanisms, Diagnosis, Treatment.'' Philadelphia: Lea and Febiger, 1984, pp 451–473.
153. Denniss AR, Johnson DC, Richards DA, et al.: Effect of excision of ventricular myocardium on delayed potentials detected by signal-averaged electrocardiogram in patients with ventricular tachycardia. Am J Cardiol 59:591–595, 1987.

154. Guiraudon GM, Klein GJ, Gulamhusein S, et al.: Total disconnection of the right ventricular free wall: Surgical treatment of right ventricular tachycardia associated with right ventricular dysplasia. Circulation 67:463–470, 1983.
155. Haung SK, Messer JV, Denes P: Significance of ventricular tachycardia in idiopathic dilated cardiomyopathy. Observations in 35 patients. Am J Cardiol 51:507–512, 1983.
156. Francis GS. Development of arrhythmias in the patient with congestive heart failure: Pathophysiology, prevalence, and prognosis. Am J Cardiol 57:3B–7B, 1986.
157. Roberts WC, Siegel RJ, McManus BM: Idiopathic dilated cardiomyopathy: Analysis of 152 necropsy patients. Am J Cardiol 60:1340–1355, 1987.
158. Marchlinski FE : Use of the automatic implantable cardioverter-defibrillator in patients with ventricular arrhythmias and dilated cardiomyopathy (abstract). PACE 12:450, 1989.
159. Stevenson LB, Fowler BM, Schroeder JS, et al.: Poor survival of patients with idiopathic cardiomyopathy considered too well for transplantation. Am J Med 83:871–876, 1987.
160. Copeland JG: Cardiac transplantation. Curr Prob Cardiol 13:159–224, 1988.
161. Kemkes B: Heart transplantation for end-stage malignant ventricular arrhythmias. International Workshop on The Patient at Risk of Sustained Ventricular Tachyarrhythmias, Munich, 1986.
162. Kowey PR, Eisenberg R, Engel TR: Sustained arrhythmias in hypertrophic cardiomyopathy. N Engl J Med 310:1566–1569, 1984.
163. Mohr R, Schaff HV, Danielson GK, Puga FJ, Pluth JR, Tajik AJ: The outcome of surgical treatment of hypertrophic cardiomyopathy. J Thorac Cardiovasc Surg 97:666–674, 1989.
164. Guiraudon G, Fontaine G, Frank R, Leandri R, Barra J, Cabrol C: Surgical treatment of ventricular tachycardia guided by ventricular mapping in 23 patients without coronary artery disease. Ann Thorac Surg 32:439–449, 1981.
165. Frank S, Johnson A, Ross J Jr: Natural history of valvular aortic stenosis. Br Heart J 35:41–46, 1973.
166. Chizner MA, Pearle DL, deLeon AC: The natural history of aortic stenosis in adults. Am Heart J 99:419–424, 1980.
167. Cameron JS, Myerburg RJ, Wong SS, Gaide MS, Epstein K, Alvaraz TR, Gelbond H, Guse PA, Bassett A: Electrophysiologic consequences of experimentally induced left ventricular pressure overload. J Am Coll Cardiol 2:481–487, 1983.
168. Olshausen KV, Schwarz F, Apfelbach J, Rohrig N, Kramer B, Kubler W: Determinants of the incidence and severity of ventricular arrhythmias in aortic valve disease. Am J Cardiol 51:1103–1109, 1983.
169. Olshausen KV, Witt T, Schmidt G, Meyer J: Ventricular tachycardia as a cause of sudden death in patients with aortic valve disease. Am J Cardiol 59:1214–1215, 1987.
170. Klein RC: Ventricular arrhythmias in aortic valve disease: analysis of 102 patients. Am J Cardiol 53:1079–1083, 1983.
171. McLenachan JM, Henderson E, Morris KI, Dargie HJ: Ventricular arrhythmias in patients with hypertensive left ventricular hypertrophy. N Engl J Med 317:787–792, 1987.
172. McLenachan J, Henderson E, Kindop GB, Dargie HJ: Sudden death in hypertension: A possible mechanism. Br Heart J 57:572, 1987.
173. Pantley G, Morton MJ, Rahimtoola SH: Effects of successful, uncomplicated valve replacement on ventricular hypertrophy, volume, and performance in aortic stenosis and aortic imcompetence. J Thorac Cardiovasc Surg 75:383–391, 1978.
174. Henry WL, Bonow RO, Borer JS, et al.: Evaluation of aortic valve replacement in patients with valvular aortic stenosis. Circulation 61:814–825, 1980.
175. Rahimtoola SH: Valvular heart disease: a perspective. J Am Coll Cardiol 1:199–215, 1983.
176. Czer LSC, Gray RJ, Steward ME, DeRobertis M, Chaux A, Matloff JM: Reduction in

sudden late death by concomitant revascularization with aortic valve replacement. J Thorac Cardiovasc Surg 95:390–401, 1988.

177. Winkle RA, Lopes MG, Popp RL, Hancock EW: Life-threatening arrhythmias in the mitral valve prolapse syndrome. Am J Cardiol 60:961–967, 1976.
178. Wei JY, Bulkley BH, Schaeffer AH, Greene HL, Reid PR: Mitral valve porolapse syndrome and recurrent ventricular arrhythmias. Ann Intern Med 89:6–9, 1978.
179. Deal BJ, Miller SM, Scagliiotti D, Prechel D, Gallastegui JL, Hariman RJ: Ventricular tachycardia in a young population without overt heart disease. Circulation 73:1111–1118, 1986.
180. Buxton AE, Waxman HL, Marchlinski FE, Simson MB, Cassidy DL, Josephson ME: Right ventricular tachycardia: Clinical and electrophysiological characteristics. Circulation 68:917–927, 1983.
181. Palileo EV, Ashley WW, Swiryn S: Exercise provokable right ventricular outflow tract tachycardia. Am Heart J 104:185–193, 1982.
182. Pietras RJ, Lam W, Bauernfeind, Sheikh A, Palileo E, Strosberg B, Swiryn S, Rosen KM: Chronic recurrent right ventricular tachycardia in patients without ischemic heart disease: Clinical, hemodynamic, and angiographic findings. Am Heart J 105:357–366, 1983.
183. Rosenthal ME, Hamer A, Gang ES, Oseran DS, Mandel WJ, Peter T: The yield of programmed ventricular stimulation in mitral valve prolapse patients with ventricular arrhythmias. Am Heart J 110:970–976, 1985.
184. Ross A, de Weese JA, Yu PN: Refractory ventricular arrhythmias in a patient with mitral valve prolapse: Successful control with mitral valve replacement. J Electrocardiol 11: 289–295, 1978.
185. Cobbs BW, King SB: Ventricular buckling: A factor in the abnormal ventriculogram and hemodynamics associated with mitral valve prolapse. Am Heart J 93:741–758, 1977.
186. Kay HJ, Krohn BG, Hoffman RL: Surgical correction of severe mitral valve prolapse without mitral insufficiency but with pronounced cardiac arrhythmias. J Thorac Cardiovasc Surg 78:259–268, 1979.
187. Garson A, McNamara DG, Cooley DA: Tetralogy of Fallot. In Roberts WC (ed): "Adult Congenital Heart Disease." Philadelphia: F.A. Davis, 1987, p 493.
188. Garson A: Sudden death in a pediatric cardiology population 1958–1983. In Morganroth J, Horowitz LN (eds): "Sudden Cardiac Death." Orlando, FL: Grune and Stratton, 1985, p 47.
189. Garson A, Porter CBJ, McNamara DG: Induction of ventricular tachycardia during electrophysiologic study after repaired tetralogy of Fallot. J Am Coll Cardiol 1:1493–1502. 1983.
190. Horowitz LN, Vetter VL, Harken AH, Josephson ME: Electrophysiologic characteristics of sustained ventricular tachycardia occurring after repair of tetralogy of Fallot. Am J Cardiol 46:446–452, 1980.
191. Sullivan ID, Presbitero P, Gooch VM, Aruta E, Deanfield JE: Is ventricular arrhythmia in repaired tetralogy of Fallot an effect of operation or a consequence of the course of the disease? Br Heart J 58:40–44, 1987.
192. Fellows CL, Bardy GH, Ivey TD, Werner JA, Draheim JJ, Green HL: Ventricular dysrhythmias associated with congential left ventricular aneurysms. Am J Cardiol 57: 997–999, 1986.
193. Fellows CL, Weaver WD, Greene HL: Cardiac arrest associated with coronary artery spasm. Am J Cardiol 60:1397–1399, 1987.
194. Garson A, Gillette PC, Titus JL, et al.: Surgical treatment of ventricular tachycardia in infants. N Engl J Med 310:1443–1445, 1984.
195. Kearney DL, Titus JL, Hawkins EP, Ott DA, Garson A: Pathologic features of myocardial hamartomas causing childhood tachyarrhythmias. Circulation 75:705–771, 1987.

196. Garson A, Smith RT, Moak JP, Kearney DL, Hawkins EP, Titus JL, Cooley DA, Ott DA: Incessant ventricular tachycardia in infants. Myocardial hamartomas and surgical care. J Am Coll Cardiol 10:619–626, 1987.
197. Engle MA, Ebert PA, Redo SF: Recurrent ventricular tachycardia due to resectable cardiac tumor. Circulation 50:1052–1057, 1974.
198. Sirinelli A, LeGuludec D, Laine JF, Sebag C, Gourguignon M, Slama M, Davy JM, Motte G: Ventricular tachycardia revealing a hydatid cyst. Am Heart J 114:656–659, 1987.
199. Selle JG, Svenson RH, Sealy WC, et al.: Successful clinical laser ablation of ventricular tachycardia: A promising new therapeutic method. Ann Thorac Surg 42:380–389, 1986.
200. Svenson RH, Gallagher JJ, Selle JG, et al.: Neodymium: YAG laser photocoagulation: a successful new map-guided technique for the interoperative ablation of ventricular tachycardia. Circulation 76:1319–1327, 1987.
201. Epstein SE, Quyyumi AA, Bonow R: Sudden cardiac death without warning: Possible mechanisms and implications for screening asymptomatic populations. N Engl J Med 321:320–324, 1989.

Chapter 11

Life Style: Its Effect and Modification for the Prevention of Sudden Cardiac Death

Robert Allan, Ph.D., and Stephen Scheidt, M.D.

Division of Cardiology, The New York Hospital—Cornell Medical Center, New York, New York 10021

> On October the 16th, 1793, [John Hunter] . . . went to St. George's Hospital [London] and, meeting with some things which irritated his mind, and not being perfectly the master of the circumstances . . . withheld his sentiments, in which state of restraint he went into the next room, and turning around . . . gave a deep groan, and dropt down dead.
>
> It is a curious circumstance that, the first attack of these complaints was produced by an affection of the mind, and every future return of any consequence arose from the same cause . . . and as his mind was irritated by trifles, these produced the most violent effects on the disease. His coachman being beyond his time, or a servant not attending to his directions, brought on the spasms, while a real misfortune produced no effect [1].

Prior to his dramatic sudden cardiac death (SCD), Hunter had been quoted as stating that his life was "in the hands of any rascal who chooses to annoy or tease me" [2]. Hunter's first biographer, Everard Home, was his

The Prevention of Sudden Cardiac Death, pages 261–294

brother-in-law and disciple. Home also performed Hunter's autopsy and observed: "the symptoms of . . . Hunter's complaint, for the last twenty years of his life, may be considered as those of angina-pectoris, and form one of the most complete histories of that disease on record" [1]. John Hunter was an eminent scientist and surgeon, a fellow of both the Royal Society of Science and the Royal Society of Medicine, a person who achieved considerable fame and glory in his day. Yet, despite Hunter's worldly success, his personality might be characterized as a bit heartless. Home observed, "his temper was very warm and impatient, readily provoked, and when irritated, not easily soothed. His disposition was candid, and free from reserve, even to a fault . . . in conversation he spoke too freely, and sometimes harshly of his contemporaries . . ." [1].

Despite this anecdote, with its suggestion of causality, the relationship between lifestyle and SCD is controversial. In recent years, however, data from a number of divergent approaches to this question appear to strengthen the link between how we live and our ultimate destiny. This chapter examines several areas that bear on possible relationships between life style and sudden cardiac death.

1. Since most cases of SCD are thought to be precipitated by cardiac arrhythmia, we will touch on studies linking behavior or stress to arrhythmia. There is little or no information on behavioral links to atrial arrhythmia or conduction defects and little information on bradyarrhythmia and behavior in general; for the most part, we will discuss preliminary information attempting to link behavior or stress to ventricular arrhythmia, almost certainly the final precipitant of most cases of SCD.

2. SCD, although triggered by a cardiac arrhythmia, most often occurs in a setting of acute or chronic cardiac disease. Although there are many different types of cardiac pathology that predispose to SCD, notably, dilated cardiomyopathy and congestive heart failure of any etiology, the most common anatomic substrate for ventricular arrhythmia and SCD is atherosclerotic coronary artery disease. Acute myocardial ischemia, sometimes but not always the early stages of acute myocardial infarction (MI), often plays an important role. Determinants of myocardial ischemia have recently come under intense scrutiny with the realization that much ischemia is not perceived by the patient as angina or MI but instead is silent, yet this so-called silent ischemia can now be diagnosed with various modalities, including ambulatory electrocardiogram (ECG) (Holter) monitoring. The ability to monitor continuously for ischemia during everyday activities has introduced a whole new dimension into the search for precipitants of myocardial ischemia, and we discuss new work clearly implicating mental stress as one such precipitant of ischemia, often of the silent variety. This may have major ramifications for causality of SCD.

3. A certain amount of work exists that attempts to link behavioral or

stress factors with SCD without reference to biologic mechanisms. Two areas in particular will be summarized: the literature on acute behavioral precipitants for SCD, and the evidence that social support (or the lack thereof) is a major factor in morbidity and mortality from many causes, including heart disease and SCD.

4. Since SCD so often occurs in the setting of coronary artery disease, we will summarize the current status of research linking behavior or stress to atherosclerosis. By far the most information concerns type A behavior (TAB) and its possible relation to the initial development or recurrence of coronary heart disease (CHD). Aside from the status of TAB as a risk factor for CHD, many other "standard" risk factors for atherosclerosis are powerfully influenced by behavioral factors, and this may be the most important link of all between behavior and SCD.

BEHAVIORAL FACTORS AND CARDIAC ARRHYTHMIA

> . . . My father told me of a careful observer, who certainly had heart disease and died from it, and who positively stated that his pulse was habitually irregular to an extreme degree yet to his great disappointment it invariably became regular as soon as my father entered the room.
>
> —Charles Darwin (1872) [3]

Most research relating behavioral factors to arrhythmia has concentrated on ventricular arrhythmia, since it is widely believed that SCD is most often caused by ventricular tachycardia (VT) leading to ventricular fibrillation (VF). In 1976, Lown et al. [4] described a 39-year-old man with CHD who had ventricular premature contractions (VPCs) that were provoked by psychological stress and could be reduced by meditation. β-adrenergic blockade was successful at controlling VPCs, implicating the sympathetic nervous system in arrhythmogenesis. Wellens et al. [5] described a young woman in whom ventricular tachycardia or fibrillation could be regularly precipitated by the ringing of an alarm clock.

Lown [6] reported interesting experiments in patients with ventricular ectopic activity who were subjected to psychological stress testing. In one series, 19 patients were stressed in three ways: mental arithmetic under time pressure; Stroop color cards (which promote confusion by asking the subject to read the name of a color from a card of a different color); and an emotionally charged interview, which included discussion of current illness, job-related stress, marital problems, and fear of death [6]. In 11 of the 19 patients, VPCs increased by a factor of two or more, with the frequent appearance of couplets and paroxysms of ventricular tachycardia.

TABLE 11–1. Theoretical Formulation of Relationship Between Behavioral Factors and Cardiac Arrhythmia

Anatomic/physiologic substrate
Myocardial electrical instability
often ischemic heart disease
sometimes acute ischemia/MI
reeentry pathways
cardiomyopathy/CHF
Psychologic state
often long-lasting
frequently depression, hopelessness
"Trigger"
often psychologic, mental stress, "higher nervous activity"

A 1981 report [7] described a "higher nervous activity" task force created by the Lown group, consisting of psychiatrists, psychologists, and members of a cardiovascular team. Of 117 patients with life-threatening ventricular arrhythmia followed closely by the task force, 25 (21%) had psychological precipitants, 15 (25%) within 1 hour of the arrhythmia onset. Triggers included interpersonal conflicts, public humiliation, threat of marital separation, bereavement, business failure, loss of job, and nightmares. Personality testing, however, was unable to discriminate "trigger" patients from others in the study [6]. According to Lown, three sets of conditions contribute to the occurrence of ventricular arrhythmias.

1. Myocardial electrical instability, most often resulting from ischemic heart disease
2. An acute triggering event, often related to mental stress or "higher nervous activity"
3. A chronic, pervasive, and intense psychological state (often including depression and hopelessness)

The proposed interaction of these variables is shown in Table 11–1.

There seems little doubt that "triggering" of ventricular arrhythmia, when this phenomenon occurs, is related to autonomic imbalance, either increased sympathetic or decreased parasympathetic tone. In a series of animal experiments, Verrier [8] showed the following.

1. Psychologic stress (aversive conditioning with mild electric shocks while an animal is confined in a sling) or anger substantially reduces the threshold to repetitive ventricular extrasystoles.
2. Psychologic stress increases the incidence of spontaneous VF after experimental coronary artery occlusion and reperfusion.

3. β-Adrenergic blockade diminishes or blocks the adverse effects of psychologic stress in the above situations, suggesting that sympathetic overactivity is causal.

4. Vagal blockade substantially increases the adverse effects of psychologic stress, suggesting that parasympathetic underactivity also plays a role.

The role of the autonomic nervous system in modulating ventricular arrhythmia and SCD is further highlighted by recent studies of autonomic tone after MI. In animal work done with several hundred animals over a 7 year period, Schwartz and coworkers in Oklahoma City and Milan, Italy, have assessed parasympathetic function by studying baroreflex sensitivity (BRS) [9]. Reduced BRS (less slowing in heart rate for a given rise in arterial blood pressure), an indication of diminished vagal tone, was an important predictor of SCD in dogs after experimental MI. In addition, MI itself substantially reduced BRS in most dogs (approximately three-fourths of the group); the animals with the most severely depressed BRS were at greatest risk for SCD. Most intruigingly, by studying animals before and after experimental MI, a group was identified that had lower BRS *even before the infarct,* and this group had the greatest risk after MI for SCD. This raises the possibility of *identifying in advance* a group at special risk for SCD (those with less vagal tone at the outset).

Immediate clinical confirmation of the importance of these animal findings came from La Rovere and coworkers [10], who found that BRS was lower among patients who had inferior MI, triple-vessel disease, VT, and reduced exercise tolerance, and, over a 24 month follow-up period, markedly reduced BRS was strongly associated with mortality. These data are entirely consistent with reports from the Multicenter Post-Infarction Research Group [11] demonstrating that reduced vagal tone as measured by another index, decreased heart rate variability on 24-hour Holter monitoring, was a powerful predictor of increased mortality including SCD in 808 patients over 31 months after MI. Table 11–2 lists possible physiologic mechanisms linking behavioral factors to cardiac arrhythmia.

Aside from acute behavioral stimuli, so-called "triggers" that appear related to sympathetic/parasympathetic imbalance, there have also been suggestions that a more chronic psychologic state of some sort might influence the propensity to arrhythmia or SCD. Table 11–3 lists several studies [12–15] that have examined this issue.

Engel [12] categorized the "life settings" of 170 sudden deaths reported in newspapers over a 6 year period (mostly in the Rochester, New York, area). Although the methodology is questionable, it is nonetheless interesting to note that Engel found only a limited number of themes: death of a loved one; grief; mourning; loss of a close person, status, or esteem; personal danger or relief from such danger; reunion; triumph; or happy

TABLE 11–2. Possible Physiologic Mechanisms Linking Behavioral Factors to Cardiac Arrhythmia

Increased sympathetic stimulation
Cardiac sympathetic nerves
Left stellate ganglion stimulation
Circulating catecholamines
Indirect effects of sympathetic stimulation
β_1-Epinephrine-mediated hypokalemia
Prolonged QT interval
Increased ischemia (increased HR, BP, contractility)
Increased platelet aggregability
Thrombosis
Coronary spasm
Decreased parasympathetic stimulation
??Increased parasympathetic stimulation for bradyarrhythmia or tachyarrhythmia
Decreased brain serotonin
Other

TABLE 11–3. Chronic Psychologic State and Sudden Death

Engel (Rochester NY), newspaper reports of SCD: many ''overwhelming excitation'' and/or ''giving up'' [12]
Greene et al., 26 spouse interviews: many depressed [13]
Rahe et al., Helsinki, Recent Life Change Questionnaire: marked elevations in RLC scores within 6 months before SCD [14]
Follick et al., transtelephonic monitoring post-MI: significant relationship between VPCs and distress scores [15]
Loss of spouse: major increase in short term mortality in many studies [34–36,38]

ending. Common to all such ''life settings'' is ''overwhelming excitation or giving up or both.'' A number of Engel's categories have received more systematic scrutiny, and some have achieved a degree of scientific validity in recent years.

Greene et al. [13] subsequently interviewed the spouses of 26 sudden death victims in an early effort to make some sense of behavioral parameters in SCD. Curiously, many spouses (all wives) were furious at the deceased, who was described as foolish for not having consulted a physician earlier. Prodromal symptoms were clearly evident to the wives in nearly every case. Furthermore, most of the wives characterized their husbands as depressed. The authors suggested a hypothesis that SCD may occur in a basically depressed man at high risk for CHD who succumbs to an overwhelming level of arousal. Despite its lack of statistical validation, this work is congruent with the current concepts of ''cardiac denial'' and the arousal-seeking inherent in compulsive, hard-driven TAB.

In an early attempt to bring empirical data into this area of study, Rahe et al. [14] introduced the Recent Life Change (RLC) questionnaire. The RLC has come to be a nearly ubiquitous measure in the popular literature on stress. It seeks to classify the *intensity* of life changes. Events such as the death of a spouse, marriage, divorce, and loss of a job are given high scores, whereas life changes such as working hours, trouble with in-laws, and vacation receive low scores. The RLC was administered to 279 survivors of documented MI and to the spouses of 226 cases of SCD in Helsinki, Finland. Marked elevations in RLC scores were seen for most cases of MI or SCD during the 6 months prior to the event. The data were particularly impressive for SCD.

Follick et al. [15] conducted a prospective examination of 125 post-MI patients equipped with a transtelephonic ECG monitor. Patients were followed over a 1 year period after being administered the SCL-90, a questionnaire thought to measure psychological distress. A significant relationship was found between VPCs and distress scores after controlling for cardiac risk, age, and use of beta-blocking drugs.

A few investigators have attempted to identify an ''arrhythmogenic personality'' or behavior patterns that might identify those at high risk. Using Swedish men, Orth-Gomer et al. [16] reported a relationship between the Emotions Profile Index (a self-administered questionnaire) and ventricular arrhythmias in healthy men, but not in men with documented ischemic heart disease or those with a risk factor profile for ischemia. Katz et al. [17] studied 102 patients with a history of arrhythmia. Patients with frequent VPCs (more than 30/hour) without MI were more psychologically symptomatic than age- and sex-matched medical-surgical patients with whom they were compared. Significant subscales for the arrhythmogenic patients were: high anxiety, less moral orientation, depression and alienation, and an inhibited and low respectful style. These variables were combined into a discriminant function that the authors claim accounted for 54% of the variance between the arrhythmia and control groups and could correctly predict group membership in 83% of the cases.

Regarding nonventricular arrhythmias, very little research has been done on relationships, if any, between behavioral factors and such arrhythmia. Little is known, for example, about any possible effect of behavioral factors or stress on atrioventricular conduction (e.g., influence on heart block), on the sinus node (e.g., influence on sick sinus syndrome and severe bradyarrhythmia), or on depolarization or repolarization (e.g., influence on the QT interval) in spite of the obvious influence of the nervous system on cardiac electrophysiologic events including but not limited to automaticity, irritability, and conduction.

Based on the few available studies, psychological stress appears to be a trigger for ventricular arrhythmias in some people. Animal research provides some support for a link between arrhythmia and life events. However, the foremost problem with human research on behavioral factors and arrhythmia is a lack of sensitivity and specificity. Most investigators have been unable to identify specific psychological traits that discriminate arrhythmia-prone patients from the cardiac population or the population at large [6,7,16]; currently, it appears that general psychological "distress" is the best available marker for those at risk. There is no uniformity in the types of stressors that have produced arrhythmia, and it seems likely that stressors in life vary widely in their ability to induce arrhythmia according to the behavioral make-up of the subject, the underlying extent of cardiac disease, and other poorly understood factors. Finally, although many reports in this area have demonstrated links between behavior or stress and arrhythmia, it is by no means clear that stress-induced arrhythmia always or even often has clinical consequences, whether SCD or other manifestations.

BEHAVIORAL FACTORS AND MYOCARDIAL ISCHEMIA

Behavioral factors or stress might be linked to SCD not through precipitation of arrhythmia but instead through behavior- or stress-linked induction or exacerbation of myocardial ischemia. In general terms, myocardial ischemia occurs whenever myocardial oxygen demand exceeds available supply. The long-term, chronic problem is usually the slow and insidiously progressive atherosclerotic narrowing of coronary arteries. Whether stress, behavior, or both are related to long-term risk of development of CHD is still debated; particularly heated is the controversy over the TAB pattern as a possible major risk factor either for the initial development of CHD or for recurrent events after CHD's initial manifestation (see below).

Regarding the acute event that causes immediate clinical consequences in the setting of chronic coronary artery narrowings, possibilities include increases of myocardial oxygen demand or decreases in myocardial oxygen supply. The most common cause of transient increased myocardial oxygen demands is physical exercise, and many ischemic episodes are classically triggered by exertion. However, stress can also raise myocardial oxygen needs. The three major determinants of myocardial oxygen needs, heart rate, blood pressure, and contractility, all increase with stimulation of the sympathetic nervous system, an almost universal response of the body to internal or external stress. What is less certain but increasingly likely is that myocardial oxygen supply might also be affected by internal or external stress. α-Adrenergic coronary artery vasoconstriction has recently been demonstrated to occur after a number of stressors, particularly in atherosclerotic coronary artery segments [18].

Research on stress and myocardial ischemia has recently become much more interesting since the discovery that ischemia need not always be perceived as angina but is often silent to the patient (so-called silent ischemia). The first study on stress and silent ischemia was reported only in 1984. Deanfield et al. [19] studied a series of patients with CHD and chronic stable angina using positron emission tomography. Patients were subjected to a mental arithmetic test that was not intended to frustrate or upset them and were compared with normal, non-CHD controls. There was an association between mental activity and myocardial ischemia in 12 of the 16 (75%) patients studied. Most instances of ischemia were not accompanied by angina or electrocardiographic changes. It is of note that these results were produced with mental arithmetic, a relatively mild stressor.

A similar link between silent ischemia and mental arousal was reported by Rebecca et al. [20], who followed 21 patients with chronic stable angina for 891 hours of Holter monitoring in order to measure episodes of ST depression. Most ischemic episodes were silent (87%), and 75% of these occurred in association with tasks demanding routine mental work (conversation, routine office work, reading, watching television). Transient ischemia was more commonly associated with activities demanding mental arousal than with exertion.

Freeman et al. [21] studied 30 consecutive patients awaiting the results of coronary angiography. Ambulatory ST segment Holter monitoring was performed for two 48 hour periods: the first 6 days after outpatient coronary arteriography, which included the time just prior to the results (and the possible need for coronary bypass surgery) being discussed with the patient, and the second monitoring period, an average of 66 days later, after the patient had had time to adjust to the treatment plan. Anticipation of results from the angiogram was expected to serve as a naturally occurring life stressor of considerable magnitude.

Psychological stress was assessed by measurement of urinary cortisol and catecholamine (noradrenalin) levels during the first 24 hours of each monitoring period and completion of the General Health Questionnaire (GHQ) and a diary in which patients recorded episodes of chest pain and feelings of emotional upset. There were 515 episodes of myocardial ischemia, 174 associated with pain and 341 asymptomatic. Silent ischemia was significantly more frequent and of greater duration during the first monitoring than the second and was associated with higher urinary cortisol and catecholamine excretion, higher scores on the GHQ, and more reports of emotional upset in the diaries.

Some of the most impressive findings linking emotional stress with silent ischemia were recently reported by Rozanski et al. [22]. The authors subjected CHD patients and controls to a series of mental and physical tasks: arithmetic, reading, Stroop color word test, and "simulated public speaking," during which subjects gave a 5 minute talk to two observers about their personal faults and undesirable habits. Quite dramatically, the magnitude of ischemic cardiac dysfunction (measured by radionuclide ventriculography) induced by the simulated public speaking was similar to that observed during bicycle exercise. Of the patients with CHD, 59% had wall motion abnormalities during periods of mental stress, and 36% had a fall in left ventricular ejection fraction (LVEF) of more than 5%. Mentally induced ischemia was silent in 83% of the patients with wall motion abnormalities and occurred at lower heart rates than did exercise-induced ischemia. These results suggest a causal association between mental stress and myocardial ischemia, which is often silent, in CHD patients. Rozanski et al. conclude that, since mental stress occurs more frequently than stress from exercise in daily life, it could represent an important factor in the precipitation of clinical coronary events.

Finally, the role of silent ischemia in SCD has recently received some scrutiny. Scheidt [23] reviewed 65 SCD patients who died while 24 hour ambulatory monitoring was in progress. Although prior authors have concentrated on premonitory arrhythmias occurring shortly before the final event, usually VF, at least 20% of patients demonstrated prior ischemia, often silent (Table 11–4). The actual number of patients with ischemia just prior to death is almost certainly higher, since many authors either did not search for ischemia or did not report their ECG findings in sufficient detail for reliable assessment of silent ischemia occurring just prior to monitored SCD.

The psychological implications of silent ischemia are considerable. Most salient is that the individual is deprived of conscious awareness about the organism's vulnerability. Since most ischemia is silent for those patients manifesting this condition, cognitive information other than the angina pectoris must come to serve as a monitor for emotional and physical limitations. This represents a dangerous situation for individuals who have some impairment in their ability to assess their physical and emotional capacity. Persons who make extensive use of denial and those exhibiting extreme levels of compulsive, hard-driven TAB might be a particularly vulnerable subgroup. Such patients might even trigger their own demise unaware of their myocardial insufficiency.

Although the importance of such findings for SCD remains unclear, the following facts are striking.

1. Much myocardial ischemia is silent, to the patient as well as the physician, so that patient perception of chest pain is not a reliable measure of whether ischemia is occurring. Diagnostic tests such as 24 hour Holter monitoring are needed to assess ischemia occurring during activities of daily living.
2. Many mental tasks that hardly seem objectively stressful can indeed cause considerable ischemia in those with preexisting coronary artery disease, in some cases producing ischemia of magnitude similar to that caused by vigorous physical exercise.
3. The role of ischemia, especially silent ischemia, just prior to SCD may be substantial, and many cases of SCD might have as a precipitating factor some sort of heretofore unappreciated mental stress.

Thus our current perception that many cases of SCD occur without

TABLE 11–4. Prodromal Findings in Sudden Death During 24 Hour Ambulatory ECG Monitoring[a]

Author[a]	Patients	ST changes before arrest	Ventricular arrhythmia before arrest: VPBs/VT	Ventricular arrhythmia before arrest: R on T	Activity before arrest, comments
Bleifer	1	1 ST ↑		1	1
Hinkle	1	1 ST ↓	1	1	Sitting after exercise
Gradman	1	1 ST ↑	1	1	Exciting TV
Pool	2	1 ST ↓	2		Washing car
Lahiri	3	None	3	3	
Bissett	1	None	1	1	"Limited activity"
Denes	5	None	5	2	All on quinidine, with long QT
Salerno	1	1 ST ↓ then ↑	—	—	
Nikolic	6	1 T ↓ , 1ST-T ↓	5	3	Bed 2, sitting 1, walking 1, 1 poss. dig/ quinidine toxicity
Pratt	15	1 More ST ↑	13	2	All VF
Panidis	15	3 ST ↑	—	—	14 In-patients 3 CHB, 2 AIVR
Lewis	12	1 ST ↑	11	9	7 Long QT, 8 past syncope
Milner	13	?	10	2	13 In-patients, all prior arrest or syncope

[a]Adapted from Scheidt [23], with permission of the publisher. See Scheidt [23] for references. Abbreviations: VPB, ventricular premature beats; VT, ventricular tachycardia; VF, ventricular fibrillation; R on T, R on T VPBs; CHB, complete heart block; long QT, prolonged QT interval; AIVR, accelerated idioventricular rhythm; ST ↑ , ST segment elevation; ST ↓ , ST segment depression; T ↓ , T wave inversion; ST-T ↓ , ST segment depression and T wave inversion; dig, digitalis.

obvious precipitating factor may be very much in error. We cannot assess silent ischemia easily, nor do we know in many cases whether mental stress preceded the event.

ACUTE BEHAVIORAL PRECIPITANTS FOR SCD

Through the centuries there has been a fascination with the dramatic life events that seem to "trigger" SCD. In his classic paper, "'Voodoo'

Death,'' Cannon [24] identifies Soares de Souza (1587) as the first to report instances of death apparently induced by fright among South American Indians who were condemned and sentenced by a so-called ''medicine man.'' Similar observations have been reported by anthropologists living with primitive people in Africa, Australia, the islands of the Pacific, and Haiti. One instance of death apparently brought on by superstitious fear was reported by Merolla on a voyage to the Congo in 1682 and is cited by Cannon [24].

> A young negro on a journey lodged in a friend's house for the night. The friend had prepared for their breakfast a wild hen, a food strictly banned by a rule which must be inviolably observed by the immature. The young fellow demanded whether it was indeed a wild hen and when the host answered ''No,'' he ate of it heartily and proceeded on his way. A few years later, when the two met again, the old friend asked the younger man if he would eat a wild hen. He answered that he had been solemnly charged by a wizard not to eat that food. Thereupon the host began to laugh and asked him why he refused to eat it now after having eaten it at his table before. On hearing this news the negro immediately began to tremble, so greatly was he possessed by fear, and in less than twenty-four hours was dead.

Although folklore is replete with stories such as that of John Hunter, ''voodoo death,'' and the like, it was not until 1971 that investigators began to study behavioral antecedents that might be precipitants for SCD. In an attempt to link stressful events with SCD, Myers and Dewar [25] studied 100 sudden deaths in London and interviewed surviving relatives with a standardized questionnaire. Twenty-three of the sudden death victims were reported to have experienced a significant psychological stress within 30 minutes before death and another 40 within 24 hours. Examples of stressors in this sample include attacks by dogs, visits for outpatient surgery, rows over games, being informed of the finality of divorce, competing in an automobile race for the first time, and an upcoming job interview when the victim had been out of work for some months. However, as Myers and Dewar point out themselves, ''relatives are suggestible and keen to find stress factors to account for disasters as dramatic as sudden death and myocardial infarction.''

In another study from Helsinki, Rissanen et al. [26] looked at premonitory symptoms and stress factors preceding SCD. In this series of 118 patients, prodromes were often nonspecific, for example, fatigue or chest discomfort. The significance of both acute and long-standing stress was most apparent in deaths *without* a history of clinical heart disease when stress did not appear to play a role in premonitory symptoms. Information on stress was obtained from relatives and was gathered according to a uniform protocol. Of interest, 19% of patients had some acute stress preceding death. The authors report that *acute stress* was often associated with SCD and no detectable MI at autopsy. *Long-standing stress* was more frequently accompanied by a definite MI verified at autopsy.

More recently, Brodsky and associates [27] studied 80 consecutive patients who were referred for evaluation of cardiac arrest or syncope due to documented VF or VT. Nine had no evidence of structural cardiovascular disease, and six of these patients were studied extensively. (Two were excluded because they refused cardiac catheterization, and the other had possible antiarrhythmic drug exacerbation of benign arrhythmia). None had risk factors for CHD. In five of these six carefully studied patients, psychological assessment indicated profound disturbances, including major depression, escape from the traumas of war, loss of a loved one, unwanted pregnancy, and a dysthymic disorder. The other patient did not manifest psychological disturbance.

Using data from the Recurrent Coronary Prevention Project (RCPP), Brackett and Powell [28] reviewed all deaths in this large-scale clinical trial for modifying the TAB pattern. After 4.5 years, there were 23 sudden deaths (within 1 hour) and 32 nonsudden deaths from among the 1,012 post-MI patients at entry. Independent multivariate predictors of SCD were anterior location of infarction (relative risk 3.1), socioeconomic status (relative risk 1.7) and type A score at entry (relative risk 1.5). Biological factors predominated in nonsudden death, and psychosocial variables were *not* found to be predictors for these cases. Brackett and Powell claim that their data demonstrate "a direct relation between stress and sudden cardiac death in a large prospective clinical study . . ." [28].

The alternate point of view, namely that SCD is a chance event and unrelated to psychological stress, has been advanced by Surawicz [29]. SCD is the rare exception even in life's most stressful conditions, such as soldiers marching into battle, parachute jumps, people on death row or in earthquakes and other panic situations affecting large groups. Hinkle [30] followed 700 individuals who may have had up to 30,000 episodes of ventricular arrhythmias over a 5–10 year period and found that death was the rare exception rather than the rule. McIntosh [31] supports a similar view, asserting that "practically nothing is known about why sudden cardiac death occurs in one but not another individual." Reviewing the data from Framingham, Kannel and Schatzkin [32] conclude that there are no specific risk factors for SCD that are independent of those for CHD.

SOCIAL SUPPORT

> Man's characteristic privilege is that the bond he accepts is not physical but moral; that is, social. He is governed . . . by a

> conscience superior to his own . . . because the greater, better part of his existence transcends the body . . . but is subject . . . to society.

These are the words of Emile Durkheim [33], the sociologist who at the turn of the century noted that *anomie,* individual deregulation with the breakdown of societal boundaries, was a factor in the increase in suicide rates. Social support, or the degree with which one is connected to others in the community, has recently emerged as a risk factor of considerable magnitude not only for CHD but for morbidity and mortality from all causes. Early work in this field was focused on widows and widowers [34,35], who had a higher death rate than the rest of the population. In a case control study, Cottington et al. [36] discovered that SCD in women was preceded by the loss of a significant other within 6 months with more than a sixfold increased frequency. (The interested reader is referred to Broadhead et al. [37] for a review of the early literature on social support.)

For many survivors of MI, the spouse is the major source of emotional support. Chandra et al. [38] studied the effects of marital status on in-hospital and long-term survival of 1,401 post-MI patients. The in-hospital fatality rate was 19.7% for married vs. 26.7% for unmarried men; for married vs. unmarried women, the rate was 23.2% vs. 37.4%. These patterns of improved survivorship in married patients were consistent for 10 years of follow-up.

Ruberman et al. [39] were the first to look at more global parameters of social connectedness as epidemiologic variables in a post-MI population. Interviews with 2,315 male survivors in the Beta-Blocker Heart Attack Trial showed that those with both high levels of social isolation and a high degree of life stress had a more than fourfold increased risk of death for 3 years following MI (Fig. 11–1). In addition, high levels of social isolation and stress were most prevalent among the least educated men and least prevalent among the best educated. The increased risk applied both to total deaths and to SCD.

In a recent analysis of five large-scale prospective studies on the impact of social relationships and health, House et al. [40] claim that social support is a risk factor of major significance. Reviewing data collected from more than 37,000 people in the United States and Europe, this analysis indicates that results rival the 1964 Surgeon General's report that first established cigarette smoking as a risk factor for moribidity and mortality from a wide range of diseases. House et al. also make an interesting point about the changing panorama of health and disease as the major cause of disability and death in industrialized countries: ''Theories of disease etiology have shifted from ones in which a single factor (usually a microbe) caused a single disease, to ones in which multiple behavioral and environmental as well as biologic and genetic factors combine, often over extended periods, to pro-

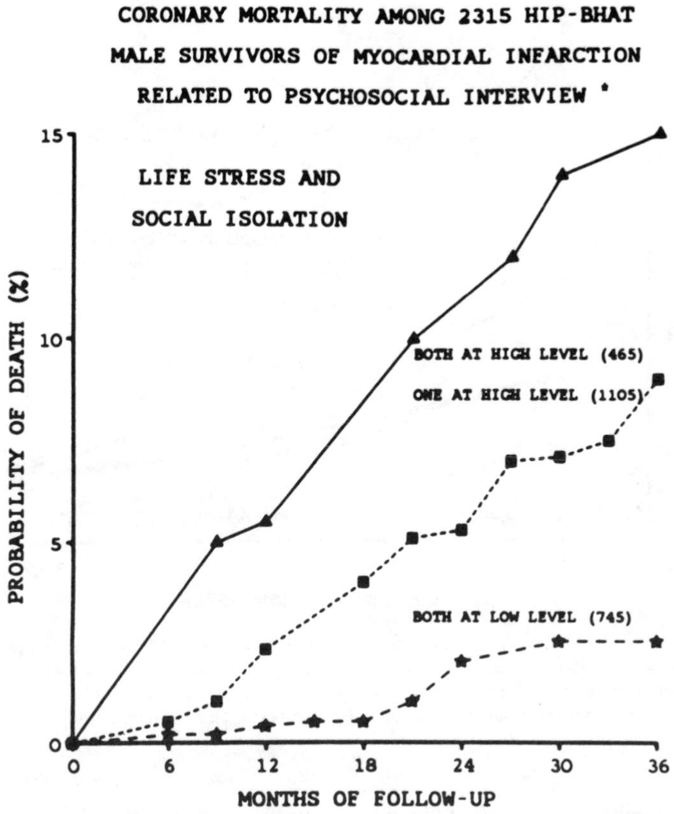

Fig. 11–1. Life table cumulative mortality according to life stress and social isolation in male survivors of myocardial infarction in the Health Insurance Plan subjects of the Beta-Blocker Heart Attack Trial. (Reproduced from Ruberman et al. [39] with permission of the publisher.)

duce any given disease, with a given factor often playing an etiologic role in multiple diseases.''

Figure 11–2 shows the relative risk ratios for mortality in the five studies reviewed by House et al. Categories of social ties are marriage, contacts with extended family and friends, church membership, and other formal and informal affiliations. The studies ranged from 8 to 13 years of follow-up and controlled for a wide range of factors. Increased risks for those with lower social support were significant for both men and women, with the relative risk ratios higher for males.

Studies on social support have tended to rely on questionnaires or ask brief interview questions about the nature and frequency of interpersonal contacts. Efforts are now underway to examine more closely the nature of social support in order to understand the underlying mechanisms that may

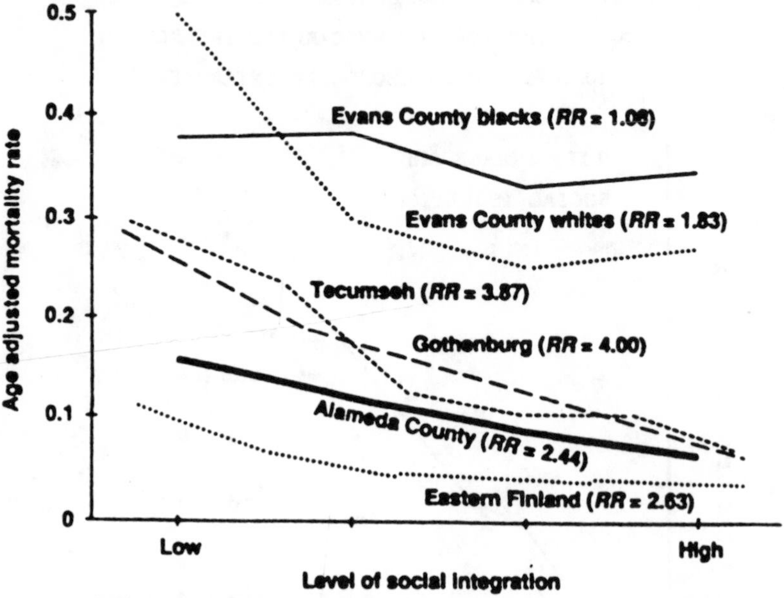

Fig. 11–2. Level of social integration and age-adjusted mortality for males in five prospective studies. RR is the relative risk ratio for mortality at the lowest vs. highest level of social integration. Evans County is in Georgia, Tecumseh is in Michigan, Alameda County is in California, Gothenburg is in Sweden. (Reproduced from House et al. [40] with permission of the publisher.)

promote health or disease. One recent study examined the differences between the structure and function of interpersonal relationships in patients undergoing coronary angiography [41]. The structural aspects of social support were defined as the number of relationships and the frequency of social contacts, and the functional aspects relate to the quality of the relationships. The results of this study indicate that it is the functional aspects of relationships and feelings of being loved that appear protective for atherosclerosis.

In an attempt to integrate the theory of TAB with social support, Blumenthal et al. [42] studied the interaction of these two effects on 113 patients undergoing coronary angiography. A Perceived Social Support Scale (PSSS) was developed for this investigation. For TAB persons in this study the extent of atherosclerosis was inversely related to level of perceived social support; that is, TAB persons with high levels of support had the least atherosclerosis. This relationship did not exist for type B persons. Blumenthal et al. argue that results are consistent with the hypothesis that social support moderates the long-term consequences of TAB.

Unfortunately, the literature on social support provides mainly an indication of large trends: mortality tends to be higher (and powerfully so) in those with less social support, but it has not yet been possible to focus on particular types of mortality (e.g., cardiovascular death or SCD), nor is there anything but speculation regarding the biologic mechanism by which this psychosocial variable might act to influence mortality or morbidity.

The major difficulty in the investigation of behavioral antecedants for SCD has been in gathering reliable, comparable, and valid psychologic data. Information has usually been obtained from relatives and others in close proximity to the victim. Methodology has varied widely. Studies were done in Finland, England, and different parts of the United States, raising the issue of whether questions about "stress" mean the same thing in each of these cultures. The field is also characterized by a lack of follow-up by the authors whose work has been the most encouraging. Rahe's Life Style Change Questionnaire appeared a promising instrument in his Helsinki study, yet there was no further research using this tool for studying SCD after his initial articles.

Research to date on acute behavioral precipitants provides provisional support for a link between acute stress and SCD *in some cases*. From the available data, it appears that the precipitant may occur in close temporal proximity to the event, although "subacute" stress (life changes several days or weeks beforehand) may also be important. There is, though, a lack of both sensitivity and specificity in identifying dangerous "target" behaviors or even thresholds of intensity for emotional or behavioral precipitants of SCD. No clear characterization of a prototypical SCD-inducing stressor has emerged. Just why some particular stress triggers SCD at some particular moment in time remains a mystery, and many patients with considerable anatomic or physiologic CHD tolerate similar stress or lifestyle changes without developing SCD.

TYPE A BEHAVIOR

The importance of the link between *psyche* and *soma* can be traced back to classical antiquity. In approximately 200 BC, Hippocrates was quoted in Plato's *Dialogues,* admonishing that "you ought not to attempt to cure the body without the soul . . . and this . . . is the reason why the cure of many diseases is unknown to the physicians of Hellas, because they disregard the whole. . . . Temperance is implanted in the soul, and where temperance comes and stays, there health is speadily imparted, not only to the head, but to the whole body" [43].

A similar sentiment about temperance was echoed in 1898 by Sir William Osler, father of internal medicine, when he observed that angina pectoris was the "Nemesis through which Nature exacts retributive justice for the transgression of her laws" [44]. Osler was perhaps the first to link life style directly with atherosclerosis: ". . . in the worry and strain of modern life, arterial degeneration is not only very common but develops at a relatively early age. For this I believe that the high pressure at which men live and the habit of working the machine to its maximum are responsible . . ." [44].

Systematic investigation of the heart and mind relationship began in the late 1950s with the pioneering work of Meyer Friedman and Ray Rosenman, two San Francisco cardiologists. In one of their early studies [45], occupational stress was linked to changes in serum cholesterol and blood clotting time, two presumed markers for susceptibility to MI. In this study of accountants, both serum cholesterol and blood clotting time were shown to rise with the pressures of the April 15 tax deadline.

The work of Friedman and Rosenman has spawned hundreds of studies, and a great deal of controversy, as scientists have argued the relative importance of *psyche* and *soma* for the development of CHD. Although little of the research on TAB has been targeted to SCD, this behavior pattern has been linked with both atherosclerosis and MI, two frequent "host" conditions for SCD. Thus TAB is important for the current inquiry into life style and SCD.

TAB is a complex clinical phenomenon. As with most manifestations of the human condition, there are tremendous variations and gradations in how TAB is expressed. Many of the subtleties and quirks of TAB are not easily predicted, nor are they readily understood by the scientist, who more typically is concerned with easily quantifiable, "hard" data. Nonetheless, the definition of the TAB pattern (TABP) is quite specific. As originally formulated by Friedman and Rosenman [46]:

> Type-A behavior pattern is an action-emotion complex that can be observed in any person who is *aggressively* involved in a *chronic, incessant* struggle to achieve more and more in less and less time, and if required to do so, against the opposing efforts of other things or other persons. It is not psychosis or a complex of worries or fears or phobias or obsessions, but a socially acceptable—indeed often praised—form of conflict. Persons possessing this pattern also are quite prone to exhibit a free-floating but extraordinarily well-rationalized hostility. As might be expected, there are degrees in the intensity of this behavior pattern. . . . For Type-A behavior pattern to explode into being, the *environmental challenge must always serve as the fuse for this explosion.*

Ten years later, Friedman and Ulmer [47] offered the psychodynamic formulation of TAB that is presented in Figure 11–3; a list of the common clinical attributes of TAB is given in Table 11–5. In the new model, insecurity and inadequate self-esteem form the nucleus of TAB. The "struggle to achieve more and more in less and less time," from the previous definition, is thought to be propelled by an *unconscious drive for self-esteem.* The individual becomes overly identified with personal achievements in a *sym-*

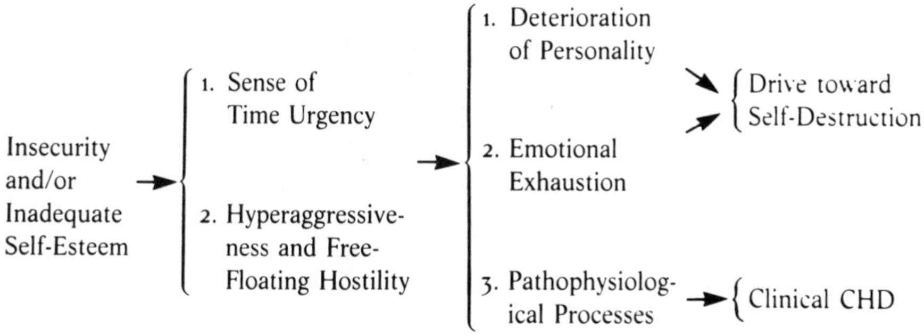

Fig. 11–3. Interrelationships between type-A behavior components and pathophysiologic processes. (Reproduced from Friedman and Ulmer [47] with permission of the publisher.)

bolic and *unattainable* search for self-worth. Typically, the *symptoms* of *time urgency* and *free-floating hostility* arise with any perceived interference with such self-defining achievements. Positive self-esteem and a sense of personal security, however, can never be attained solely by worldly accomplishment. Many, in fact, suggest that positive self-worth is related more with interpersonal connectedness and "feeling loved" than with worldly success. Thus achievement leaves the individual unfulfilled when it is motivated by an unconscious, symbolic quest for self-worth. Often, such frustration takes the form of a new round of pursuits that are "bigger and better." Ultimately, time urgency, hyperaggressiveness, and free-floating hostility become ubiquitous, with a deterioration of personality and emotional and often physical exhaustion. Over the course of several decades, it is thought that the pathophysiological processes accompanying the chronic "struggle" accelerate atherogenesis, leading to premature CHD.

The life of John Hunter, the eighteenth century surgeon, a description of whose SCD introduced this chapter, provides a fascinating illustration of the TAB paradigm. Hunter was born into a respectable Scottish family, the youngest of 10 children. He cared little for school in his childhood but displayed a very inquisitive mind about nature. At the end of his teens, John followed his older brother, Dr. William Hunter, to London, where he served very enthusiastically as an apprentice in his brother's anatomy laboratory. John had remarkable skills in dissection and anatomical preparation and quickly established himself as a lecturer in anatomy. Surgery, in the mid-eighteenth century, was a primitive affair, lacking in both anesthetics and

TABLE 11–5. Clinical Characteristics of Type A Behavior as Noted on the Videotaped Clinical Examination

Time pressure items	Hostility items
Content	
Spouse says slow down	Irritable waiting; restaurant, traffic bank
Walks, eats fast, no dawdle	
Polyphasic; bath, TV, conversation	Use of obscenity
Fetish of being on time	
Difficulty doing nothing	
Substitutes numerals for metaphors	
Behavior, motor	
Facial tautness expressing tension	Hostile facial set
Tense posture	Over-forceful gestures, i.e., clenched fist
Fast and jerky movements	
Motorization/gestures accompanying responses	Tic-like drawing back lips
Repetitive hand, arm, leg movements	
Tic-like eyebrow lifting	
Rapid eye blinking	
Expiratory sighing	
Tongue to teeth clicking	
Head nodding	
Behavior, speech	
Speech hurrying, head nodding when listening	Hostile, jarring laugh
Interrupts interviewer	Unpleasant voice; explosive, staccato, loud
Rapid speech/dysrhythmic, elision of final words	
Sucking in air during speech	
Behavior, hostile/competitive attitudes	
	Interviewer challenge; hostile response
	Angry generalizations (race, women, doctors)
	General distrust of others motives
	Competition with children
	Exhibits anger at past events
Physiological indicators	
Periorbital pigmentation	
Excessive forehead, upper lip perspiration	

antiseptics, and surgeons often had "practical," rather than medical, educations.

Although it is unusual to observe poor self-esteem directly (particularly at a distance of two centuries) there is good reason to believe that John Hunter suffered from this condition. Unlike his older brother, John had little formal education and never received a medical degree. In fact, John had an aversion to books from early childhood and, because he read so little, was often unaware of others' research on topics that he was studying. William sent his younger brother to Oxford in hope of improving his education, but John returned home after only a few weeks. Hunter practiced for more than 20 years without a proper license as a surgeon. At age 35 years, after serving in the army, he returned to a London that was deeply prejudiced against Scots. "John faced the problem of building up a private practice with few helpful connections. . . . He held no hospital appointment. He had no diploma" [48]. Everard Home, John's brother-in-law, disciple, and first biographer, described him as quite insecure about what others thought: "giving lectures was always particularly unpleasant . . . so that the desire of submitting his opinion to the world and learning their general estimation were scarcely sufficient to overcome his natural dislike to speaking in public" [1]. Before speaking in public, Hunter would often compose himself with a draught of laudanum (opium). In a similar reference to inadequate self-esteem, Home pointed out that Hunter's lectures were sometimes revised for 20 years before "giving them to press." In 1794, a less flattering biographer [49] criticized Hunter for lecturing at home, rather than at his hospital, because he "shut out everyone capable of comparing his dogmas to established doctrines." Perhaps the penultimate statement of insecurity is contained in Hunter's own words: "my life is in the hands of any rascal who chooses to annoy or tease me" [2].

Hunter was a driven man, and this, no doubt, contributed to his vast productivity. When driven by insecurity, however, productivity often takes on unreasonable proportions along with the TAB symptoms of time urgency and free-floating hostility. According to one early biographer [50], "Hunter was a great economist of time. . . . Any unnecessary discomposure of . . . engagements greatly annoyed him, and caused him to give vent to his feelings in no unmeasured terms." He demonstrated time urgency by "seldom sleeping more than four hours in the night" and by irritation when his coachman was "beyond his time" [1]. "Four hours of sleep . . . with an hour after dinner was all the time he devoted to the refreshment of his body. He had no home amusements . . . for the relaxation of his mind" [50].

Hunter's life style and pace were *hyperaggressive:* "He was generally to be found in his dissecting room before six in the morning and worked there until breakfast at nine. Then he saw patients at his house until twelve, after which he went out on his rounds. . . . He dined at four, slept an hour, and spent the evening working. At twelve the family retired to bed and the butler brought a fresh argand lamp, by the light of which Hunter continued his labors until one or two in the morning, or even later in winter. Of course, all this had the inevitable result: he broke down and had to go to Bath for a long convalescence. But the warning seems only to have made him work harder . . . and the pace grew faster'' [51].

Free-floating hostility, or the tendency to be easily angered, is perhaps the current theoretical hallmark of CHD-prone behavior. This is a quality that Hunter displayed in abundance. According to Home, ''his temper was very warm and impatient, readily provoked, and when irritated not easily soothed'' [1]. According to another biographer [51], this observation about Hunter's temper was ''confirmed by most of those who were intimately acquainted with him. An intrusion on his studies, even by one with whom he was on friendly terms, would call forth expressions of strong disgust and impatience: an object of which he was in want being misplaced would bring down all the vials of his wrath . . . and during these fits of passion he used to swear in the most outrageous manner. . . . ''

There are a number of curious incidents in the life of John Hunter that raise the issue of his *self-destructiveness,* another of the characteristics of TAB. Clearly, Hunter's hyperaggressive work habits negatively affected his health. This hard-driving manner extended to other spheres: ''By an exertion in dancing after the muscles of the leg were fatigued, he broke his tendo achillis'' [1]. Hunter collected a very wide assortment of animal species from all over the globe for his studies in comparative anatomy. ''The fiercer animals were those to which he was most partial. . . . Among these was a beautiful small bull he had received from the Queen, with which he used to wrestle and play, and entertain himself with its exertions in its own defense. In one of these contests the bull overpowered him, and got him down, and had not one of the servants accidentally come by and frightened the animal away, this frolic would probably have cost him his life'' [1].

By the time he had reached age 65 years, Hunter had become the foremost surgeon in London. His contributions to anatomy were prodigious and included the first explorations of the lymph system, and extending knowledge about the male reproductive system and the relationship between the mother and fetus during pregnancy, to name but a few. For the last 5 years of his life, Hunter's income was abundant. He had been appointed Surgeon-General to the Army, Inspector General of Hospitals and Surgeon-Extraordinary to George III, King of England. Hunter's large house was adorned with a multitude of exotic creatures and filled with more than 14,000 preparations, which were subsequently installed as the Hunterian Museum. Yet, things were not right in John Hunter's interpersonal dealings.

Many pupils were enrolled at St. George's Hospital because of Hunter's fame. Feeling that this situation was unjust and that his colleagues were not doing their fair share, John unilaterally declared that he would no longer share students' fees with his colleagues. A special court ruled against Hunter in this matter, and his colleagues subsequently rearranged hospital responsibilities such that Hunter's already overburdened schedule would become even more unmanageable. Around this same time, two young Scots without formal training applied to the hospital as pupils and appealed to Hunter's influence for their admission. Hunter took up the case of these men, who surely must have reminded him of his younger self, against ". . . a regulation, which, thirty years sooner would have excluded himself from the hospital . . ." [51]. These were the circumstances surrounding the Hospital Board meeting on October 16, 1793.

Early that morning, Hunter told a Baronet "that he was going to the hospital; that he was fearful some unpleasant recontre might ensue; and if such should be the case, he know it must be his death" [51]. The habitually punctual John Hunter arrived late and, after being contradicted by a colleague, withdrew to an adjoining room, where he expired.

It is noteworthy that a few years earlier, Hunter had been studying mechanisms of death. In 1792, he identified "death from . . . a violent affection of the mind . . . which . . . may be instantaneously produced." He declared, "every part of the body sympathizes with the mind, it must be referred to the universal influence which the mind has over the body" [52]. Referring to this passage, one of Hunter's contemporaries noted " . . . if he had not his own death in view, he has at least described its immediate cause . . . with a perspicuity which could not have been exceeded if he had attended the examination of his own corpse" [51]. Ironically, Hunter predicted his own death theoretically and then again on the very morning of its occurrence.

TAB may be understood as an inversion of *stress*. Generally, stress has been considered to arise from forces outside the individual, for instance the loss of a loved one or the demands of a difficult employer. With TAB, however, the individual *creates* stress, often in situations that can be characterized as trivial. With TAB, even the most neutral of events can be transformed into a stressful condition, particularly if the individual's goal (and hence self-esteem) is threatened. Perhaps the modern day analog to Hunter's "coachman" is automobile traffic and the "servant" a less than perfectly competent spouse or subordinate, two prototypical scenarios for the unleashing of time urgency and free-floating hostility.

TAB is also closely related to *cardiac denial,* a factor possibly important in SCD. Approximately 60% of out-of-hospital cardiac deaths occur within 2 hours of the onset of symptoms [53]. Dimsdale and Hackett [54] have defined denial as "the conscious or unconscious repudiation of all or a portion of the total available meaning of an illness in order to allay anxiety and to minimize emotional stress." There is reason to believe that the individual who makes extensive use of TAB will also tend to deny the importance of cardiac symptoms depriving himself or herself of timely medical care. Particularly with the recent emergence of thrombolysis, such individuals probably risk increased myocardial damage and possibly increase the risk of their own demise by not seeking prompt medical attention. It is important to note that an individual suffering from TAB is not a "bad" person. Rather, TAB symptoms arise because of insecurity and *as a result* of living a TAB life style.

Diagnosis of TAB

The diagnosis of TAB has been most successful with a videotaped, structured interview, now referred to as the videotaped clinical examination (VCE). Detailed instructions for the administration and scoring of the VCE are provided by Friedman and Powell [55]. Scores are obtained not only from the content responses to a series of questions but also from the manner in which the individual responds. Motorizations (unconscious movements), facial expressions, and bodily tensions are all scored manifestations of TAB. Currently, there are subscale scores for hostility and time pressure as well as a global score for TAB.

Several questionnaires have been developed for the diagnosis of TAB. The Jenkins Activity Survey (JAS) has been used most extensively but does not appear to reflect the hostility component. The Framingham Type A scale has been used successfully for the prediction of CHD, and the Bortner scale has been used extensively in Europe. The clinical examination and these questionnaires appear to measure different aspects of the TAB pattern; since many of the manifestations of TAB are beyond a subject's awareness, they are unlikely to be self-reported on a questionnaire.

Epidemiology of TAB

A number of studies that have attempted to relate TAB to CHD were reviewed by Matthews and Haynes in 1986 [56] and are summarized in Table 11–6. Briefly, the Western Collaborative Group Study (WCGS) was the first large-scale, prospective investigation of the relationship between TAB and CHD [57]. In this study, men classified as showing TAB had approximately twice the incidence of CHD of those showing type B behavior (type B behavior has generally been defined as the absence of TAB). Similar results were found for both men and women in the Framingham Heart Study.

On the other hand, several studies have failed to find a relationship between TAB and CHD in high-risk populations. The Multicenter Post-Infarction Research Program [58], the Aspirin Myocardial Infarction Study [59], and the Multiple Risk Factor Intervention Trial (MRFIT) [60] all found no relationship between TAB and CHD or CHD-related mortality.

In a follow-up to the WCGS, Ragland and Brand [61] showed that those who were diagnosed as showing TAB in 1960 and developed overt CHD had only 58% of the mortality of those diagnosed as showing type B behavior over the next 23 years. Rather than a risk factor for CHD, Ragland and Brand suggested that TAB may even be "protective" for subsequent cardiac mortality.

TABLE 11–6. Type A Behavior and Prediction of Coronary Heart Disease—Large-Scale Prospective Clinical Trials

	n	Types of subjects	Follow-up (years)	CHD incidence Type A	Type B	Risk ratio, A:B
"Primary" (no prior CHD)						
Framingham Study [56]	1,330	Subgroup at 8th or 9th biennial exam free of CHD, age 45–64 years	10			2.4 Men 2.0 Women
Western Collaborative Group Study (WCGS) [57]	3,154	Employed California men, age 35–59 years	8.5			2.24
MRFIT [60]	3,110	Subgroup of 12,866 men, age 35–57 years, in top 10–15% of CHD risk by blood pressure, smoking, serum cholesterol	7.1	4.9[a]	4.4[b]	0.99
"Secondary" (in those with diagnosed CHD)						
Case, Multicenter Postinfarct Group [58]	516	Subgroup of 866 patients within 2 weeks of acute MI	1–3	No difference in mean type A score of survivors vs. deaths		
Aspirin MI Study (AMIS) [59]	2,314	Subgroup of 2,698 patients given aspirin for prevention of recurrent CHD 30 days–5 years post-MI	3	No difference in mean type A score of those with and without coronary events		
Ragland and Brand WCGS [61]	231	231 of 257 subjects who developed angina, silent or symptomatic MI, and survived 24 hours	12	19/1,000 31.7 0.58 patient years		

[a] Type A1 behavior.
[b] Adjusted for age, blood pressure, smoking, serum cholesterol, alcohol consumption, education.

In 1987, a metaanalysis of 83 studies of TAB and CHD [62] concluded that 1) TAB does appear to be a risk factor for CHD, approximately doubling risk; 2) depression, anger, and hostility also appear related to CHD; 3) structured interview techniques are more effective for predicting disease endpoints than are questionnaires; 4) cross-sectional studies appear to be more powerful predictors than prospective studies; 5) the TAB effect has been smaller in studies published more recently than in those done in the early days of the TAB hypothesis. In a further refinement, Williams et al.

[63] noted that the TAB–CHD link was strongest in the youngest (under age 45 years) of a group of 2,289 patients undergoing coronary arteriography.

A recent trend in the research on TAB has been a search for its most toxic components. Williams [64] has coined the term "hostility complex" to describe a CHD-prone behavior pattern that includes easily aroused hostility and a cynical and pessimistic orientation to life. This variable has been assessed by the Cooke-Medley Hostility Scale of the Minnesota Multiphasic Personality Inventory (MMPI). The Cooke-Medley scale has predicted both CHD and mortality in a 25 year follow-up study of physicians [65], although a recent replication [66] failed to find similar results. Hostility too has been differentiated into a variety of components in a search for those aspects most predictive of disease endpoints. Speech stylistics [67], "neurotic" hostility [68], and anger-in (unexpressed) are some of the parameters that may help to sharpen the concept of CHD-prone behavior.

Ongoing studies in primates at Bowman-Gray University have provided experimental confirmation of the importance of behavior patterns and stress for atherosclerosis. In a series of studies recently reviewed by Clarkson et al. [69], cynomolgus monkey colonies were subjected to considerable stress by repeatedly reshuffling groups and thus breaking up a stable social structure of dominant and subordinate individuals. In some experiments, high-lipid diets were added to promote atherosclerosis; in others, the struggle was accentuated by adding a single sexually receptive female to the disorganized group. Dominant monkeys in unstable and stressful social situations developed strikingly increased coronary atherosclerosis as compared both to subordinates (who presumably did not struggle as hard to achieve dominance) and to dominant monkeys in stable (low external stress) groups. This tendency to increased atherosclerosis was prevented by beta-blockers.

The variable results of studies attempting to relate TAB to CHD may be due to a number of factors.

1. Different types of populations: "Primary prevention" (is TAB a risk factor in those without clinical CHD?) as assessed in the WCGS, MRFIT, and other studies vs. "secondary prevention" (is TAB a risk factor for *recurrent* CHD after an initial CHD manifestation, usually acute MI, has occurred?) (Multicenter Post-Infarct Program, AMIS, Ragland and Brand WCGS follow-up); TAB may be a risk factor for one group but not the other.

2. Difficulties in diagnostic methodologies: In particular, questionnaires seem less good than structured interviews in diagnosing the presumed "virulent core" of TAB, but this raises a new and highly troubling matter: interviews are highly prone to subjectivity, and claims that only certain interviewers trained by certain "experts" are capable of reliably diagnosing TAB have badly tarnished an objective assessment of the TAB hypothesis for many cardiologists.

3. Diagnostic tools may be better with general populations rather than

in those at high risk of CHD; within CHD or CHD-prone groups who may be more homogeneous than the overall population, our current diagnostic instruments for diagnosis of TAB may not be sufficiently sensitive.

4. Subsets of TAB characteristics may not be equally important; in particular, it may be that hostility is more, and time-pressured behavior less, important as a risk factor, and reliance on overall TAB scores that combine several types of psychosocial behavior may obscure relationships within one subset; for example, free-floating hostility may indeed be a powerful risk factor for development of CHD.

The current feeling, by no means universal among cardiologists, is that TAB probably is a risk factor for CHD, although the magnitude of the added risk is uncertain. There are, as yet, few data to suggest that risk for SCD can be in any way separated from risk for CHD (although in most studies in which TAB was a risk factor for total CHD it was also a risk factor for SCD).

BEHAVIORAL INFLUENCES ON OTHER RISK FACTORS FOR CHD

Regardless of one's views on TAB as a risk factor for CHD, there seems little question that behavioral factors play a major role in the prevalence and severity of the "standard" and well accepted risk factors for CHD in the population. Figure 11–4 presents our view of the risk factors for CHD described with respect to life style issues. "Coronary-prone" behavior is, at least theoretically, a matter of some choice and implies a potential benefit for living a "heart-healthy" life style. The traditional "big three" risk factors, cigarette smoking, elevated serum cholesterol, and hypertension, account for about one-half the variance for CHD, the United States' most prevalent disease [70,71]. Clearly, cigarette smoking and dietary intake of cholesterol-rich and high-saturated-fat or high-calorie foods are life choices. Some too consider hypertension to have a life style component. Thus each of the risk factors most strongly associated with CHD contains elements of behavior. Stress, social support, sedentary life style, obesity, and physical condition are all matters of how we live and represent one frontier of prevention in modern cardiology that may be expected to account for some of the missing variance in the etiology of atherosclerosis.

LIFE STYLE MODIFICATION

Awareness of risk factors for CHD is increasingly common in contemporary society. The American Heart Association estimates that, between 1964 and 1984, mortality from CHD declined 39%, an improvement thought to result to a considerable extent from risk factor modification by the general public [72]. A number of studies have systematically attempted to reduce risk factors and have reported subsequent impact on cardiac morbidity and mor-

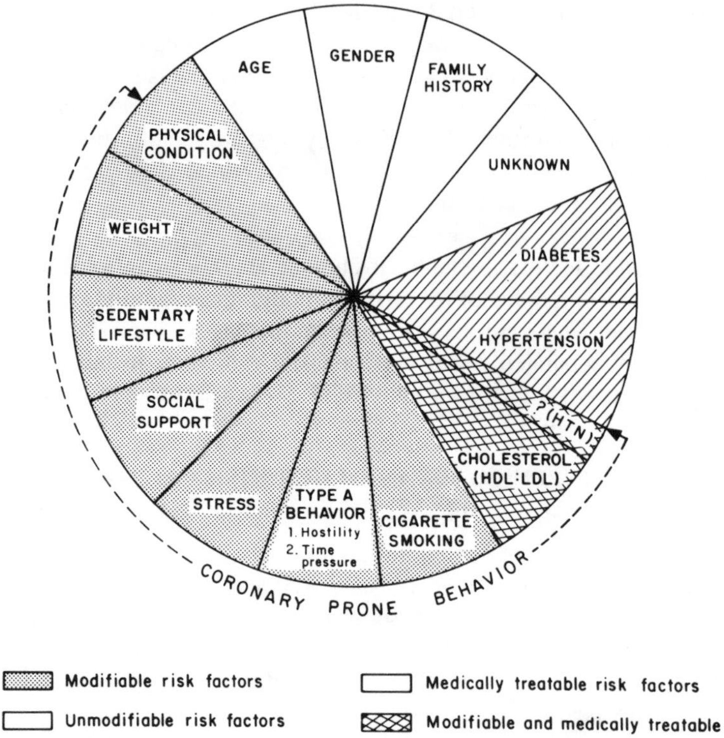

Fig. 11–4. Schematic representation of risk factors for coronary artery disease with emphasis on behavioral factors.

tality if any. Siegel et al. [73] have provided a discussion of some of the relevant theoretical issues and a summary of the limited number of clinical trials in this area. Behavioral strategies for risk factor modification have also been reviewed [74]. Some highlights from this budding research follow.

Clearly the largest life style modification study was the Multiple Risk Factor Intervention Trial (MRFIT) [60], which screened 361,662 men to form a cohort of 12,866 high-risk individuals between 35 and 57 years of age, who were assigned to special intervention (SI) programs or usual health care (UC) within the community. The SI programs consisted of counseling for cigarette smoking cessation, a stepped-care treatment for hypertension, and dietary advice for lowering blood cholesterol levels. In 1982, after an average follow-up of 7 years, risk factor levels declined in both groups, but only slightly more for SI men. Mortality was 7.1% lower for the SI group, but this difference was not statistically significant. One explanation offered by the MRFIT investigators for the disappointing results was the lower-than-expected mortality of the UC group. It may be that entry into the study itself—or perhaps even living in the risk-factor-conscious society of that time—was a significant motivator for the UC group to change their health habits. A higher-risk subgroup within the MRFIT cohort, those 12.5% of participants who had abnormal stress tests at entry, showed better results with special intervention. These high-risk participants showed a 57% reduction in CHD mortality ($P = .002$) for special intervention compared to usual care [75]. (For a review of other efforts at primary prevention of CHD, including results of interreaction directed at hypertension, cigarette smoking, and other major risk factors, see Fuchs and Scheidt [76].)

One major clinical trial has attempted to modify the TAB pattern in a post-MI population. The Recurrent Coronary Prevention Project (RCPP) [77] was a study of 1,012 post-MI patients, who were randomly assigned to groups that received counseling for CHD risk factors and those who received counseling for TAB along with CHD risk factor counseling. At the end of 4.5 years, the TAB-counseled group showed reductions in TAB as well as a significant reduction in recurrence rates for MI (12.9% vs. 21.2% for controls, $P = .005$) (Fig. 11–5). The control group was subsequently offered counseling for TAB and showed a similar reduction in recurrence rates over an additional year [78]. A further follow-up of RCPP participants [28] showed that TAB at study entry was a predictor of increased mortality for sudden, but not nonsudden, cardiac death.

Ornish et al. [79] introduced a radical life style change program that includes a vegetarian diet, stress management, exercise, and group support. In a randomized study of 23 patients and controls, subjects were treated in a secluded residential environment that was removed from usual life stressors. After 24 days, patients showed improved LVEF response to exercise, reduced frequency of angina and need for medication, lowering of blood cholesterol, and reductions in blood pressure. This work represents a very serious life style modification effort, requiring major departures from standard contemporary U.S. living. It also provides an opportunity to look into the potential benefits of life style modification at the extremes of human effort and may define the potential limits of this type of therapeutic intervention.

Atherosclerosis is a chronic, multifactorial disease. It makes little sense to diagnosis CHD and perform technologically advanced treatments such as angioplasty and coronary bypass surgery only to have patients resume an atherogenic life style. A central issue is the identification of thresholds of health and disease with the least restriction in freedom of choice. Is there a CHD-free life style that can be prescribed for the general public? Are there optimal levels of risk factors for the segment of the population already suffering from CHD? The coming decade will surely see answers to the question of the role of life style for the prevention of atherosclerosis and SCD.

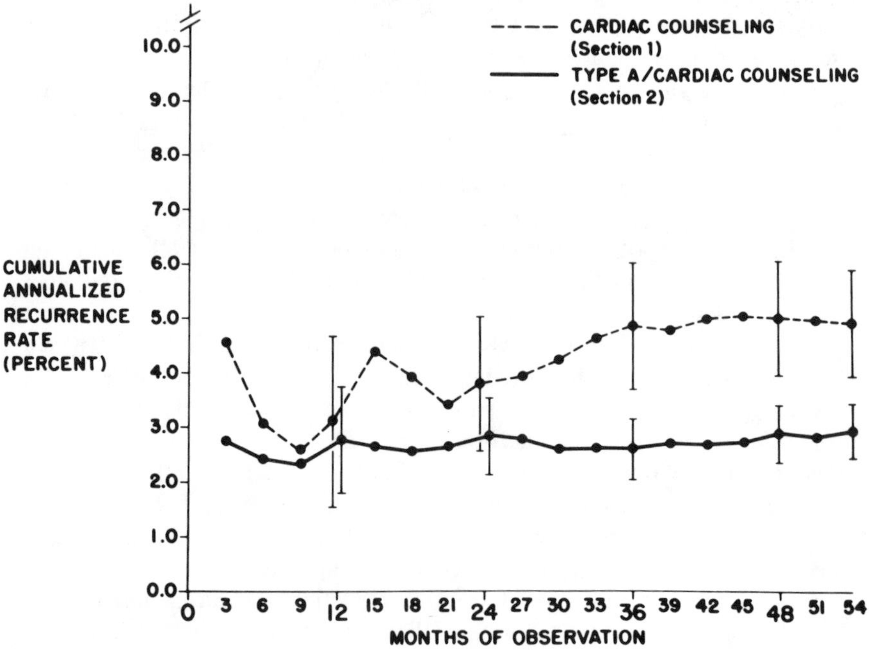

Fig. 11–5. Cumulative annualized recurrence rate of cardiac deaths and nonfatal myocardial infarction in the Recurrent Coronary Prevention Project for participants given type A behavior counselling and general cardiac risk factor counselling for 4–5 years vs. those given general counselling alone. Those given type A behavior counselling (section 2) have significantly lower recurrence rates at the end of 36 months. (Reproduced from Friedman et al. [77] with permission of the publisher.)

CONCLUSIONS

The association between behavioral, life style, or psychosocial factors and SCD is far from clear, yet there is increasing evidence from many lines of research that there are many potential links between heart and mind. Over the longer term, evidence as diverse as primate studies with social disorganization and prospective follow-up of TAB persons in several large clinical trials suggests that particular behavior patterns, perhaps interacting with certain types of external stressors, probably do constitute a substantial risk factor for increased atherosclerosis. Since SCD is most often associated with significant atherosclerosis, this alone would link behavioral and psychosocial factors to SCD.

Beyond that, though, there may be powerful influences of the mind on short-term or precipitating factors for SCD. There are numerous studies that demonstrate an influence of the central nervous system on the propensity for arrhythmia, particularly ventricular tachyarrhythmia, and either behavior pattern or internal or external stress may precipitate SCD by increasing vulnerability to or actually triggering arrhythmia. Behavioral influences on the parasympathetic portion of the autonomic nervous system are also possible and might be associated with tachyarrhythmias (from decreased parasympathetic tone) or bradyarrhythmias, heart block, or asystole (from excessive parasympathetic stimulation). It seems incontrovertible that mental stress can cause ischemia, at least in persons with coronary atherosclerosis, and, since many arrhythmias are far more dangerous, even lethal, in the presence of ischemia, the precipitation or exacerbation of myocardial ischemia is another mechanism by which behavior factors might be associated with SCD. For the moment, the associations regarding the elusive links between heart and mind are inferential and the mechanisms uncertain. The time is ripe for experimental treatment designs that are multifactorial and include a behavior component.

ACKNOWLEDGMENTS

This study was supported in part by the Nathaniel and Josephine Sokolski Foundation, the Horace W. Goldsmith Foundation, and the Terner Foundation.

REFERENCES

1. Hunter J: "A treatise on the Blood and Gun Shot Wounds With a Short Account of the Author's Life." London: John Richardson, 1794.
2. "Dictionary of National Biography." New York: Macmillan, 1908.
3. Darwin C: "Expressions of the Emotions in Man and Animals." Chicago: University of Chicago Press, 1965 (1872).
4. Lown B, Temte JV, Reich P, Gaughan C, Regestein Q, Hai H: Basis for recurring ventricular fibrillation in the absence of coronary heart disease and its management. N Engl J Med 294:623–629, 1976.
5. Wellens HJJ, Vermeulen A, Durrer D: Ventricular fibrillation occurring in arousal from sleep by auditory stimuli. Circulation 46:661–665, 1972.
6. Lown B: Sudden cardiac death: biobehavioral perspective. Circulation 76[Suppl I]:I-186–196, 1987.
7. Reich P, DeSilva RA, Lown B, Murowski BJ: Acute psychological disturbances preceding life-threatening ventricular arrhythmias. JAMA 246:233–235, 1981.
8. Verrier RL: Mechanisms of behaviorally induced arrhythmias. Circulation 76[Suppl I]: I-48–I-56, 1987.
9. Schwartz PJ, Vanoli E, Strama-Badiale M, deFerrari GM, Billman GE, Foreman RD: Autonomic mechanisms and sudden death. New insights from analysis of baroreceptor reflexes in conscious dogs with and without a myocardial infarction. Circulation 78: 969–979, 1988.
10. La Rovere MT, Specchia G, Mortara A, Schwartz PJ: Baroreflex sensitivity, clinical correlates and cardiovascular mortality among patients with a first myocardial infarction: A prospective study. Circulation 78:816–824, 1988.
11. Kleiger RE, Miller JP, Bigger JT, Moss AJ, the Multicenter Post-Infarction Research Group: Decreased heart rate variability and its association with increased mortality after acute myocardial infarction. Am J Cardiol 59:256–262, 1987.

12. Engel GL: Sudden and rapid death during psychological stress: Folklore or folkwisdom? Ann Intern Med 74:771–782, 1971.
13. Greene WA, Goldstein S, Moss AJ: Psychosocial aspects of sudden death. Arch Intern Med 129:725–731, 1972.
14. Rahe RH, Romo M, Bennet L, Siltanen P: Recent life changes, myocardial infarction, and abrupt coronary death. Arch Intern Med 133:221–228, 1974.
15. Follick MJ, Gorkin L, Capone RJ, et al.: Psychological distress as a predictor of ventricular arrhythmias in a post-myocardial infarction population. Am Heart J 116:32–36, 1988.
16. Orth-Gomer K, Edwards MR, Erhardt L, Sjogren A, Theorell T: Relation between ventricular arrhythmias and psychological profile. Acta Med Scand 207:31–36, 1980.
17. Katz C, Martin RD, Landa B, Chadda K: Relationship of psychologic factors to frequent symptomatic ventricular arrhythmia. Am J Med 78:589–594, 1985.
18. Feigl EO: The paradox of adrenergic coronary vasoconstriction, Circulation 76:737–745, 1987.
19. Deanfield JE, Kensett M, Wilson RA, et al.: Silent myocardial ischaemia due to mental stress. Lancet 1:1001–1005, 1984.
20. Rebecca GS, Wayne RR, Campbell S, et al.: Transient ischemia in coronary disease is associated with mental arousal during early life (abstract). J Am Coll Cardiol 7:239, 1986.
21. Freeman LJ, Nixon PG, Sallabank P, Reaveley D: Psychological stress and silent myocardial ischemia. Am Heart J 114:477–482, 1987.
22. Rozanski A, Bairey CN, Krantz DS, et al.: Mental stress and the induction of silent myocardial ischemia in patients with coronary artery disease. N Engl J Med 318: 1005–1012, 1988.
23. Scheidt S: Silent ischemia: incidence and prognosis. Cardiovasc Rev Rep June [Suppl], pp 14–18, 1988.
24. Cannon WB: ''Voodoo'' death. Am Anthropol, 1942 (Reprinted in Psychosom Med 1957; 19:182–190, 1957).
25. Myers A, Dewar HA: Circumstances attending 100 sudden deaths from coronary artery disease with coroner's necropsies. Br Heart J 37:1135–1143, 1975.
26. Rissanen V, Romo M, Siltanen P: Premonitory symptoms and stress factors preceding sudden death from ischaemic heart disease. Acta Med Scand 204:389–396, 1978.
27. Brodsky MA, Sato DA, Iseri LT, Wolff LJ, Allen BJ: Ventricular tachyarrhythmia associated with psychological stress. JAMA 257:2064–2067, 1987.
28. Brackett CD, Powell LH: Psychosocial and physiological predictors of sudden cardiac death after healing of acute myocardial infarction. Am J Cardiol 61:979–983, 1988.
29. Surawicz B: Neural control of the heart: Summary of discussion. J Am Coll Cardiol 5:111B–112B, 1985.
30. Hinkle LE: In Neural control of the heart: Summary of discussion. J Am Coll Cardiol 5:111B; 1985.
31. McIntosh HD: The stabilizing and unstabilizing influences of neurogenic and vascular activities of the heart as related to sudden cardiac death. J Am Coll Cardiol 5:105B–110B, 1985.
32. Kannel WB, Schatzkin A: Sudden death: Lessons from subsets in population studies. J Am Coll Cardiol 5:141B–149B, 1985.
33. Durkheim E: ''Suicide.'' New York: The Free Press, 1951 (1897).
34. Parkes CM: Effects of bereavement on physical and mental health—A study of the medical records of widows. Br Med J 2:274–279, 1964.
35. Rees WD, Lutkins SG: Mortality of bereavement. Br Med J 311:552–559, 1984.
36. Cottington EM, Matthews KA, Talbott E, Kuller LH: Environmental events preceding sudden death in women. Psychosom Med 42:567–574, 1980.

37. Broadhead WE, Kaplan BH, James SA, et al.: The epidemiologic evidence for a relationship between social support and health. Am J Epidemiol 117:320–325, 1983.
38. Chandra V, Scklo M, Goldberg R, Tonascia J: The impact of marital status on survival after an acute myocardial infarction: A population based study. Am J Epidemiol 117: 320–325, 1983.
39. Ruberman W, Weinblatt E, Goldberg J, Chaudhary BS: Psychosocial influences on mortality after myocardial infarction. N Engl J Med 311:552–559, 1984.
40. House JS, Landis KR, Umberson D: Social relationships and health. Science 241:540–545, 1988.
41. Seeman TE, Syme SL: Social networks and coronary artery disease: A comparison of the structure and function of social relations as predictors of disease. Psychosom Med 49:3541–3554, 1987.
42. Blumenthal JA, Burg MM, Barefoot J, Williams RB, Haney T, Zimet G: Social support, type-A behavior, and coronary artery disease. Psychosom Med 49:331–340, 1987.
43. Plato: "The Dialogues of Plato" (trans. B. Jowett). Oxford: Oxford University Press, 1953 (1871).
44. Osler W: "Lectures on Angina Pectoris and Allied States." New York: Appleton, 1897.
45. Friedman M, Rosenman RH, Carroll V: Changes in the serum cholesterol and blood clotting time in men subjected to cyclic variations of occupational stress. Circulation 27:852–861, 1958.
46. Friedman M, Rosenman RH: "Type-A Behavior and Your Heart." New York: Knopf, 1974.
47. Friedman M, Ulmer D: "Treating Type-A Behavior and Your Heart." New York: Knopf, 1984.
48. Kobler J: "The Reluctant Surgeon: A Biography of John Hunter." Garden City, NY: Doubleday, 1960.
49. Foot J: "The Life of John Hunter." London: T. Beckett, 1794.
50. Ottley D: "The Life of John Hunter, F.R.S." In Palmer JF (ed): "The Complete Works of John Hunter." Philadelphia: Barrington and Haswell, 1841.
51. Adams J: "Memoirs of the Life and Doctrines of John Hunter." London: J. Callow, 1817.
52. Hunter J: "Observations on Certain Parts of the Animal Oeconomy, 2nd Ed." London: Nicol, 1792.
53. Albarran-Sotelo R, Flint LS, Kelly KJ: "Health Care Provider's Manual for Basic Life Support." Dallas: American Heart Association, 1988.
54. Dimsdale JE, Hackett TP: Effect of denial on cardiac health and psychological assessment. Am J Psychiatry 139:1477–1480, 1982.
55. Friedman M, Powell LH: The diagnosis and quantitative assessment of Type-A behavior: Introduction and description of the videotaped structured interview. Integr Psychiatry 2:123–129, 1984.
56. Matthews KA, Haynes SG: Type-A behavior pattern and coronary disease risk: Update and critical evaluation. Am J Epidemiol 123:923–960, 1986.
57. Rosenman RH, Brand RJ, Jenkins CD, Friedman M, Straus R, Wurm M: Coronary heart disease in the Western Collaborative Group Study: Final follow-up experience of 8 1/2 years. JAMA 233:872–877, 1975.
58. Case RB, Heller SS, Case NB, Moss AJ: Type-A behavior and survival after acute myocardial infarction. N Engl J Med 312:737–741, 1985.
59. Shekelle RB, Gale M, Norusis M: Type-A score (Jenkins Activity Survey) and risk of recurrent coronary heart disease in the Aspirin Myocardial Infarction Study. Am J Cardiol 56:221–225, 1985.
60. Skekelle RB, Hulley SB, Neaton JD, et al.: The MRFIT behavior pattern study II. Type-A behavior and incidence of coronary heart disease. Am J Epidemiol 122:559–570, 1985.

61. Ragland DR, Brand RJ: Type-A behavior and mortality from coronary heart disease. N Engl J Med 318:65–69, 1988.
62. Booth-Kewley S, Friedman HS: Psychological predictors of heart disease: A quantitative review. Psychiatr Bull 101:343–362, 1987.
63. Williams RB, Barefoot JC, Haney TL, et al.: Type-A behavior and angiographically documented coronary atherosclerosis in a sample of 2,289 patients. Psychosom Med 50:139–152, 1988.
64. Williams RB: Refining the Type-A hypothesis: Emergence of the hostility complex. Am J Cardiol 60:27J–32J, 1987.
65. Barefoot JC, Dahlstrom WG, Williams RB: Hostility, CHD incidence, and total mortality: A 25 year follow-up of 255 physicians. Psychosom Med 45:59–63, 1984.
66. McCramie EW, Watkins LO, Brandsma JM, Sisson BD: Hostility, coronary heart disease (CHD) incidence and total mortality: lack of association in a 25-year follow-up study of 478 physicians. J Behav Med 9:119, 1986.
67. Dembrowski TM, MacDougall JM: Beyond global Type-A: relationships of paralinguistic attributes, hostility and anger-in to coronary heart disease. In Field T, McAbe P, Schneiderman N (eds): "Stress and Coping." Hillsdale, NJ: Lawrence Erlbaum, 1985.
68. Siegman AW, Dembrowski TM, Ringel N: Components of hostility and the severity of coronary artery disease. Psychosom Med 49:127–135, 1987.
69. Clarkson TB, Kaplan JR, Adams MR, Manuck SB: Psychosocial influences on the pathogenesis of atherosclerosis among nonhuman primates. Circulation 76[Suppl I]:I-29–I-40, 1987.
70. Weiss SM: Introduction and overview. In Matthews KA, Weiss SM, Detre T, Dembrowski TM, Falkner B, et al. (eds): "Handbook of Stress, Reactivity and Cardiovascular Disease." New York: Wiley, 1986.
71. Chesney MA, Ward MM: Biobehavioral treatment approaches for cardiovascular disorders. J Cardiopulmonary Rehab 5:226–232, 1985.
72. American Heart Association: "Heart Facts 1987." Dallas: AHA.
73. Siegel D, Grady D, Browner WS, Hulley SB: Risk factor modification after myocardial infarction. Ann Intern Med 56:323–392, 1988.
74. Heaton RK: Introduction to the special series (cardiovascular disease). J Consulting Clin Psychiatry 56:323–392, 1988.
75. Multiple Risk Factor Intervention Trial Research Group: Exercise electrocardiogram and coronary heart disease mortality in the multiple risk factor intervention trial. Am J Cardiol 55:16–24, 1985.
76. Fuchs R, Scheidt SS: Prevention of coronary atherosclerosis. Cardiovasc Rev Rep 4: 671–695, 791–811, 1983.
77. Friedman M, Thoresen CE, Gill JJ, et al.: Alteration of Type-A behavior and its effect on cardiac recurrences in post myocardial infarction patients: Summary results of the Recurrent Coronary Prevention Project. Am Heart J 112:653–665, 1986.
78. Friedman M, Powell LH, Thoresen CE, et al.: Effect of discontinuance of Type-A behavioral counseling on Type-A behavior and cardiac recurrence rate of post myocardial infarction patients. Am Heart J 114:483–490, 1987.
79. Ornish D, Sherwitz LW, Doody RS, et al.: Effects of stress management training and dietary changes in treating ischemic heart disease. JAMA 249:54–59, 1983.

Index